Advance Praise for *Skills for Communic[...]*

"Finally! Drs. Kurtz and Adams have created a muc[...] [...]rehensive, clear and concise, evidence-based guide for all of us working in the veterinary field. No matter what stage in your career, whether you are a student, educator, practitioner, manager or other practice team member, you will find this book extremely useful. *Skills for Communicating in Veterinary Medicine* has the potential to move the practice of veterinary medical communication forward by twenty years if enough of us read it and sharpen our communication skills. We are all experts in communication just as we are all excellent drivers. Remember that just because we've been communicating all of our lives, it doesn't mean we've been doing it right, and it doesn't mean we can't improve our skills! Another beautiful thing about improving our communication skills is we can use them in our personal relationships as well. This book is a wonderful gift being handed to the veterinary profession! Please take advantage of it!"

—Michael T. Cavanaugh, DVM, DABVP, Chief Executive Officer,
American Animal Hospital Association

"This comprehensive and highly readable book will be valued by all who teach, learn, and use communication skills and knowledge in veterinary medicine. Our clients and patients will be better served by those who have benefited from the authors' thorough and thoughtful approach to the discipline."

—Peter Conlon, BSc(Agr), MSc, DVM, PhD, Med, Professor and Associate Dean,
Students, Director, Hill's Pet Nutrition Primary Healthcare Centre,
Ontario Veterinary College, University of Guelph, Canada

"Congratulations on this great achievement. I have never ever read such a thorough overview of all literature available on communication skills. In my opinion, the book:
- is essential knowledge for every veterinarian and vet-to-be, to keep animals healthy, large and small
- makes the difference between an average vet, and an excellent vet
- has real life examples of typical conversations with clients and how to improve them
- shows that even communication science in veterinary practice can be evidence based
- teaches the best way to perform a client-oriented consultation
- improves the perceived emotional quality of the veterinary profession
- applying these techniques does help to prevent miscommunication and accompanying consequences like lawsuits
- as a vet, to keep animals healthy, the animal species you need to know most about is the human being
- offers a very thorough analysis of communication skills needed for an effective consultation
- provides an extensive review on veterinary consultation skills
- is a must read, oh no, a must apply, for every vet and vet-to-be.
- supplies a missing piece in veterinary education
- fulfills a need of many working in the veterinary industry
- adds value to the veterinary profession, and helps animal owners to see that added value

All in all, a great overview of how to perform a perfect consultation."

—Jolanda Jansen, PhD, MSc, St Anna Advies, Nijmegen,
the Netherlands, communication and behavioral change specialist
in animal health and in the agricultural and veterinary industry, author of
Communication in Practice, The Vet's Manual on Clienthusiasm

"This is the first textbook which provides a comprehensive overview of the science demonstrating that 'communication matters' in all branches and specialties of veterinary medicine. The authors clarify the research evidence and weave countless practice examples showing the connection between communication practices and quality client and patient care outcomes. This text will serve as a reassuring go-to for veterinary students, residents and seasoned veterinarians who want to strive for professional and rewarding relationships with clients, patients, and veterinary teams."

—Kathleen A. Bonvicini, MPH, EdD, Chief Executive Officer, Institute for Healthcare Communication, New Haven, CT, USA

"The practice of veterinary medicine is often regarded as an animal health care industry, when in fact it's really a customer service industry that uses animal health care as its platform. In any service-based industry, successful outcomes, including content and satisfied clients, and confident and assured staff team members, are based on multiple criteria, but communication is the pivotal centre for success in all contexts of veterinary practice. This impactful publication, *Skills for Communicating in Veterinary Medicine*, is a unique resource in that it will not only help the reader understand the process and nature of the communication process, but acts as a coaching tool, aid, and teaching tool for all practice team members, regardless of their role in the practice.

Skills for Communicating in Veterinary Medicine uses practical contexts and applicable examples and scenarios supported by research and years of immersion in the profession by Drs. Adams and Kurtz to provide meaningful direction and advice for the practice and its team members. It is a 'must have' resource in the increasingly complex and demanding business and customer service environment to help you, the reader, on your own path to success.

Congratulations to Dr. Adams and Kurtz for identifying and meeting a priority need for the changing and evolving veterinary profession."

—John Tait, MS(Finance), DVM, MBA, CFP, Certified in Business Valuation, Certified in Mediation and Negotiation, Past President, American Animal Hospital Association

"Like its counterparts, *Skills for Communicating in Veterinary Medicine* is a key reference book for teaching and learning veterinary communication, including definitions of core communication skills, example phrasing, and importantly, providing evidence-based rationales for why to put communication into practice in veterinary medicine."

—Jane R. Shaw, DVM, PhD, College of Veterinary Medicine and Biomedical Sciences, Colorado State University, Fort Collins, CO, USA

"If every practitioner knows how important communication with the pet owner is, very few know that there is a lot of evidence-based data in this area. In Cindy and Suzanne's book, you'll discover that a good consultation requires 73 identified skills or steps! You'll learn also that closed questions are a disaster in communication with the pet owner, at least at the beginning of the consultation. We all know from various surveys that the compliance is very poor in veterinary medicine, and this book should help making progress in this area."

—Philippe Marniquet, DVM, dip. ESSEC, Veterinary Communication Director, Montpellier, France, Royal Canin Global

Skills for Communicating in Veterinary Medicine

Cindy L Adams

Suzanne Kurtz

Forewords by

Warwick Bayly
Christoph K.W. Mülling
Anthony L. Suchman

Otmoor Publishing
Oxford
Dewpoint Publishing
New York

Otmoor Publishing
Oxford OX5 2RD
United Kingdom
www.otmoorpublishing.com

Dewpoint Publishing
114 Old Bloomfield Avenue
Parsippany, NJ 07054
USA
www.dewpointpublishing.com
info@dewpointpublishing.com

Printed in the United States of America (for books sold in the US and Canada)
Printed in the United Kingdom (for books sold in the UK)
May be printed in other regions for books sold in those regions
First edition, 2017

Every effort has been made to ensure that the information in this book is accurate. This does not diminish the requirement to exercise clinical judgment, and neither the publisher nor the authors can accept any responsibility for its use in practice.

British Library Cataloguing in Publication Data
A catalogue record for this book is available from the British Library.

ISBN (paperback): 978-0-9977679-0-2
ISBN (mobi): 978-0-9977679-1-9
ISBN (epub): 978-0-9977679-2-6
ISBN (epdf): 978-0-9977679-3-3

Grateful acknowledgement is made to Radcliffe Publishing and to Jonathan Silverman and Juliet Draper for permission to create a veterinary medicine version of *Skills for Communicating with Patients, Third Edition* by Jonathan Silverman, Suzanne Kurtz, and Juliet Draper, Radcliffe Publishing, 2013.

Grateful acknowledgement is made to Julie Cary and Jason B. Coe for permission to use their practical examples of communication skills in action. Julie Cary, DVM, MS, DACVS-LA, Director, Clinical Communication Program and Clinical Simulation Center, Washington State University, College of Veterinary Medicine, USA. Jason B. Coe, DVM, PhD, Associate Professor, Department of Population Medicine, Ontario Veterinary College, University of Guelph, Canada.

Text design and typesetting by Darkriver Design, Auckland, New Zealand

Significant discounts for bulk sales are available.
Please contact info@dewpointpubilshing.com

Grateful acknowledgement is made for permission to use the following:

[Fig 1.1] Jeffrey Bryan and Julie Cary, "The Clinical Method Map," 2010. Unpublished course materials for the Clinical Communication Program, College of Veterinary Medicine, Washington State University. Used with permission.

[Figs 1.6, B.1, B.2, B.3] Jack Wilson, Darlene Donszelmann, Emma Read, Michel Levy, Gord Krebs, Tom Pittman, Gord Atkins, Renaud Leguillette, and Ashley Whitehead, "Historical Investigation Pyramids: Dairy, Beef, Equine, Small Animal." Unpublished course materials for the Clinical Communication Program and Clinical Skills, University of Calgary, Veterinary Medicine. Used with permission.

[Fig 6.1] Vincent M. Riccardi and Suzanne M. Kurtz, "Trilevel Model," adapted from the model as it appears in Riccardi VM and Kurtz SM (1983), *Communication and Counseling in Health Care*, Charles C Thomas Publisher, Springfield, IL. Used with permission.

[Fig 6.2] Nancy K. Janz and Marshall H. Becker, "The Health Belief Model: A Decade Later," *Health Education & Behavior* (Vol. 11, Issue 1), pp. 47, copyright © 1984 by SAGE Publications, Reprinted by Permission of SAGE Publications, Inc.

Contents

Forewords

Given the widespread recognition of the importance of communication in daily lives, from a retrospective perspective it is surprising that it has taken so long for a book of this kind to be published. Effective communication is acknowledged as being essential to success in corporate organizations, business transactions, personal relationships, politics, and team-based sporting competitions to give just a few examples of situations in which short- and long-term outcomes are heavily influenced by the quality of communication. How often do we hear that the hallmark of a great leader is her or his skill as a highly effective communicator? Therefore, in hindsight it is chastening to realize that it has taken the veterinary profession as a whole so long to accept that, along with discipline-based knowledge and well-developed physical procedural skills and problem solving abilities, the possession of effective communication skills is the fourth essential requirement for the practice of high quality medicine.

There is no place on the veterinary health care team where excellent communication skills are not essential. They are integral to building any good practice. Unfortunately, not only did it take our profession too long to acknowledge this, but it also had to accept that these skills could be taught. The caliber of an individual's communication abilities was not dependent on what was learned as a child from parents and other family members while sitting around the dinner table. As the contents of this book thoroughly demonstrate, effective medical communication is a cognitive skill that can be taught and must be regularly practiced in order to develop proficiency; just like any other veterinary skill.

I met Cindy Adams and Suzanne Kurtz at the 1st International Conference on Communication in Veterinary Medicine (ICCVM) in Ontario in 2004. Cindy was a faculty member at the Ontario Veterinary College, University of Guelph, and Suzanne was a member of the faculty in the Faculty of Medicine at the University of Calgary. The timing was perfect. For the previous couple of years some of the leadership group at Washington State University's College of Veterinary Medicine had been discussing the importance of so-called "non-technical" skills in the successful delivery of veterinary services, and whether it was possible to incorporate the teaching of these skills into an already overcrowded veterinary curriculum. There had also been healthy debate regarding the advisability of such a consideration and the lack of specific evidence supporting the contention that medical communication should be regarded as an essential cognitive skill and/or that it could be effectively taught. Attending that ICCVM and meeting Cindy and Suzanne convinced me and others that we in veterinary medicine had to commit to improving the communication skills of our new graduates and that there was emerging evidence to support such a move. Furthermore, it was apparent that, no matter how full the curriculum appeared to be, provision had to be made to teach clinical communication to veterinary students in a practice-like setting. Also, it had to be classified as a core course and woven into the overall fabric of the whole curriculum to the extent possible. It could not be put into a box like the "-ologies" and treated as a heavily didactic course that was assigned a semester in which it was to be "taught". Finally, we could not have just anyone teach it. It quickly became apparent that experience did not make one an effective teacher of communication. Specific methods for teaching communication had to be developed and documented and they then had to be engaged, evaluated and further refined along evidence-based lines if veterinary schools were ever to effectively teach clinical communications.

Since that time in 2004, Suzanne has joined the veterinary faculty at Washington State University while continuing to work closely with Cindy, who is now on the veterinary faculty at the University of Calgary and the rest, as they say, is history. The body of evidence indicating that clinical communication is a teachable and learnable skill has grown substantially and curricula have been developed and improved. Recognition of the importance of teaching clinical communication to future veterinarians and helping existing ones improve their competencies is now recognized globally. So it seems logical, as another sign of the natural progression of these developments, that Drs Adams and Kurtz have now written *Skills for Communicating in Veterinary Medicine*. It is the first book to address this specific subject from such a heavily evidence-based and conceptual point of view and it is only fitting that they, as members of a very small core group that was there at the beginning of this emergent process, should be the ones to have authored it.

This book is not just for veterinary students. There is a growing recognition that even the most experienced of veterinary practitioners can benefit from periodic objective evaluations of their effectiveness as clinical communicators. Individuals are always changing, even if they don't know it. Change in style and manner of communication is frequently unnoticed by the communicator and these changes are not always for the best, which is why this book is not just for future veterinarians. There is much in it that practitioners can utilize on a recurring basis. As such it should be regarded by everyone on the veterinary health delivery team as a text that is as valuable as any discipline-based one. Every practice should have at least one copy.

Warwick Bayly **BVSc MS PhD Dip ACVIM**
Professor, Department of Veterinary Clinical Sciences
Dean, 2000–2008, College of Veterinary Medicine
Washington State University, USA
May 2016

What one does not understand one owns not [Goethe].

The unique, evidence-based *Skills for Communicating in Veterinary Medicine* opens the gate in one sentence for understanding communication and developing ownership of this essential veterinary skill. Without a trace of a doubt, communication is an essential clinical skill without which excellent veterinary medicine is virtually impossible. "If you can't communicate it doesn't matter what you know" - this phrase clearly highlights the great importance of communication not exclusively but in particular in our profession. We have strong evidence for the significance and indispensibility of communication in veterinary medicine. Communication is a clinical and beyond that a practical core competence and a foundational part of modern evidence-based veterinary medicine.

In this context *Skills for Communicating in Veterinary Medicine* is a long expected and urgently needed book for the veterinary profession and the global community of veterinarians in whatever field or context they may work. It is authored by two leading authorities in veterinary and medical communication, Cindy Adams and Suzanne Kurtz. I had the privilege of working with Cindy Adams for three years setting up and integrating communication into the curriculum at the University of Calgary, Faculty of Veterinary Medicine. And on several occasions I had the pleasure of meeting with Suzanne Kurtz to exchange thoughts and ideas around clinical communication. The high level of professionalism, knowledge and extensive experience, the dedication and passion of the authors for the topic, is present and tangible in every single paragraph throughout the book.

This book employs a highly evidence-based approach for enhancing communication skills in veterinary medicine. This book is practical, truly comprehensive and certainly applicable across contexts in veterinary medicine as well as within the veterinary community across the globe. It is based on and constituted around the Calgary–Cambridge Guides, an evidence-based, structured and practical instrument for teaching and learning communication skills in medicine. The Guides are well established and widely used in medical and veterinary curricula. A cornucopia of practical examples illustrates the knowledge, techniques and theories covered in the different chapters.

Communication is key for a successful professional – and private – life. This is particularly true in veterinary medicine. As our patients cannot communicate verbally we rely, often critically, on successful communication with their owners. As a matter of fact we cannot deliver quality veterinary diagnoses and treatments without skilled communication. Clinical communication is highly technical. In order to develop these skills profound technical knowledge, guided and coached training, and continuous practice are essential. *Skills for Communicating in Veterinary Medicine* provides the foundations, detailed technical knowledge and guidance for the initiation of this process in the novice as well as the guidance and advanced knowledge for ongoing lifelong development and improvement of communication skills no matter whether we teach, work in practice or at a University.

Clinical communication deserves and requires great attention by the global veterinary community. This handbook is an extremely rich, comprehensive resource for all veterinarians and a standard reference for teaching and learning veterinary medical communication. Beyond this it will spark enthusiasm, infecting everyone who has an interest in learning or improving his or her communication skills. And once infected, with the help of this book, you will develop a deep dedication to communication and the desire to continuously improve your skills. This book will become a deeply appreciated companion you will never want to be without.

Communication is key for a successful and sustainable relationship between the veterinarian and the client and beyond that for the quality of the veterinary medicine applied to the patient. Communication is a core clinical competence essential for high quality veterinary medicine in any country. This is equally true for human medicine. In the era of globalization and the concept of *One World, One Health, One Medicine*, it is important to emphasize that this book integrates the human and veterinary literature throughout.

As stated earlier this book is a long needed and awaited resource for the veterinary profession, not only in North America but also in Europe and across the world. We need advocates around the world to become the voice for the uptake of clinical communication. I would like to congratulate Cindy and Suzanne on this outstanding masterpiece, this unique, comprehensive and very practical resource for learning and teaching skills for communicating in veterinary medicine. This is a new standard, a reference for learners, teachers, students and coaches, and all veterinarians no matter what they do or where they work. With the help of this work we can understand and ultimately own communication.

Skills for Communicating in Veterinary Medicine is applicable across the variety of veterinary contexts and across the globe. It will also facilitate integration of communication between medicine and veterinary medicine and substantially contribute to developing and continuously improving communication skills in One Medicine. *Skills for Communicating in Veterinary Medicine* is poised to change how future generations of veterinarians will communicate with their peers and clients. I am confident that this book will make a difference in our profession.

May the story of *Skills for Communicating in Veterinary Medicine* be a successful one and may this book make a difference to our medicine and our profession.

Prof. Dr. med. vet. **Christoph K.W. Mülling**
Professor of Veterinary Anatomy
Institute of Veterinary Anatomy,
Faculty of Veterinary Medicine, Leipzig University
An den Tierklinken 43, D-04103 Leipzig/Germany
May 2016

My wife and I love our veterinarian. He cares for Lulu (our aging and increasingly frail cockapoo) and for us with skill and compassion. He listens in a way that leaves us feeling understood and respected; he explores symptoms and conducts examinations carefully; he explains treatments and prepares us to be partners in care; and he organizes his office visits efficiently. In short, he does everything described in this book. And it works really well.

Throughout all of health care there is a growing awareness that relationships matter, that what used to be dismissed as touchy-feely or soft is absolutely critical to achieving good clinical outcomes, keeping care safe, reducing waste and maximizing efficiency, giving clients or patients a satisfying experience, and – now more urgently important than ever – maintaining the health and well-being of the health-care workforce.

Just as interest in healthcare relationships is crescendoing, along comes *Skills for Communicating in Veterinary Medicine*. This book is truly a *tour de force*. It describes and synthesizes the evidence that relationships matter – an important achievement in its own right, establishing a strong foundation for further scholarship in this area. But it goes much farther, and in a very practical clinical direction. It provides detailed guidance – also evidence-based – on what you can do or say in each moment to establish effective relationships with clients to get the clinical work done in a way that is satisfying for them and uplifting for you.

While the book is structured around the sequential steps of a typical clinical encounter, the methods for listening, inquiring, negotiating, planning and organizing apply at all levels of veterinary care. They can improve teamwork in an office practice as veterinarians, technicians and front office staff collaborate to provide successful and satisfying episodes of patient care and reduce daily wear and tear in the office. They can help executives and managers in a multi-group practice or a veterinary college to take a relational approach to management, fostering a culture of engagement and co-creation, autonomy support and peer accountability. Again, more motivation and meaning at work, less burnout and turnover. And at the highest level of organization, One Health requires the capacity for multi-stakeholder perspective taking and outstanding collaboration skills as people work together across institutions, disciplines and paradigms. This, too, rests on the fundamental communication skills described in the pages that follow.

I want to appreciate the authors, Cindy Adams and Suzanne Kurtz, for their achievement in bringing this landmark book into being. And I want to appreciate you, the reader, for taking relationships seriously and seeking to strengthen this core capacity in yourself. I wish you every success in your studies and your work; the wisdom in this book will give you a huge head start.

Dr. Anthony L. Suchman MD MA
Senior Consultant and Founder, Relationship Centered Health Care, LLC
Clinical Professor of Medicine
University of Rochester School of Medicine and Dentistry, USA

Preface

Skills for Communicating in Veterinary Medicine is a handbook that provides a detailed, evidence-based exploration of the communication skills that make a difference in the practice of veterinary medicine. We examine how to use specific communication skills effectively in veterinary contexts and provide the research evidence that both validates the importance of these skills and documents the potential gains to all of the parties involved. This book presents:

- the individual communication skills that make a difference in all veterinary contexts and that form the core content of communication skills teaching and learning programs
- an overall structure to the veterinary consultation that helps organize the skills and our learning and teaching about those skills regardless of whether learners are experienced veterinarians or veterinary students early in their training
- a detailed description and rationale for the use of each of these core skills in veterinary consultations
- principles, concepts and research evidence that validate the importance of the skills and document the potential gains for veterinarians, their staffs, and the clients and patients they serve
- suggestions and examples for how to use each skill in practice
- discussions of the major role that these core communication skills play in tackling communication issues and challenges.

Our book is the veterinary version of *Skills for Communicating with Patients, 3e* (2013), a book originally written for communication in human healthcare and one of a set of two companion books on improving communication in medicine that veterinary communication educators, researchers, practitioners and students have been using as resources for many years. The companion, *Teaching and Learning Communication Skills in Medicine*, examines how to construct an evidence-based communication skills curriculum at all levels of professional education and explores in depth the specific learning and teaching methods employed in this unique field of medical education.

We are deeply grateful to Drs. Jonathan Silverman FRCGP and Juliet Draper FRCGP, MD, co-authors of both companion books with Dr. Kurtz, for their important contributions here and for their generous permission to make use of their work in this veterinary version of the book. Working across disciplinary lines – interacting with colleagues in both professions ourselves and connecting these colleagues with each other – has been particularly helpful not only for assistance offered and insights gained as we all continue to develop clinical communication in each profession, but also because this integration of effort has helped us to think more deeply about how these two professions might engage with each other to move local, national and global health forward.

In writing this new book, we have added significant research and conceptual literature regarding communication in veterinary medicine, incorporating it with relevant concepts and research from the literature on communication in human medicine. Based on their veterinary, teaching and research experience, Drs. Julie Cary DVM, MS, DACVS-LA and Jason Coe DVM, PhD have provided insightful suggestions and contributed practical examples and dialogue throughout the book illustrating how veterinarians and their staff use specific communication skills in practice. They have added invaluable perspective to the book.

We have retained the layout, organizational structure, conceptual framework, relevant insights and research evidence, and much of the language found in *Skills for Communicating with Patients, 3e*. Now also serving as a companion to our veterinary book, the *Teaching and Learning* book offers:

- an overall rationale for communication skills teaching – the "why," the "what" and the "how" of teaching and learning communication skills in medicine
- the individual skills that constitute effective communication in healthcare
- a systematic approach for presenting, learning and using these skills in practice
- a detailed description of appropriate teaching and learning methods including:
  — innovative approaches to analysis and feedback in experiential teaching sessions
  — key facilitation and coaching skills that maximize participation and learning
- principles, concepts and research evidence that substantiate the specific teaching and learning methods used in communication skills programs
- strategies for constructing a communication skills curriculum and program in practice.

Together, the *Skills* book and the *Teaching and Learning* book provide a comprehensive approach to teaching and learning communication that works across the gamut of veterinary specialties from the early student years through continuing professional education and beyond. We encourage our readers to study both volumes.

While at first glance it would appear that this volume might be exclusively for learners and our companion volume exclusively for teachers, this is far from our intention:

- Communication teachers and coaches need as much help with "what" to teach as "how" to teach. We demonstrate how in-depth knowledge of the use of communication skills and of the accompanying research evidence is essential if these facilitators wish to maximize learning in their experiential teaching sessions.
- Learners need to understand "how" to learn as well as "what" to learn. Understanding the principles of communication skills teaching will enable learners to maximize their own learning throughout the communication curriculum, improve their own participation in that learning, understand the value

of observation and rehearsal, provide constructive feedback and contribute to the formation of a supportive climate.

In communication skills teaching there is a fine line between teachers and learners. Teachers will continue to make discoveries about communication throughout their professional lives and to learn from their students. Learners not only teach their peers and other colleagues but soon become the communication skills teachers of the next generation of clinicians, whether formally, informally or as role models. No veterinarian can escape this responsibility.

Cindy Adams and Suzanne Kurtz
January 2016

About the Authors

Cindy Adams, MSW, PhD is Professor in the Department of Veterinary Clinical and Diagnostic Sciences at the University of Calgary, Veterinary Medicine, where she developed and implemented the Clinical Communication Program in Calgary's new veterinary school. She honed her professional understanding of human-animal relationships serving from 1980–1992 as a social worker in child welfare, women's shelters and the justice system. Animals were frequently involved in that work. Combining the very different perspectives gained from her experiences in social work and a doctorate in veterinary epidemiology, she became a faculty member at the Ontario Veterinary College, University of Guelph (1996–2006). There she designed and directed the first veterinary communication curriculum in North America and pioneered a research program regarding communication in veterinary medicine. She helped initiate the Institute for Healthcare Communication, Bayer veterinary communication project. Her research has focused on communication education and veterinary–client communication in large and small animal contexts. She has also done research on services dogs and autism, therapeutic riding programs, animal death and human grief and has investigated policy regarding animals in urban settings, and animals' contribution to human health. Founder of the International Conference on Communication in Veterinary Medicine, she has presented widely and advised veterinarians and veterinary practice teams throughout North America, Europe and the Caribbean. In 2015, the *Journal of the American Veterinary Medical Association* recognized her for early contributions to the literature regarding the human–animal bond and the significance of communication in veterinary medicine.

Suzanne M. Kurtz, PhD, is Professor Emerita, University of Calgary, Canada, where she served the Faculties of Education and Medicine from 1976 through 2005, and directed the Faculty of Medicine's communication program. Beginning in 2006, she became Nestlé Purina Professor of Clinical Communication and founding director of the Clinical Communication Program, College of Veterinary Medicine, Washington State University. Her career has focused on improving communication and educational practices in the professions and in the community, and on developing communication curricula; she has worked with veterinarians and physicians across the specialties, students and residents, nurses, allied health professionals in both disciplines, patients, clients, educators, administrators, industry partners, lawyers, government agencies and professional organizations. Co-developer of Pfizer's FRANK program, she also co-organized seven International Conferences on Communication in Veterinary Medicine. She received the 2014 Distinguished Achievement Award from the Washington State Veterinary Medical Association and the 2015 Lynne Payer Award for outstanding contributions to literature on effective healthcare communication from the American Academy on Communication in Healthcare. Contributing across diverse cultural and disciplinary lines, she continues to consult nationally and internationally at all levels of medical and veterinary practice and education and has collaborated on several health-related international development projects. Her publications include two books co-authored with J Silverman and J Draper: *Skills for Communicating with Patients* (Radcliffe Publishing, 3e-2013) and *Teaching and Learning Communication Skills in Medicine* (Radcliffe Publishing, 2e-2005), a book co-authored with VM Riccardi entitled *Communication and Counseling in Health Care* (Charles C. Thomas, 1983) and many articles and chapters.

Acknowledgements

We could not have written this book without the assistance and contributions of those who have taught and influenced us across the years. First and foremost are veterinary practitioners, veterinary and graduate students, learners from other disciplines, clients with their animals, others responsible for the care of animals, and research and teaching colleagues from around the world.

Numerous people have helped us with their ideas, time and support, in particular our families and those we have worked with regularly, including coaches (faculty and community) in our communication programs, case authors, simulated clients, and veterinary and audiovisual technicians.

We particularly want to acknowledge faculty members, administrators and administrative assistants at our home institutions past and present for their ongoing and substantial collaboration and encouragement to us personally and to the development of communication education in veterinary medicine. At University of Calgary, Veterinary Medicine: Nigel Caulkett, Alastair Cribb, Johanna Holm, Debbie Mowat, Christoph Mülling, Carl Ribble, Kimberly Way, Jack Wilson. At University of Guelph, Ontario Veterinary College: Al Binnington, Jason Coe, Peter Conlon, Betty Power, Jane Shaw, John Tait, Julie Tremblay-Audet, Lorna Wyllsun. At Washington State University, College of Veterinary Medicine: Warwick Bayly, Gilbert Burns, Julie Cary, Steve Hines, Karen Hornfelt, Rachel Jensen, Dale Moore, Kathy Ruby, Bill Sischo, Bryan Slinker. Simulated client coordinators Brian Gromoff, Daniel Haley, and Pamela Yenser have provided significant expertise across institutions. We extend special thanks to Richard DeBowes at Washington State and Lynda Ladner at Guelph and Calgary for their crucial contributions to the beginnings and ongoing development of communication programs in veterinary medicine.

We especially appreciate our industry partners for their support and belief in this work. Our thanks to Mike Cavanaugh, Malcolm Kram, Brent Matthew, Fiona McLellan, Johanne Pelletier, Rick Sipple, Kristina Wahlstrom, and Kurt Venator.

For their advice and commitment to communication in veterinary medicine we also thank Cass Bayley, Brenda Bonnett, Kathleen Bonvicini, John Boyce, Doug Jack, Mike Paul, Anthony Suchman, and Donal Walsh.

We are grateful to Jonathan Silverman, Julie Draper and all those from human medicine who have provided us with foundational material for this book, including patients, medical practitioners, learners, coaches, simulated clients, and research and teaching colleagues.

We also want to thank two individuals who have made important contributions to the preparation of this book. Lorraine Toews initiated a substantive literature search regarding the evidence on communication in veterinary medicine. Her expertise and advice as a medical reference librarian were essential. Deanne Jeffery's meticulous work integrating the human and veterinary medicine reference lists together and formatting the example boxes was indispensible.

Sincere thanks to Lynne Feldman who generously contributed her painting, "After the Rain," for our book's cover. Her work speaks eloquently to the relationship between humans and other animals that is central to this book.

We acknowledge with deep appreciation the contributions of our valued colleagues, Julie Cary, an equine surgeon and director of the Clinical Communication Program and Clinical Simulation Center (College of Veterinary Medicine, Washington State University), and Jason Coe, a mixed animal veterinarian, communication researcher and educator (University of Guelph, Ontario Veterinary College). Based on their substantial and varied experience, Drs. Cary and Coe wrote the practical examples found throughout this book demonstrating how to apply communication skills in veterinary practice and also provided their expert insights, suggestions, and ideas for enhancing early drafts of the manuscript.

Finally, we gratefully acknowledge Gillian Nineham, Martin Hill, Rachel Inger, Steve Bonner, Vivianne Douglas and all the team at Otmoor Publishing, Dewpoint Publishing, and Darkriver Design for their invaluable expertise, assistance, suggestions and encouragement.

Individuals from all of these contexts and perspectives have been instrumental in the creation of this book. We owe each of them a debt of gratitude.

Dedication

We dedicate this book to our families and families-by-affection who have taught us the importance of animals to livelihood, health and well-being and the value of relationships and communication between people and with other animals.

To my mother and father Shirley and Larry Adams, my husband David Schieck, our children Camille, Kal, and Charlotte.

To my grandparents John and Erla Myer and Michael and Annie Kurtz, who farmed in Pennsylvania, my parents Earl and Esther Kurtz, and Dot and Winnie Heisey, in loving memory; to Kathy (Kurtz) and Sam Frankhouser, John Kurtz and Ellen Manobla, my niece and nephews and their spouses and children.

And to the animals who have been in our lives.

Introduction and guide to using this book

An evidence-based approach

The practice of excellent veterinary medicine is inextricably linked with skilled communication – you cannot have one without the other. This is true no matter what role you play in the profession of veterinary medicine, no matter whether you work in rural or urban settings, primary or specialty care, small animal, equine, production animal, exotics or public health.

During the past dozen years, interest in communication in veterinary medicine has sharply increased among veterinary practitioners, researchers, educators and students. McDermott et al. (2015) administered a survey looking at veterinarians' perceptions of the importance of communication skills to personal and practice success;1774 small, farm, equine, mixed and other UK and US veterinarians responded to the survey. Ninety-eight percent agreed that communication skills were as important as or more important than clinical knowledge. A study assessing the attributes that constitute a good veterinarian found that the 300 large and small animal veterinarians in Britain who participated ranked communication as the most important out of 20 attributes (Mellanby et al. 2011). Walsh et al. (2009) asked veterinarians in the United States to assess how important several key competencies were to the practice of veterinary medicine. The 1714 respondents had 3 to 19 years of experience and worked across the range of veterinary contexts. They ranked clinical reasoning and client communication skills most highly, giving both the maximum score possible (19 out of 19). The next highest competencies (business skills and physical examination skills across species) were ranked at 14. Martin and Taunton (2006) found that all 415 small animal veterinarians who participated in their study ranked communication skills first in importance out of 10 skills associated with veterinary practice. A Canadian study involving 217 veterinary students (years 1 to 4) showed that students have also recognized the importance of communication – 99% of them had concerns about their ability to communicate effectively with clients, 65% said they did not receive enough training in communication, and 100% wanted more training in this area (Adams et al. 2004).

Professional organizations and veterinary medical education councils have acknowledged and taken on communication training as an essential component of the curriculum. For example, the American Veterinary Medical Association Council on Education (Accreditation Policies and Procedures of the AVMA Council on

Education. Standard 11, Outcomes Assessment 2012) lists client communication as an essential outcome of the Doctor of Veterinary Medicine program and states that graduating students must be able to demonstrate communication competency. The North American Veterinary Medical Education Consortium (NAVMEC 2011) agreed on nine competencies in which North American veterinary students must be proficient and confident upon graduation – one of these competencies is communication. In Australia veterinary educators from across the country agreed that communication is one of the key attributes for Australian veterinary graduates (Collins and Taylor 2002). The Royal College of Veterinary Surgeons in the United Kingdom and the European Association of Establishments for Veterinary Education are also focusing on ways to develop and implement communication curricula.

Veterinary educators in many countries have begun to include communication teaching in the veterinary curriculum and are offering continuing education. Many have published material about what they are doing (e.g. Prescott et al. 1994; Heath 1996; Mills 1997; Radford et al. 2003; Adams and Ladner 2004; Institute for Health Care Communication, Veterinary Communication Project (2004); Brandt and Bateman 2006; Adams and Kurtz 2006; Kurtz 2006; Shaw and Ihle 2006; Mills et al. 2006; Radford et al. 2006; Gray et al. 2006; Cornell and Kopcha 2007; Chun et al. 2009; Hafen et al. 2009; Baillie et al. 2010; Gray and Moffett 2010; Klingborg 2011; Shadle 2011; Hecker et al. 2012; Artemiou et al. 2013; Everitt et al. 2013; Hafen et al. 2013; Hodgson et al. 2013; McArthur and Fitzgerald 2013; Artemiou et al. 2014; Wessels et al. 2014; Frank communication training from Pfizer Animal Health/Zoetis 2015).

Clearly many in the profession believe in the importance of communication skills in veterinary medicine. But even strong belief is not enough to produce sustained change in veterinary practice and professional education. Without evidence to back claims that improving communication skills in veterinary medicine results in better outcomes for patients, clients and practitioners, we cannot expect this relatively new field of communication in veterinary medicine to make substantial inroads into already crowded curricula and busy practices. The communication between humans and animals is certainly also important in veterinary medicine and we discuss it in general terms at various points; however, the primary focus of this book is on human-to-human communication in veterinary contexts.

So our overarching objective in writing this book is to provide an evidence-based approach for enhancing communication skills in veterinary medicine. We wish not only to demonstrate how to use communication skills effectively in veterinary practice, but also to provide the research evidence that validates the importance of these skills and documents the potential gains to veterinarians, clients, and animals. Evidence-based findings and concepts should now inform our educational processes and drive our communication practices forward in the profession. (Stewart and Roter 1989; Makoul 2003; Suchman 2003; Adams and Kurtz 2006; Gray et al. 2006; Kurtz 2006; Radford et al. 2006; Street et al. 2009; Artemiou et al. 2013; Adams and Kurtz 2016; Cake et al. 2016).

This book strives to:

- enhance the communication skills of students, interns, residents, veterinary staff and practitioners of veterinary medicine and provide them with a common language for conceptualizing and applying communication skills across all veterinary contexts
- provide veterinary practitioners, clinical faculty, learners and program directors with the research evidence and knowledge to understand, teach, learn and apply this vital subject at a professional level of competence
- convince veterinary educators and administrators of the importance of developing extensive, evidence-based communication skills teaching at all levels within their institutions and organizations
- provide accrediting and other professional organizations with evidence-based standards of practice regarding clinical communication in veterinary medicine
- provide researchers with foundations for future research.

We hope you will find this handbook to be a useful resource throughout your career as you encounter communication opportunities and challenges in your own education and practice and also as you develop or teach in educational programs or conduct research projects.

A skills-based approach

This book deliberately takes a predominantly skills-based approach to enhancing communication in veterinary medicine rather than an attitude- or issues-based approach. We believe it is important to address both skills and attitudes and to continue to develop the underlying values, beliefs and intentions that motivate them. However, only the skills-based approach provides the communication skills that enable learners to put values, beliefs and intentions into practice. We also devote considerably more attention to core communication skills than to specific communication issues and challenges such as managing anger, breaking bad news, responding to ethical dilemmas, dealing with financial issues, resolving disagreements or conflicted situations, etc. Core communication skills are again of fundamental importance; once individuals understand and develop competence in applying the skills, issues and challenges can be much more readily tackled. We wish to provide a secure platform of core skills that will serve as the primary resource for dealing with all communication challenges. There is no need to invent a new set of skills for each issue. Instead, we need to be aware that although most of the core skills are still likely to pertain, we will need to use some of them with greater intention, intensity and awareness. Doing this requires that we deepen our understanding of these core skills and enhance the level of mastery with which we apply them. The core skills that we describe in this book represent the foundations for effective clinical communication in all circumstances.

An approach incorporating research and concepts from human and veterinary medicine

Why do we use conceptual and research evidence from both human and veterinary medicine to substantiate communication skills to be used in veterinary contexts? The first answer is that we are eager to build on the foundations that are already in place. Those foundations draw upon an extensive body of literature on clinical communication in human medicine that has been developed over the past 45 years. Veterinary researchers, educators and practitioners have been using findings and insights from this literature to advantage for many years. The foundational evidence we rely on also comes from the more recent and growing literature on clinical communication in veterinary medicine, including research on large and small animal contexts. Communication research in veterinary medicine is most definitely progressing, yet there is still much work to do. The literature from human medicine offers insights and practical approaches that fill some of the gaps or provide a useful foil against which to compare and contrast what we are doing with respect to communication in veterinary practice, education and research. Colleagues in human medicine will find that the veterinary literature provides them with similar insights and benefits.

The rationale for incorporating both literatures goes back to basics – we are talking about human-to-human communication in both instances. This is not to say that human and veterinary communication are exactly the same. Certainly the content of what veterinarians and physicians say differs and we are talking on the one hand of animal health and illness and on the other of human health and illness. However, the goals of communication in both fields are closely aligned: enhanced accuracy, efficiency and supportiveness; relationships characterized by collaboration; and improved outcomes of care. As we shall see in Chapter 1, the actual communication process skills and underlying capacities and values that are needed to achieve these goals are essentially the same for both human and veterinary medicine.

There is increasing pressure from consumers of veterinary services and those funding the research that the practice of veterinary medicine be evidence based and that the best available research findings will be translated into practice and inform clinical decision making. These are additional reasons for writing this book and for so intentionally synthesizing communication research from human medicine with what is available in veterinary medicine.

On a related note Toews (2011) compared the information infrastructures supporting evidence-based veterinary medicine with those supporting human medicine (i.e. systematic reviews, indexing of clinical intervention research, clinical filters for MEDLINE, point of care decision support information resources). She found that veterinary medicine is significantly underdeveloped in its information infrastructure. She concluded that this lack of development creates barriers to the timely translation of veterinary medical research into practice and further research. Although this book will not solve our information infrastructure issues, it helps by consolidating the research on communication in human and veterinary medicine in one place.

Research on communication in veterinary medicine can benefit from incorporating human health literature by building on qualitative and quantitative research methods and designs previously used in human medicine (Shaw et al. 2004a). The human health communication literature will continue to contribute to the development of research questions and study designs for communication research in veterinary medicine. The converse is also true. As we develop and deepen this area of research in veterinary medicine, this work will inform communication research and practice in human medicine. In fact this has already begun to happen. Veterinary professionals have published in the human medical literature and presented at human health conferences on communication topics and vice versa (Frankel 2006; Adams and Frankel 2007; Shaw et al. 2010; Cary and Kurtz 2013).

For all of these reasons, this book intentionally draws on literature from both professions. While we have kept considerable research from human medicine, we have also removed some of this research regarding specific topics or issues that do not seem relevant to veterinary contexts. If you wish to access the studies we have deleted, please see *Skills for Communicating with Patients, 3e* (Silverman et al. 2013). We have also added literature regarding topics in veterinary medicine that are less applicable to human medicine.

The way we integrate communication concepts and research from both human and veterinary medicine in this book and use them to arrive at a set of core skills that is essentially the same for both professions leads to a final, perhaps less obvious, purpose for this book. Proponents of One Health[1] have been talking about it for some 20 years, yet many professionals and educators in the various disciplines involved have been slow, possibly even resistant, to making the changes that seem necessary to move One Health forward. If One Health is to succeed, interprofessional communication must advance to a higher level of competence than is currently the case at local, national and international levels (Rock et al. 2009; Buntain et al. 2015). Enhancing communication competence must of course begin with individuals. Using language appropriate for all the disciplines involved, this book sets forth an organized set of evidence-based communication skills and concepts already proven to be effective in both veterinary and human medicine. This skill set enhances communication not only between clinicians and their clients or patients in either profession but also between colleagues within their own professions and, significantly for One Health, across disciplines. Here again these skills are relevant whenever accuracy, efficiency, supportiveness, relationships characterized by collaboration and improved outcomes are important. Therefore the skill sets presented in this book have considerable potential for becoming a template for the interprofessional communication that is so critical if we are serious about One Health initiatives.

A unified approach throughout veterinary medical training and beyond

At this stage in the development of veterinary communication learning and teaching, it is crucial that we tie together our efforts regarding communication skills training

---

1   The American Veterinary Medical Association defines One Health as "… the integrative effort of multiple disciplines working locally, nationally, and globally to attain optimal health for people, animals, and the environment." Source: https://www.avma.org/kb/resources/reference/pages/one-health.aspx

from the early years of veterinary school through internship, residency and beyond into continuing education and professional development. In our own work, we teach the same principles and core skills across all of these levels (Adams and Kurtz 2016). We wish to demonstrate the need for a continuing, coherent program of communication skills teaching that extends throughout all levels of veterinary medical education, the need to both review and reiterate previous learning, and the importance of moving on to more complex situations and challenges as learners move from one level to the next. The curriculum of core skills that we offer provides a common foundation for communication programs throughout all levels of learning.

A unified approach to communication skills teaching and learning applicable to the full range of veterinary contexts

Some commentators have suggested that it is not possible for a text on clinical communication skills teaching and practice to be appropriate to the wide range of settings found in veterinary medicine as these different contexts require very different skills. We disagree with this point of view. The authors have considerable experience in teaching communication across a wide range of contexts, including general and specialty practice, small animal, food animal, equine medicine, One Health and others. Conferences representing a variety of veterinary contexts feature workshops and presentations on communication; for example, conferences for the American College of Veterinary Internal Medicine, American Association of Equine Practitioners, Primary Care Veterinary Educators, Academy of Dairy Veterinary Consultants, Association of Veterinary Technician Educators, etc. This broad range of veterinary contexts and specialties is represented in international conferences as well.

While different veterinary contexts may require a shift in emphasis, our overwhelming common experience is that the similarities far outweigh the differences and that the underlying principles and core communication skills remain essentially the same; the differences between veterinary contexts are more in subject matter than in communication skills. This book presents research evidence from a variety of diverse veterinary contexts that lends additional support to this unified approach across contexts.

A unified approach to communication skills teaching and learning that is applicable across cultures

It has also been said that there are such important differences in culture, client expectations, veterinary training, clinical management and approaches to veterinary medicine between Europe, North America and other countries that it is very difficult to write a book on communication skills that appeals to such a wide audience. Again, we disagree. In human medicine, the book on which this book is based and the companion teaching and learning book have been taken up in many countries and the books as well as the guides that delineate the core skills (a centerpiece of both books) have now been translated into several languages and used in many countries worldwide.[2] In veterinary medicine, the authors and many others have applied these same methods and principles of learning and taught the same clinical communication skills to veterinarians and veterinary students from a variety of countries, and the uptake from this variety of learners has been overwhelmingly positive.

Strangely, research and theory have not always travelled well across the oceans in any direction and teaching programs tend not to take account of the progress made elsewhere. Consensus statements in human and veterinary medicine (Simpson et al. 1991; Makoul and Schofield 1999; Participants in the Bayer-Fetzer Conference on Physician-Patient Communication in Medical Education 2001; Gray et al. 2006; von Fragstein et al. 2008; Bachmann et al. 2012;), major international conferences on communication in healthcare (including seven International Conferences on Communication in Veterinary Medicine), and international organizations (e.g. the American Association of Communication in Healthcare, European Association for Communication in Healthcare, and International Research Centre for Communication in Healthcare) have begun to break down these international and cultural barriers, as did the books. Many additional conferences that include international participants have included pieces on communication in human and veterinary medicine, including the North American Veterinary Conference, Ottawa Conferences, International Association for Medical Education (AMEE) conference, Western Veterinary Conference, International Veterinary Simulation in Teaching, Veterinary Education Worldwide, International Conference on Udder Health and Communication, and International Association of Human–Animal Interactions Conference. We would like to continue the process with the veterinary version of this book.

Who is the intended audience for this book?
Learners at all levels of veterinary education

This book is intended as core material for learners in communication skills programs at all levels of education and experience. We are keen for learners to read this book to complement their experiential training and independent learning. We emphasize, however, that reading and deepening understanding by themselves are not likely to change learners' behavior in the consultation – experiential methods are required to cement into place learning from knowledge-based methods and ensure skill development. On the other hand, knowledge does allow learners to understand more fully just what each skill involves, the evidence for each skill leading to improved outcomes in the consultation, and the issues behind communication skills teaching and learning. Intellectual understanding can greatly augment and guide our use of skills and aid our exploration of attitudes.

So learners in formal communication education programs are part of our intended audience. This book is also intended for learners who are not involved in any formal

---

2   The books have been translated into Dutch, French, Arabic, Italian and Korean and are currently being translated into Spanish, Russian and Polish. The Calgary–Cambridge Guides have been translated into some 25 languages.

education program, including those who might support such programs or those engaged in lifelong independent learning whose work might benefit directly from a deeper understanding of communication in veterinary medicine. Such learners include:

- practicing veterinarians across all contexts
- veterinary technicians and other allied health professionals in veterinary medicine
- practice managers
- veterinary educators who teach elsewhere in the veterinary curriculum
- interns and residents
- administrators of veterinary colleges and hospitals
- members of governing bodies who regulate or set practice policies and standards
- industry partners who support veterinary education or run workshops themselves
- researchers
- communication specialists
- psychologists, social workers and lawyers who are connected to veterinary medicine.

Communication coaches and program directors

Another major audience for our book are the coaches and program directors who wish to teach, plan and develop communication skills training programs at any educational level. Ideally this group also includes clinicians who teach learners in their practices or who model communication, whether in the veterinary teaching hospital or in the community. As discussed in the companion book, coaches and program directors need help with both the "what" and the "how" of communication skills teaching. Although this is beginning to change, most veterinarians who are becoming coaches and program directors were themselves educated in an era when communication skills were hardly taught at all. Too often it has been assumed that coaches through their very practice of veterinary medicine will have gained sufficient knowledge of the specific skills involved in veterinary communication – the "what" of communication skills teaching – and that all they need to learn is "how" to teach this subject. We place equal emphasis on training coaches and program directors in the "what" and the "how." Both are vitally important. The companion book tackles "how" to teach. In this book we help coaches and program directors to increase their knowledge of "what" to teach and to understand the research basis of communication in veterinary medicine.

We recognize that coaches and program directors are not a uniform group. Some will have little if any communication training while others will have extensive training; some are just developing an interest in communication in healthcare while others have already made a commitment to it that they want to strengthen and build upon. Coaches and directors may in fact come from very diverse backgrounds. Both groups will find confirmation as well as challenge in these books.

Newer additional audiences consist of learners, practitioners, educators and researchers in One Health, global animal health, linguistics and pharmacy who are using the lessons from research and experience concerning communication skills in veterinary medicine as a foundation for their increasing efforts to enhance clinical communication, and communication between colleagues. Hopefully readers will understand that we are not implying that all coaches and teachers are or should be veterinarians. The interdisciplinary nature of communication in veterinary and human medicine has strengthened and enriched the field.

Veterinary education administrators, funders, industry partners and politicians

It is vital that the importance of communication skills teaching and research is understood by those in positions of authority and power, including department heads and deans of veterinary education institutions, hospital directors, politicians, and administrators or agents of health authorities, food and drug administrations, veterinary medical societies and associations, funding agencies, and industry partners. It is also vital that these audiences appreciate the complexity of the communication curriculum and the scholarship that underpins and validates this subject.

How have we addressed style issues in a book intended for the European, North American and wider international market?

A particular problem of this book has been how to write a book for a diverse audience. So many words and phrases have subtly different meanings that we have had to tread carefully to avoid unnecessary confusion. Throughout the book, we have decided to use certain words consistently: we apologize for this shorthand and hope that readers will be able to translate our convention to fit their own context. For instance:

When referring to both human and veterinary medicine, we use:

- *clinicians* when referring to both *physicians* and *veterinarians*
- *consultation*, *visit* or *interview* interchangeably
- *learner* to refer to *students at all levels* from veterinary school through continuing education and self directed professional development
- *student* to refer to *learners who have not yet received their professional degree*
- *resident* rather than *registrar* or *trainee*
- *office* or *clinic* rather than *surgery*
- *follow-up visit* rather than *review*
- *coach*, *teacher* or *facilitator* rather than *preceptor* or *small group leader*.

When referring to veterinary medicine, we use:

- *veterinarian* to refer to *generalists, specialists, primary care, tertiary care, etc.*
- *veterinarian* rather than *veterinary surgeon*
- *veterinary team* or *practice team* interchangeably
- *technician* rather than *nurse*
- *practice* rather than *hospital* or *care centre* to refer to *private practices*
- *teaching hospital* to refer to *university veterinary centers.*

When referring to human medicine, we use:

- *specialist* rather than *consultant*
- the British term *general practice* and the North American term *family medicine* to mean the same, despite their different meanings in North America.

Generally *client* refers to *veterinary client* and *patient* means *human patient*; however, as the context will make clear, *patient* will also sometimes refer to *animal patient*.

Finally, *we* is meant to be inclusive, referring to *we in veterinary medicine* or *we in human medicine* rather than only *we who are veterinarians or physicians*. Sometimes *we* refers to the *authors* of this book, as the context will make clear.

CHAPTER 1

Defining what to teach and learn about communication in veterinary medicine

The next six chapters of this book follow through the sequence of the veterinary consultation and provide an in-depth understanding of each individual skill of clinical communication. First, however, to make the skills easier to understand and use, this chapter presents the scaffolding that helps us think more critically and clearly about what we are trying to do with communication in veterinary medicine, what we are trying to teach and learn. The chapter explores several key questions:

- **What is the rationale for teaching and learning communication skills in veterinary medicine?** Why bother? What is the significance of communication in veterinary medicine? Isn't it just a social skill that we already have? Can you really learn communication skills – isn't it more of a personality trait or question of personal style?
- **What are the skills that make a difference?** Is it possible to break down such a complex, important task as the interaction between veterinarians and those they serve into its individual components? Can we identify and define the individual skills that together constitute clinical communication and that we wish to include in communication curricula? How do we decide what communication skills to teach and learn?
- **How do the skills fit together?** Can we present the skills within an overall conceptual framework that enables learners and teachers to make sense of the skills themselves and how they relate to the consultation as a whole?
- **Is there evidence that these skills make a difference in veterinary medicine?** What is the theoretical and research basis that justifies the inclusion of the skills in our clinical communication programs? Is there good evidence for the efficacy of these skills in veterinary practice or is it all subjective opinion?

The overview presented in this chapter of what it takes to learn and teach communication skills that you intend not just to understand but to actually make use of in practice is needed to make optimal use of the rest of the book.[3]

---

3   How to teach and learn communication effectively and the extensive evidence on which we base our approach is found in much greater detail in this book's companion volume, *Teaching and Learning Communication Skills in Medicine* (Kurtz et al. 2005) and in Adams and Kurtz (2016, 2012).

Why bother?

What do we gain by improving communication in veterinary medicine? What does the combined evidence in veterinary and human medicine show we get if we invest in enhancing communication? As the rest of this book demonstrates, the evidence-based bottom line is that improving communication leads to all the benefits in Box 1.1:

Box 1.1 Evidence-based benefits gained from skilled communication

- More effective consultations for client(s), veterinarian(s), and patient(s):
  — greater accuracy
  — heightened efficiency
  — enhanced supportiveness and trust
  — relationships characterized by collaboration and partnership.
- Better coordination of care with clients, colleagues, team members, etc.
- Improved outcomes:
  — greater satisfaction for everyone involved
  — better understanding and recall
  — improved adherence and follow-through
  — greater patient safety and fewer errors
  — better outcomes for patients
  — reduced conflicts, complaints and malpractice claims.

More effective consultations

Throughout this book, we return to the benefits outlined in Box 1.1 and examine how the communication skills that we discuss can produce more *effective* consultations for both veterinarian(s) and client(s). We show how communication skills can make history taking and problem solving more *accurate* and explore how attention to communication skills helps us to be more *supportive* to clients, regardless of the context in which we see them. In particular, we stress how the appropriate use of communication skills enables us to be more *efficient* in day-to-day practice. We are not interested in promoting skills that are inappropriate given the time constraints within which we have to practice veterinary medicine in the real world. We argue throughout this book that using the suggested communication skills will enhance efficiency and we take pains to provide evidence to validate our assertions.

Improved outcomes

If more effective communication improves accuracy (including what we understand, what the client understands, diagnostic accuracy, etc.) and follow-through (including client adherence and our own ability to follow up), it stands to reason that coordination of care will be better and ultimately that outcomes for patients, clients and veterinarians will improve. To substantiate these claims for improvements, this book takes *an evidence-based approach* to communication skills that not only identifies the skills and demonstrates their use in the consultation but also provides the research and theoretical evidence that validates their importance and documents the potential gains for all parties involved, including everything in Box 1.1.

Not least, effective communication plays a significant role in preventing complaints. Dinsmore and McConnell (1992), writing on behalf of the American Veterinary Medical Association Professional Liability Insurance Trust, indicate that significant numbers of malpractice claims are triggered by veterinarian–client communication breakdowns that fall into one or more of the following categories where the client:

- was not made aware of or was unable to understand the prognosis of the case
- lacked comprehension of examination findings
- received inadequate explanation of procedures needed for a definitive diagnosis
- was shocked and surprised over charges at the conclusion of treatment
- failed to receive complete instructions for aftercare
- suffered anger and hostility from unrealized expectations or unexpected, unfortunate results
- was made to feel uncomfortable by the veterinarian's response to the client's request for a second opinion.

Johnson and Ellis, from the same organization, estimated that 75–85% of all veterinary malpractice claims are related to breakdowns in communication (pers. comm. 2006). Nunalee and Weedon (2004) point out that breakdowns in communication cause many problems between veterinarians and clients and that societal trends make veterinarians increasingly vulnerable to legal issues. Commentaries in equine medicine also suggest a relationship between effective veterinarian–client communication and decreased malpractice risk (Bonvicini 2006; Meagher 2005). Oxtoby et al. (2016) found that deficiencies in communication contribute to veterinary error.

In an important study in human medicine, Tamblyn et al. (2007) have demonstrated that scores achieved in patient–physician communication in the Canadian national licensing examination significantly predict complaints to medical regulatory authorities with a linear relationship over a 12-year follow-up period.

A collaborative partnership

Taken together the skills that we describe in this book support both *client-centered* and *relationship-centered approaches* that promote *collaborative partnership* between the veterinarian and all the other people who are involved in the care of the animal(s). This is not because of our own subjective opinion or personal beliefs – we take this approach because the communication skills that enable these views of veterinary–client–patient relationships to be realized have been shown both in practice and in research to produce better outcomes for all concerned. The concept of a collaborative partnership implies a more equal relationship between all parties and a shift in the balance of power away from veterinarian-centered and toward a more mutual, collaborative partnership (Roter and Hall 1992; Coulter 2002; Shaw et al. 2006). This book explores the communication skills that veterinarians can employ to enhance their clients' ability to become more involved in the consultation and to take part in a more balanced relationship.

We do not mean to imply that directive or veterinarian-centered communication is never useful; a life or death emergency, for example, often requires a directive approach. The question is not which paradigm is best – veterinarian-centered or the more collaborative client- or relationship-centered care – but rather which is most appropriate at any given moment. As Lussier and Richard (2008) point out, the answer to that question depends on the specific context and nature of the problem at a given moment, as well as the needs of the patient and the needs and preferences of the client and the clinician at that time.

There is a further dimension of equal importance that is beyond the scope of this book; namely, what clients can do in the interview to influence communication and their animals' care. Far from being passive recipients of changes that veterinarians make regarding communication in the consultation, clients have a major part to play in the process of the consultation. How individual clients can participate differently in the consultation, take responsibility themselves to alter the veterinary–client–patient relationship, or adopt a more active role in the interview are questions that equally deserve attention and investigation. This book touches on the value of providing clients with skills to enable them to adopt a more active role in the veterinary consultation, but here we concentrate on what veterinarians can do in the interview to facilitate their clients' involvement.

Underlying rationale for communication training

The companion to this book, *Teaching and Learning Communication Skills in Medicine*, presents a detailed rationale for communication skills training that we have been applying in veterinary medicine for many years. The rationale shows that:

- **veterinary–client communication is central to clinical practice**
  - — veterinarians engage in thousands of consultations in a professional lifetime so it is worth struggling to get it right
  - — there are problems and therefore opportunities regarding communication between veterinarians and clients
  - — effective communication is essential to high quality medicine: it improves client and veterinarian satisfaction, recall, understanding, adherence, follow-through and patient health
- **communication is a core *clinical* skill, an essential component of clinical competence**
  - — knowledge base, clinical communication skills, physical examination, other procedural skills, and clinical reasoning are the essential components of clinical competence, the very essence of good clinical practice
  - — communication skills are not an optional add-on extra; without appropriate clinical communication skills, our knowledge and intellectual efforts are easily wasted
  - — communication turns theory into practice – how we communicate is just as important as what we say

- **communication needs to be taught and learned**
  - communication is a series of *learned* skills that can be effectively taught and retained – it is not just a personality trait
  - experience alone can be a poor teacher of communication skills – it tends too often to be a great reinforcer of communication habits without discerning whether what we do habitually is effective or counterproductive
  - clinical communication needs to be taught with the same rigor as other core clinical skills
  - technological advancements, client access to information, developments in how we perceive our relationship with animals, and shifts in the nature of veterinary care and practice amplify the need for even experienced veterinarians to continually enhance their communication skills and knowledge
- **specific teaching and learning methods are required in communication skills training**
  - a skills-based approach is essential to change learners' skills and behavior
  - experiential learning methods incorporating repeated observation, feedback and rehearsal are required
  - a problem-based approach to communication skills learning is necessary in which learners work through real veterinary scenarios and cases – preferably with both simulated clients and patients and real clients and patients
  - cognitive and attitudinal learning and ongoing development of values and capacities such as compassion, integrity and mindfulness complement a skills-based approach and vice versa.

We hope that the foundations we lay throughout this chapter and in the companion book will convince readers not only that teaching and learning communication skills is of the utmost importance but also that appropriate teaching and learning methods can produce effective and long-lasting change in communication skills.

How do we decide what to teach and learn about communication skills in veterinary medicine?

So if communication is an essential clinical skill worth teaching and learning, how do we decide what to focus on? How do we define "effective communication"? What do we need to understand and do in order to actually communicate more effectively in the end? These questions can be approached from several angles.

First principles of effective communication

One way to decide what communication skills to focus on is to work from "first principles" that characterize effective communication (Kurtz 1989; Dance and Larson 1972; Dance 1967). As with first principles of surgery, when in doubt about what communication skills would be most useful or effective, go back to first principles.

Applicable to any setting, these principles help us to understand what exactly it is that constitutes effective communication (Kurtz 1989). Interestingly, these same principles characterize effective teaching.

Box 1.2 Principles that characterize effective communication

Effective communication:

1. Ensures an interaction rather than a direct transmission process
If communication is viewed as a direct transmission process, the senders of messages can assume that their responsibilities as communicators are fulfilled once they have formulated and sent a message. However, if communication is viewed as an interactive process, the interaction is complete only if the sender receives feedback about how the message is interpreted, whether it is understood and what impact it has on the receiver. Just imparting information or just listening is not enough: giving and receiving feedback about the impact of the message becomes crucial. The emphasis moves to the interdependence of sender and receiver, and the contributions and initiatives of each become more equal in importance (Dance and Larson 1972). The aim of communication becomes the establishment of mutually understood common ground (Baker 1955). Establishing common ground and confirmation (or acknowledgment) of the other's perspectives both require interaction.

2. Reduces unnecessary uncertainty
Uncertainty distracts attention and interferes with accuracy, efficiency and relationship building. Unresolved uncertainties in any area can lead to lack of concentration or anxiety, which in turn can block effective communication. For example, clients may be uncertain about what to expect during a given interview, about the significance of a line of questioning, about the role of a particular member of the veterinary team, or about the attitudes, intentions or trustworthiness of the other individual. Reducing uncertainty about diagnosis or expected outcomes of care is obviously important, although living with some uncertainty is often a necessity in medical situations. However, even then, openly discussing areas where knowledge is lacking or no one is certain what the best choice is can help reduce uncertainty by establishing mutually understood common ground.

3. Requires planning and thinking in terms of outcomes
Effectiveness can only be determined in the context of the needs of the patient and the outcomes you and the client are working toward at any given point. If I am angry and the outcome I seek is to vent emotion, I proceed in one direction. However, if the outcome I want is to resolve any problem or misunderstanding that may have caused my anger, I must proceed in a different way to be effective.

4. Demonstrates dynamism
What is appropriate for one situation is inappropriate for another, as different individuals' needs and contexts change continually. What the client understood so clearly yesterday seems beyond comprehension today. Dynamism underscores the need not only for flexibility but for responsiveness and involvement, for being fully present and engaging with the client and patient. Dynamism has the added benefit of indicating

how important or salient one individual is to the other – the more responsive and engaged I am, the more important you consider yourself to be in my eyes (Mehrabian and Ksionsky 1974).

5. Follows the helical model
The helical model of communication (Dance 1967) has two implications. First, what I say influences what you say in spiral fashion so that our communication gradually evolves as we interact. Second, reiteration and repetition, coming back around the spiral of communication at a little different level each time, are essential for effective communication.

Goals of communication in veterinary medicine

Thinking in terms of outcomes (the third principle above) provides a second way to conceptualize what skills to focus on. In keeping with the evidence base and first principles, the goals of communication in veterinary medicine include:

- ensuring increased accuracy, efficiency and supportiveness
- enhancing client *and* veterinarian satisfaction
- improving outcomes of care
- promoting collaboration and partnership (relationship-centered care).

The point of communication training – and of this book – is to enhance communication skills and capacities to a professional level of competence in veterinary medicine so as to ensure that all veterinarians can accomplish these goals consistently in all circumstances of practice. Professional competence implies heightened awareness, greater ability to reflect accurately and articulate with precision, heightened intentionality in choosing what to do, and more consistent performance across all situations. Moreover, professional communication competence in veterinary medicine is evidence based.

Types of communication skills

Another way to decide what to focus on is to define communication more precisely. Whether enhancing our own clinical communication skills, assisting others, or designing communication education programs, it is helpful to distinguish between *three types of clinical communication skills*:

- *Content skills* – what you communicate, e.g. the substance of your questions and responses, the information you gather and give, the issues and treatments you discuss.
- *Process skills* – how you communicate, e.g. how you go about discovering the history or providing information, how you structure interactions, ask and respond to questions, relate to clients and patients, use nonverbal skills, involve clients in decision making.
- *Perceptual skills* – what you are thinking and feeling, e.g. your internal decision

making, clinical reasoning and problem-solving skills; attitudes and values; personal capacities[4] for compassion, mindfulness, integrity, respect, flexibility; your awareness of feelings and thoughts you have about the patient, about the client, and the problems or other issues that may be concerning them; what you do with your own feelings and those of your clients; awareness of your own self-concept and confidence, of your own biases, assumptions and distractions.

Content, process and perceptual skills are inextricably linked: a weakness or strength in one set of skills translates into a weakness or strength in all. These three types of communication skills cannot be considered in isolation. We must give attention to all three when trying to teach and learn effective clinical communication (Riccardi and Kurtz 1983; Beckman and Frankel 1994; Kurtz et al. 2003. Windish et al. 2005; Adams and Kurtz 2006; Kurtz 2006; Kurtz and Adams 2009; Silverman 2009; Adams and Kurtz 2012).

Although particular content skills, such as the questions that constitute the review of systems or that need to be asked to investigate a specific problem, are vitally important, these aspects of content are well described in many textbooks and so we devote less space to them here. The same can be said of the clinical reasoning and medical problem-solving aspects of perceptual skills. On the other hand, communication process skills and the ways in which the three types of skills interact receive considerably less attention in medical curricula. Therefore, this book focuses primarily on process skills, devotes attention to significant aspects of content and perceptual skills that relate to communication in veterinary practice, and looks carefully at how all three types of skills influence each other.

A few examples help to demonstrate the interdependence between process, content and perceptual skills.

EXAMPLE 1

Say you ask a series of closed questions (process) early on in the consultation about one specific area (content). This apparently efficient way of obtaining answers to closed questions can lead to problems in effective diagnosis by preventing you from considering the wider picture (perceptual). Questioning skills used inappropriately (process) can lead directly to poor hypothesis generation (perceptual):

Compare

Client: *"Tuffy had diarrhea for the past few days."*
Veterinarian: *"OK:*
How frequent is the diarrhea?
What color is it?

---

4 We credit David Sluyter (2004, pers. comm.), a past officer of the Fetzer Institute and editor of a book on emotional intelligence, for contributing the notion of personal capacities. As he suggests, "… it is really necessary to have both the capacity … and the skills to communicate that capacity to others …".

> Have you noticed any blood in it?
> Does she seem to be straining?" etc.

with

> Client: "She's had diarrhea for the past few days."
> Veterinarian: "Yes ... "
> Client: "It is pretty foul smelling and seems to hit her at a moment's notice."
> Veterinarian: "Ah ha."
> Client: "My husband has also been really sick – he took our dog camping a couple of weeks ago. My husband's physician says he caught giardia from drinking the lake water. Do you think she could get it too?"

EXAMPLE 2

It is fascinating to examine the link between inner thoughts and feelings and outward communication. Thoughts and feelings about a client or patient (perceptual) can interfere with our normal behavior and block effective communication. For instance:

- Irritation with a client's comment about the cost of veterinary care (perceptual) can interfere with listening and lead us to miss important cues (process).

EXAMPLE 3

Unchecked erroneous assumptions (perceptual) can block effective information gathering (process) and lead us into the wrong area for discussion (content). For instance:

- Assuming that a client has brought their animal back or called the veterinarian out for a routine check of an ongoing problem can prevent us from finding out until late in the proceedings that the client has a more important concern to discuss.

The Clinical Method Map (Bryan and Cary 2010) in Figure 1.1 offers a practical way to conceptualize the significant role that communication plays in veterinary medicine and to underscore the interdependent relationship between communication process, content and perceptual skills.

Considering points on the map where communication process and content skills impact what veterinarians and others are doing with clients and animals helps learners visualize just how frequently veterinarians rely on communication skills during clinical practice. Asking learners to then discuss the points on the map at which communication process and content skills impact their clinical reasoning and what that impact is – or to consider how what they are thinking at any given point impacts how they are communicating with clients or patients – helps learners to realize how these skills influence each other.

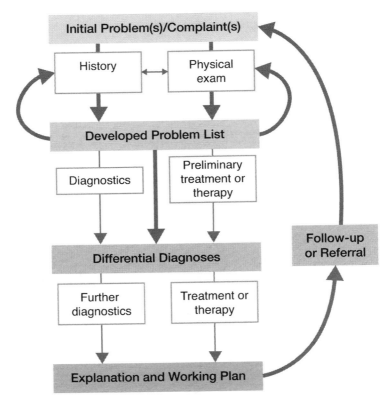

FIGURE 1.1 The Clinical Method Map. Bryan and Cary 2010. Used with permission

Reporting on a workshop in which a large international group of clinicians and medical educators participated, Cary and Kurtz (2013) provide a detailed example of a skills-based approach that integrates the teaching of communication skills, clinical reasoning, attitudes and issues. Using a well-chosen, simulated, longitudinal, veterinary surgical case (i.e. a case that unfolds across several months, but through simulation can be presented in a matter of hours) in a problem-based learning exercise that can be adapted for use with students, specialty residents, faculty or practicing clinicians, the article demonstrates how to teach:

- the interconnectedness of content, process and perceptual skills
- the influence of these three types of skills on clinical reasoning
- follow-up with clients and their significant others over time
- ways to integrate the teaching of communication with clinical reasoning and with a variety of issues, including cognitive errors, clinicians' response to such errors, clinical uncertainty and delivering bad news.

We discuss the relationship between clinical reasoning, communication skills and medical problem solving in more detail in Chapter 3.

The problem of separating content and process skills in teaching and learning about the medical interview[5]

Clearly, content, process and perceptual skills must be integrated: all are essential clinical skills. Yet too often these three types of skills have been artificially divided in veterinary education to the detriment of learners. Separating content and process skills in teaching learners how to get a history and arrive at a diagnosis has proven to be particularly problematic. One unfortunate result is that learners have been confronted with two apparently conflicting approaches to the veterinary interview. The first is the more "traditional" veterinary history which details a framework for the information that students are generally expected to obtain when taking a clinical history and to consider when formulating a diagnosis. This is the *content* of the veterinary medical interview.

Box 1.3 The more "traditional" history

- chief complaint
- signalment
- history of the present complaint or issue
- past medical history
- genetic and familial history
- current medications and allergies
- functional inquiry or systems review.

The second approach that learners face has to do with the communication *process* skills that they learn in communication and professionalism courses or programs. These communication process skills detail how veterinarians structure interviews, develop rapport, obtain the required information described in the more traditional medical history and then discuss their findings and management alternatives with clients.

Confusion over process

When confronted with these two approaches (i.e. the more traditional history describing content, and communication skills describing process), it is all too easy for learners to think of them as alternatives and to confuse the approaches' respective roles. Too often, students disregard their communication process skills learning and use the more traditional medical history model as a guide not just to the content but also to the process of the medical interview. Unfortunately this leads learners to use the framework of the more traditional medical history as their process guide, reverting to closed questioning and a tight structure to the interview dictated by the search for biomedical information.

---

5   Concepts in this section were originally published in Kurtz, Silverman, Benson and Draper (2003).

Confusion over content

Another source of confusion has to do with content. Although communication approaches are commonly perceived to focus solely on process skills, many of us have introduced a new area of content to history taking, namely the client's perspective of the issues or problems (McWhinney 1989; Adams et al. 2005; Coe et al. 2008; Jansen et al. 2010; Nogueira Borden et al. 2010). As we describe in detail in Chapter 3 of this book, the more traditional veterinary medical history concentrates on pathological disease at the expense of understanding the highly individual needs and perspectives of each client. As a consequence, much of the information required to understand and deal with the patient's problems and the client's perspectives is never elicited. Studies in human and veterinary medicine regarding satisfaction, adherence, recall and physiological outcome validate the need for a broader view of history taking that encompasses the client's perspective as well as the clinician's biomedical perspective (Stewart et al. 1995; Kanji et al. 2012; Shaw et al. 2012a).

The fact that clients' ideas, concerns and expectations are not a component of the more traditional medical history has all too often resulted in their omission in everyday clinical practice (Tuckett et al. 1985; Shaw et al. 2006) and has led communication process guides to include this area of content as a counterbalance. However, if different areas of content appear in traditional history-taking question lists and communication skills guides, learners may think they need either to discover clients' ideas and concerns *or* to take a full and accurate biomedical history, when in fact they need to do both.

Marrying content and process

In the next sections of this chapter, we discuss ways to resolve the above dilemmas. We demonstrate a unified model of the veterinary medical interview that highlights both process and content components of the consultation and combines the "old" content of the biomedical history with the "new" content of the client's perspective.

The Calgary–Cambridge Guides: evidence-based skills that make a difference

Thinking in terms of first principles, goals and types of skills helps us conceptualize more systematically and intentionally what to focus on as we work toward enhancing communication skills. But still, just what are the specific communication skills that enable everything else? Ask any group of clinicians, learners or clients and they quickly come up with a convoluted list of clinical communication skills they deem important. Although it may seem counter-intuitive, groups of veterinarians from across the spectrum of veterinary practice and learners at all levels come up with remarkably similar lists. How do we combine their long lists with research findings and translate it all into a comprehensive yet manageable and memorable delineation and definition of skills that can be put into practice in the real world?

One answer to these questions is the *Calgary–Cambridge Guides*, a proven instrument for teaching and learning clinical communication skills that has been evolving since the early 1980s when the guides were originally developed for the University of Calgary (Canada) medical school. Drawing on the work of many individuals and

their earlier communication models, the guides have gone through several itera-
tions.[6] In the mid 1990s Jonathan Silverman, a physician who had been working in
the Cambridge and East Anglian region to advance communication in the UK, came
to Calgary for a sabbatical with Suzanne Kurtz. As a result of their collaboration the
guides evolved yet again and became known as the Calgary–Cambridge Guides. As
a resource for education, research and practice, the Guides are widely recognized
and used worldwide. Many clinicians from across all specialties, students and residents, faculty and other medical educators who teach communication, and a variety
of patients from many cultures, have added their feedback and ideas. Nonetheless,
the primary resource behind this instrument continues to be the research evidence.

First published in two companion books in 1998 (Kurtz et al. 1998; Silverman et
al. 1998), the current version of the *Calgary–Cambridge Guides – Communication
Process Skills* has changed only slightly since then. This despite the explosion of
research on clinical communication since 1998 and the books' authors' concerted
efforts to identify evidence-based changes in the skills or new skills to add as they
updated the literature in the second (Kurtz, Silverman and Draper 2005; Silverman,
Kurtz and Draper 2005) and third (Silverman, Kurtz and Draper 2013) editions of
their books. Since 2003, the Calgary–Cambridge Guides have included both a process and a content guide (Kurtz et al. 2003). The content guide outlines a patient- and
relationship-centered approach to structuring the content of the medical history,
explanation and planning and the medical record.[7]

How did we come to use the Guides in veterinary medical education, practice
and research? When formal communication skills teaching and learning became an
interest in veterinary medicine in the late 1990s, Cindy Adams – who was then at
the Ontario Veterinary College – was on the leading edge of this movement. Seeking
a substantive approach for designing and implementing what was arguably the first
communication curriculum in veterinary medicine, Adams discovered the work of
Kurtz and her colleagues at the University of Calgary in human medicine and, in
1998, arranged an exploratory visit to Calgary with one of her colleagues, Dr. Harold
Chapman. Having examined numerous resources and programs in human and veterinary medicine and in consultation with veterinary educators and practitioners, Prof.
Adams chose the Guides as the centerpiece of her veterinary communication program because they were so highly evidence based and provided a coherent, unified
scaffold upon which to build communication programs, assessment strategies, and
research efforts. Virtually all that was needed to "translate" the Guides from human
to veterinary medicine was to replace "bedside" with appropriate alternatives and
substitute "veterinarian" for "physician" and, where appropriate, "client" for "patient."

---

6   We are indebted to Drs. Rob Sanson-Fisher in Australia, Peter Maguire in England, Don Cassata and Paula
    Stillman in the US, for their contributions to parts of the original guide; to Drs. Vincent Riccardi in the US
    and Cathy Heaton and Meredith Simon in Canada, who were joint authors with Dr. Suzanne Kurtz of earlier
    versions, and to Dr. Jonathan Silverman in England. Riccardi and Kurtz published an earlier version (Riccardi
    and Kurtz 1983; Kurtz 1989.

7   For more detailed explanations and substantiation of the Calgary–Cambridge Guides (human medicine ver-
    sion), *see* Kurtz, Silverman, Benson and Draper (2003); Kurtz, Silverman and Draper (2005); Silverman, Kurtz
    and Draper (2013).

From those early meetings on, Adams and Kurtz have collaborated. For 20 years we, along with many others, have tested the applicability of the skills on the Guides across the gamut of veterinary education and practice settings. We adapted the Guides for veterinary medicine in 2000, and their use in this profession has also continued to evolve (Adams et al. 2000; Adams and Ladner 2004; Radford et al. 2006; Adams and Kurtz 2006; Gray et al. 2006; Shaw and Ihle 2006; Latham and Morris 2007; Greenhill et al. 2011; Hecker et al. 2012; Artemiou et al. 2013; Englar et al. 2016).

The Calgary–Cambridge Guides are the centerpiece of this book and its companion volume on teaching and learning communication skills. Currently summarizing hundreds of studies in terms of 58 highly evidence-based communication process skills plus another 15 process and content skills related to common focuses in explanation and planning, the Guides provide a comprehensive set of communication skills that make a difference in veterinary and human medicine. Equally suited to small group, one-to-one, and self-directed learning, the Guides have two broad aims: to help learners at all levels conceptualize and structure their communication learning and practice, and to assist clinical teachers and communication program directors in their efforts to establish more effective communication training programs at all levels of education for both learners and those facilitating the learning.

Although only a few pages in length, the Guides:

- delineate and describe the individual skills that make up effective clinical communication
- provide a framework for organizing the skills of clinical communication that corresponds directly to the structure of the consultation and therefore aids teaching, learning and practice
- provide a comprehensive repertoire of skills that is validated by research and theoretical evidence
- summarize and make more accessible the literature regarding veterinary–client and physician–patient communication skills
- form the foundation of a comprehensive clinical communication curriculum in both human and veterinary medicine, providing learners, facilitators and program directors alike with a clear idea of the curriculum's learning objectives
- provide a concise summary of the skills for facilitators, learners and practitioners which they can use on an everyday basis during teaching sessions and in their practices as an accessible aide-memoire and a way to structure observation, feedback and self-assessment
- provide a common language for labeling and referring to specific skills and behaviors
- provide a sound basis for facilitator training programs, creating coherence and consistency in the teaching of the large number of facilitators required in communication programs
- provide a common foundation for communication programs at all levels of training by specifying a comprehensive set of core clinical communication skills equally valid and applicable in all veterinary contexts.

Three diagrams: the framework for the Calgary–Cambridge Guides

In both human and veterinary medicine, we have found it useful to introduce the guides to learners by first showing them three diagrams, one at a time, that graphically show what the Guides include. The three diagrams introduce the framework around which the communication skills on the Guides are organized and place the skills within a comprehensive, integrated clinical method. Seeing the diagrams makes it easier for learners and teachers to conceptualize first, what is happening in a consultation and, second, how the skills of communication and physical examination work together in an integrated way.

The basic framework

Figure 1.2 is a graphic representation of the veterinary consultation. Including both communication tasks and physical examination, this bare bones map corresponds directly to how clinicians structure veterinary consultations and depicts the flow of these tasks in real-life veterinary practice. The diagram helps learners conceptualize the clinical communication process more accurately as well as the relationships between the various tasks that comprise it.

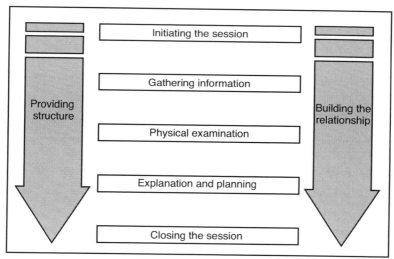

FIGURE 1.2 The basic framework

Veterinarians carry out five tasks – initiating, gathering information, physical examination, explanation and planning, and closing – more or less sequentially. The remaining two tasks – providing structure and building relationship – are essential to successful completion of the sequential tasks and are undertaken throughout the consultation. Physical examination could, of course, be included as a part of gathering information, but depicting it separately enables learners to see the fit between physical examination and the other communication tasks more readily.

The expanded framework

Figure 1.3 expands the basic framework by identifying the objectives to be achieved within each of the tasks. The expanded framework of tasks and objectives provides an overview that helps the learner organize and apply the numerous communication process skills that are delineated in the Calgary–Cambridge Guides themselves. Using the organizational structure provided in the expanded framework, the guides themselves then present the specific, evidence-based skills needed to accomplish each objective.

The complete guides include an additional "options" section under explanation and planning that is not depicted in the expanded framework. The options section includes 15 content and process skills that are related to three of the most common focuses of explanation and planning: discussing investigations and procedures; discussing the doctor's opinion and significance of problems; and negotiating a mutual plan of action. The communication skills associated with ensuring respectful conduct and keeping the client appropriately informed during the physical examination are incorporated under relationship building, structuring, and explanation and planning.

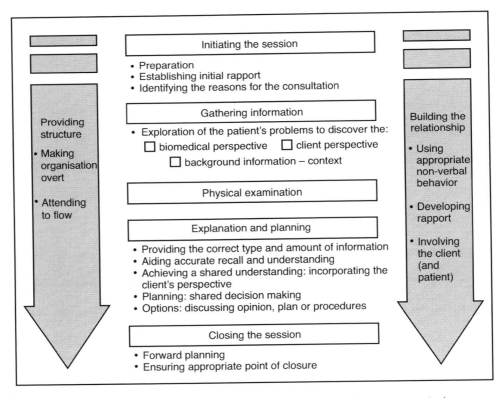

FIGURE 1.3 Expanded framework for the Calgary–Cambridge Guides (veterinary version). Adapted from Kurtz et al. (2003)

An example of the interrelationship between content and process

The third diagram (Figure 1.4) takes one task – gathering information – as an example and shows an expanded view of how content and process specifically interrelate in the medical interview.

Gathering information

Process skills for exploration of the patient's problems

- Client's narrative
- Question style: open-to-closed cone
- Attentive listening
- Facilitative response
- Picking up cues
- Clarification
- Time-framing
- Internal summary
- Appropriate use of language
- Additional skills for understanding
  the client perspective

Content to be discovered

BIOMEDICAL PERSPECTIVE

    Sequence of events
    Analysis of signs
    Relevant systems review

CLIENT PERSPECTIVE

    Ideas and beliefs
    Concerns and feelings
    Expectations
    Effects on life
    Relationship between animal
    and client, others

BACKGROUND INFORMATION – CONTEXT

    Environment and lifestyle
    Past medical history
    Current medications, adverse drug reactions, allergies
    Genetic and familial background
    Behavioral/social history
    Review of systems

FIGURE 1.4 An example of the interrelationship between content and process. Adapted from Kurtz et al. 2003

Together, the diagrams in Figures 1.2, 1.3 and 1.4 form a framework for conceptualizing the tasks of a medical encounter and the way they flow in real time. This framework helps learners (and those faculty who are less familiar with communication teaching) visualize and understand the relationships between the discrete elements of communication content and process.

Increasingly, communication programs in veterinary medicine are rightly attempting to extend communication training beyond formal communication courses and integrate it into other courses where clinical skills are taught and into clinical rotations or externships, internship or residency programs, and other clinical teaching settings. For a more detailed account of how this might be done in veterinary contexts, see Adams and Kurtz (2012, 2016). Clinical faculty and community preceptors vary in their own training and knowledge base regarding communication as well as in their expertise and comfort with teaching communication skills. The three diagrams above offer ways to conceptualize communication skills in veterinary medicine that clinical teachers and role models outside the formal communication course can relate to and use more easily.

In our experience, learners and clinical faculty who first understand the framework in Figures 1.2 to 1.4 are better able to understand and assimilate the true complexity of veterinary clinical communication as detailed in the Calgary–Cambridge Guides' many individual skills, which we present next.

Calgary–Cambridge Guides: communication process skills

The veterinary literature that we have integrated throughout this book clearly supports the applicability of the Calgary–Cambridge Guides for veterinary medicine. This literature shows that veterinarians make effective use of many skills. It also identifies problems and omissions in veterinary clinical communication for which the Guides offer a way forward. As will become evident throughout the book, effective use of the skills on the Guides impacts significant outcomes in veterinary medicine just as it does in human medicine. We want to re-emphasize that the same frameworks and the same skills comprise both the human and veterinary versions of the guides. The literature published on communication in human and veterinary medicine since the Guides were introduced in 1998 continues to validate and deepen the evidence base for the skills on the Guides, thus reinforcing those skills, rather than suggesting changes in interpretation or new skills to add.

For the sake of convenience, we use "client," "patient" and "veterinarian" in the singular throughout the Guides. When applying the Guides to the full range of veterinary contexts, you will need to broaden the bandwidth regarding the definition of "client" to include multiple owners, family members, employees on farms, and others. Similarly, where appropriate, broaden "patient" to include flock, herd or other multiple animal units and "veterinarian" to include veterinary practice teams. The "aims" written into the Explanation and Planning section below were included at the request of residents in human medicine who repeatedly asked us to clarify what they needed to accomplish within each sub-section.[8]

---

8   You can access both veterinary and human versions of the Calgary–Cambridge Guides at www.CCP.vetmed.wsu.edu/resources

Calgary–Cambridge Guides: Communication Process Skills Veterinary Medicine

INITIATING THE SESSION
Preparation
1. **Puts aside last task**, attends to self-comfort
2. **Focuses attention** and prepares for this consultation

Establishing initial rapport
3. **Greets** client and patient and obtains names
4. **Introduces** self, role and nature of visit; obtains consent if necessary
5. **Demonstrates respect** and interest, attends to client's and patient's physical comfort

Identifying the reason(s) for the consultation
6. **Identifies problem list** or issues client wishes to address with appropriate **opening question** (e.g. "What would you like to discuss?" or "What questions did you hope to get answered today?")
7. **Listens** attentively to the client's opening statement without interrupting or directing client's response
8. **Confirms list and screens** for further problems (e.g. "So that's updating vaccinations and Max seems more tired than usual; anything else?" or "Do you have some other concerns you'd like to discuss today?")
9. **Negotiates agenda** taking both client's and own perspectives into account

GATHERING INFORMATION
Exploration of problem(s)
10. **Encourages client to tell story** of problem(s) from when first started to the present in own words (clarifying reason for presenting now)
11. **Uses open and closed questioning** technique, appropriately moving from open to closed
12. **Listens attentively**, allowing client to complete statements without interruption and leaving space for client to think before answering or go on after pausing
13. **Facilitates client's responses verbally and nonverbally**, e.g. by using encouragement, silence, repetition, paraphrasing
14. **Picks up verbal and nonverbal cues** (e.g. body language, facial expression); **checks out and** acknowledges as appropriate
15. **Clarifies client's statements** that are unclear or need amplification (e.g. "Could you explain what you mean by sore?")
16. **Periodically summarizes** to verify understanding of client's comments, invites client to correct interpretation or provide further information
17. **Uses** concise, **easily understood questions and comments**; avoids or adequately explains jargon
18. **Establishes dates and sequence of events**

Additional skills for understanding the client's perspective

19. **Actively determines and appropriately explores**:
    - Client's **ideas** (beliefs regarding cause)
    - Client's **concerns** (worries) regarding each problem
    - Client's **expectations** (goals, help client expects, cost issues, urgency)
    - **Effects on client's and animal's life**
    - **Relationship** between client, animal, and others
20. **Encourages client to express feelings**

PROVIDING STRUCTURE TO THE CONSULTATION
Making organization overt

21. **Summarizes at end of a specific line of inquiry** (e.g. current history) to confirm understanding and ensure no important data was missed; invites client to correct
22. **Progresses** from one section to another **using signposting, transitional statements**; includes rationale for next section

Attending to flow

23. **Structures** consultation in **logical sequence**
24. **Attends to timing** and keeping consultation on task

BUILDING RELATIONSHIP
Using appropriate nonverbal behavior

25. **Demonstrates appropriate nonverbal behaviour**
    - eye contact, facial expressions
    - posture, position, gestures and other movement
    - vocal cues (e.g. rate, volume, intonation, pitch)
26. **If reads, writes** notes or uses computer, does so **in a manner that does not interfere with dialogue or rapport**
27. **Demonstrates** appropriate **confidence**

Developing rapport

28. **Accepts legitimacy** of client's views and feelings; **is not judgmental**
29. **Uses empathy** to communicate understanding and appreciation of client's feelings or situation; overtly **acknowledges client's views and feelings**
30. **Provides support**: expresses concern, understanding, willingness to help; acknowledges efforts and appropriate care; offers partnership
31. **Deals sensitively with embarrassing or disturbing topics and animal's pain**, including when associated with physical examination

Involving the client

32. **Shares thinking** with client to encourage client's involvement (e.g. "What I am thinking now is …")
33. **Explains rationale** for questions or parts of physical examination that could appear to be non-sequiturs

34. When **doing physical examination, explains process, findings**

EXPLANATION AND PLANNING
Providing the correct amount and type of information

Aims: to give appropriate information, neither restricting nor overloading
  to assess individual client's information needs

35. **Chunks and checks**: gives information in manageable chunks; checks for understanding; uses client's response as a guide to how to proceed
36. **Assesses client's starting point**: asks for client's prior knowledge early on when giving information; discovers extent of client's wish for information
37. **Asks** client **what other information would be helpful** (e.g. etiology, prognosis)
38. **Gives explanation at appropriate times**: avoids giving advice, information or reassurance prematurely

Aiding accurate recall and understanding

Aims: to make information easier for clients to remember and understand

39. **Organizes explanation**: divides into discrete sections; develops logical sequence
40. **Uses explicit categorization or signposting** (e.g. "There are three important things that I would like to discuss. First ... Now we shall move on to ...")
41. **Uses repetition and summarizing** to reinforce information
42. **Uses** concise, **easily understood language**, avoids or explains jargon
43. **Uses visual methods of conveying information**: diagrams, models, written information and instructions
44. **Checks client's understanding of information given** or plans made (e.g. by asking client to restate in own words; clarifies as necessary)

Achieving shared understanding – incorporating the client's perspective

Aims: to provide explanations and plans that relate to the client's perspective
  to discover the client's thoughts and feelings about the information given
  to encourage an interaction rather than one-way transmission

45. **Relates explanations to client's perspective**: to previously elicited beliefs, concerns, and expectations
46. **Provides opportunities/encourages client to contribute**: to ask questions, seek clarification or express doubts, responds appropriately
47. **Picks up, responds to verbal and nonverbal cues** (e.g. client's need to contribute information or ask questions, information overload, distress)
48. **Elicits client's beliefs, reactions and feelings**: regarding information given, decisions, terms used; acknowledges and addresses where necessary

Planning: shared decision making

Aims: to allow clients to understand the decision-making process
to involve clients in decision making to the level they wish
to increase clients' commitment to plans made

49. **Shares own thoughts**: ideas, thought processes and dilemmas
50. **Involves client**
    - offers suggestions and choices rather than directives
    - encourages client to contribute their own ideas, suggestions
51. **Explores management options**
52. **Ascertains** level of **involvement client wishes** regarding decision making
53. **Negotiates mutually acceptable plan**
    - signposts own position of equipoise or preference regarding available options
    - determines client's preferences
54. **Checks with client**
    - if accepts plans
    - if concerns have been addressed

CLOSING THE SESSION
Forward planning
55. **Contracts with client** regarding steps for client and veterinarian
56. **Safety nets**, explaining possible unexpected outcomes, what to do if plan is not working, when and how to seek help

Ensuring appropriate point of closure
57. **Summarizes session** briefly and clarifies plan of care
58. **Final check** that client agrees and is comfortable with plan and asks if any correction, questions or other items to discuss

OPTIONS IN EXPLANATION AND PLANNING
If discussing opinion and significance of problem
59. **Offers opinion** of what is going on and names if possible
60. **Reveals rationale** for opinion
61. **Explains** causation, seriousness, expected outcome, short and long term consequences
62. **Elicits client's beliefs, reactions and concerns** (e.g. if opinion matches client's thoughts, acceptability, feelings)

If negotiating mutual plan of action
63. **Discusses options** (e.g. no action, investigation, medication, non-drug treatments, fluids, surgery, behavioral consult, preventative measures, euthanasia/cull)
64. **Provides information** on action or treatment offered
    a) name

b) steps involved, how it works
c) benefits and advantages
d) possible side effects, risks

65. **Obtains client's view of need** for action, **benefits, barriers, motivation**; accepts and advocates alternative viewpoint as needed
66. **Accepts** client's views; advocates alternative viewpoint as necessary
67. **Elicits client's understanding, reactions and concerns** about plans and treatments, including acceptability
68. **Takes client's lifestyle, beliefs**, cultural **background** and **abilities into consideration**
69. **Encourages client to be involved** in implementing plans and **to follow through**
70. **Asks about client support networks**, discusses other options

If discussing investigations and procedures

71. **Provides clear information on procedures** including what client might experience and how client will be informed of results
72. **Relates procedure to treatment plan**: value and purpose
73. **Encourages questions and expression of thoughts** regarding potential anxieties or negative outcome

At this point we can almost hear readers saying: "You must be joking ... seventy-three skills to learn, assimilate and master. Does it really need to be that complicated? Couldn't we reduce the numbers or amalgamate a few items?" We admit without apology that the comprehensive list of skills is long, but effective communication in veterinary medicine is complex. The combined research on it in veterinary and human medicine is extensive and cannot be summed up in a few broad generalizations or acronyms. If we wish to identify, master and assimilate new behaviors into our practice of veterinary medicine, it is essential to break the consultation down into these individual skills. All of the skills on the Guides can be of great value to the process of the consultation, all (as we shall see throughout the rest of this book) have been validated by theory and research, and all will repay our attention.

There is an additional reason to invest the time required to master the skills on the guides; namely, that all of the skills – with the obvious exception of physical examination – are applicable not only to communication with clients but also to interaction between teachers and learners, with colleagues or within teams. In other words, this is the comprehensive delineation of skills that make a difference wherever accuracy, efficiency, supportiveness and collaboration are needed. Taken individually the skills appear to be disarmingly straightforward. Keeping the repertoire of skills in mind, using them consistently and appropriately while doing everything else veterinarians need to do, integrating them effectively with the other clinical skills in both difficult and routine circumstances – that becomes more complex.

Of course, no one will use every skill on the Guides in every consultation. Which clinical communication skills are needed depends on the situation, on the specific outcomes veterinarian and client are trying to achieve at any given moment in the consultation and the needs of the patient at that point. The good news is that the skills are highly adaptable. Applicable to the gamut of contexts where veterinarians practice, the skills are useful regardless of how routine or complex the circumstances are. Context changes and with it the content of what you say as well as the level of intensity, intention and awareness that you need to employ. But the repertoire of communication process skills you need remains the same. A sports analogy is helpful: playing good basketball requires a full repertoire of well-developed skills and you do have to stay focused – but that doesn't always require the intensity of a full-court press.

Communication skills and individuality

Each process skill listed in the Guides is only a clue to learners and facilitators that this is an area where specific behaviors and phrases need to be developed. The list by itself is not enough; each learner has to discover their own way to put each skill into practice. While the guides identify the skills that have emerged from research and practice as being of value in veterinarian–client communication, they do not attempt to specify exact or recommended ways of accomplishing these skills. An important task of communication skills teaching is to give participants opportunities to try out phrases and behaviors that fit their own individual personalities and to extend the repertoire of skills with which each participant is comfortable.

- **Structure:** where am I in the consultation and what do I want to achieve at this point? What is the client trying to achieve at this same point?
- **Specific communication skills:** how do I get there with the client?
- **Phrasing/behavior:** how can I incorporate the skills into my own style and personality?

A second task of communication teaching and learning is for individuals to develop their capacity for *flexibility* so that they can apply the skills and relate to the client in different ways at different times as appropriate. Flexibility requires development not only of communication skills and various ways to apply them but also of the individual's capacity for mindfulness, including their ability to be fully present with each client and patient, to reflect with accuracy on what is needed at any given moment, and to decide on how to apply the needed skills most appropriately. What is called for will vary from client to client, across time, and even within a single visit depending on the nature of the problem, the context, and the needs and preferences of the client and of the clinician as well as what the patient requires (Lussier and Richard 2008).

Going beyond specific skills into individuality is the real challenge of experiential learning (Skelton 2005). We cannot and should not be prescriptive about the best way to proceed in any circumstance. We must recognize that there are enormous variables that influence what is best in a given situation. However, we must also recognize that we can now advocate certain skills that are likely to be more effective than others (Silverman et al. 2011).

It is the repeated trying out of alternatives in rehearsal and feedback, role-playing with other learners or practicing with simulated or real clients and patients that allow us to reconcile the two concepts of skills and individuality. The list of skills is in itself only a start. To learn how to use each skill requires practice and further feedback. Through this process of repeated practice, feedback and rehearsal, each learner stamps their own individuality on the communication process. Appendix A presents the Calgary–Cambridge Guides: Communication Process Skills in a format that we use in our teaching and observation. The format includes space for writing in feedback comments as you observe others' interactions or video recordings of yourself.

Calgary–Cambridge Guides: communication content

The content aspect of the Guides offers an alternative method of conceptualizing and recording information during the consultation and in the medical record. The more traditional ways of recording medical information are retained but enhanced by including explicitly:

- a list of the problems or issues that the client wishes to address (rather than one concern or "chief complaint")
- the progression or sequence of events
- the "new" content regarding the client's perspective
- possible treatment alternatives considered by the veterinarian
- a record of what the client has been told
- the plan of action that has been negotiated.

With these additions, the content guide (Figure 1.5) reflects recent research and current thinking about what makes for more effective interactions in veterinary medicine. For use in practice, each item in the content guide would be followed by a space where learners can write in the appropriate information as they make notes during the interview and later write up their notes in the medical record (history up to physical exam on one page, physical exam and planning on another).[9]

The headings on the content guide and the sequential tasks of medical interviewing correspond closely:

- patient's problem list corresponds to initiation
- signalment corresponds to initiation and gathering information
- exploration of patient's problems corresponds to gathering information
- physical examination is the same in both frameworks
- the rest of the Content Guide's headings correspond to explanation and planning.

Thus, the Content Guide is closely aligned with the specific skills of the Calgary–Cambridge Process Guide. As a result, the two guides reinforce each other and encourage integration of content with process skills.

While the Calgary-Cambridge Content Guide offers a useful way to structure any given veterinary consultation from start to finish, we find that veterinary students

---

9   With respect to the veterinary version of the Calgary–Cambridge Guides – Content, we are indebted to Drs. Julie Cary, Richard DeBowes and John Gay (US) and to Drs. Aubrey Webb, Jack Wilson and Ms. Lynda Ladner (Canada).

CONTENT GUIDE

Signalment
(animal ID, breed, age, sex, reproductive status, animal's purpose, etc.)

List of problems/issues with regard to patient, herd, flock, etc.

Exploration of patient's problems (including flock, herd issues)

Biomedical perspective:	Client perspective:
• Sequence of events	• Ideas and beliefs
• Analysis of signs	• Concerns and feelings
• Relevant systems review	• Expectations
	• Effects on life (of animal and client)
	• Relationship between animal and client, others

Background information – context
- Environment and lifestyle
- Past medical history
- Current medications, adverse drug reactions, and allergies
- Genetic and familial background
- Behavioral/social history
- Review of systems

Physical examination

Differential diagnosis – hypotheses
- Veterinarian's and client's ideas

Veterinarian's plan of management
- Investigations
- Treatment alternatives

Explanation and planning with client
- What the client has been told
- Plan of action negotiated

FIGURE 1.5 The Calgary–Cambridge Guides: Content (veterinary version). Adapted from Kurtz et al. (2003)

who are just beginning to learn history taking frequently appreciate additional direction regarding pertinent details of history they need to gather. Wilson et al. (2012) have developed four species-specific "pyramids" showing the details to use with the Calgary–Cambridge Content Guide. Figure 1.6 offers an example of the pyramid for small animal investigations.

Developed using the template in Figure 1.6, the other species-specific "pyramids" pertain to beef, dairy and equine investigations and are presented in Appendix B. With all of the pyramids, the specific content to be gathered is always dependent on

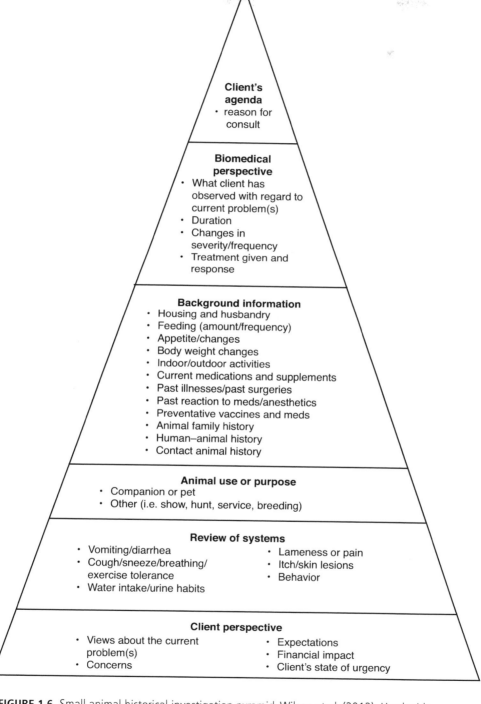

FIGURE 1.6 Small animal historical investigation pyramid. Wilson et al. (2012). Used with permission

the species and the nature of the problem(s) or issue(s) at hand. Like the Calgary–Cambridge Guides, the pyramids are based on the premise that the best patient care can be delivered if veterinarians identify not just "chief complaint" but all of the patient's problems or issues as well as the client's perspectives.

The need for a clear overall structure

An important element of the skills-based clinical communication teaching and learning that we have described here is the provision of a clear overall structure within which the individual communication skills are organized. In both this and the companion book, we refer repeatedly to the importance of the structure so explicitly provided by the framework of the Calgary–Cambridge Guides. Why place so much value on defining such an overt structure?

An understanding of the structure has benefits to practitioners, learners and coaches alike:

- **For practitioners**, an awareness of the structure prevents the consultation from wandering aimlessly and important points from being missed. Communication skills are not used randomly; different skills need to be deployed purposefully and intentionally at different points in the consultation. Practitioners therefore need to keep the structure in mind so that they can remain aware of the distinct phases of the interview as they proceed. For instance, if the veterinarian does not recognize that the gathering information phase of the interview involves developing an understanding of the client's perspective as well as the clinical aspects of the patient's problems or issues, the veterinarian may enter the explanation and planning phase of the interview prematurely and fail to address the client's actual concerns. Of course an awareness of structure in the consultation has to be combined with flexibility – consultations do not have a fixed path that can be dictated by the veterinarian without reference to the patient and the client. But without structure, it is all too easy for communication to be unsystematic and unproductive.
- **For learners at all levels**, a list of the individual communication skills alone is not sufficient. There are too many skills to remember if they are simply listed without categorization. Learners need an overall conceptual model to help organize the evidence-based skills into a memorable and useful whole. In Chapter 3 of the companion to this book, we discuss the importance of experiential methods in producing change in learners' communication skills. However, experiential learning is intrinsically random and opportunistic – the feedback and suggestions can be difficult to pull together. Providing a structure into which skills can be placed as they arise helps learners to order the skills that they discover opportunistically in experiential work and to see how the individual pieces fit together into the consultation as a whole.
- **Coaches** may also lack a clear idea of how to pull together the individual skills or skill sets that they recognize as important learning areas. Without an overall conceptual model, the numerous skills of the veterinary consultation can appear to be a disorganized bag of tricks. Coaches can find it difficult to link the

different skills together in their teaching. Providing them with a clear and overt structure can help overcome this problem. Structure has the added advantage of enabling facilitators to take an outcome-based approach in their communication skills teaching. Structure establishes an overview enabling facilitators to ask two central questions of learners at any given point: "Where are you in the consultation?" and "What are you trying to achieve?" Having established a direction, the individual skills then help with the next question, "How might you get there?" The coach can also use the structure to ask similar questions with respect to the patient and the client: "Where is the client in the consultation?", "What is the client trying to achieve at that given moment?", "What does the patient need at this point?" "How might you discover this information and then use communication skills to respond?"

We use the conceptual framework that the diagrams and Guides provide to structure communication learning and effort in much the same way that experienced clinicians use schema in clinical reasoning: to access and apply knowledge or skills systematically, to aid memory, to impose coherence and order on what would otherwise be unusable and random pieces of information. Learners can use the Guides to develop their learning agenda for a given consultation and as the basis for observation and feedback in small group teaching; coaches can assign individual observers to focus their attention and feedback on different sections or subsections of the Guides. At the beginning of the communication course, it is useful to introduce veterinary students to the whole of the Guides but then focus on developing their initiation skills first and add in a focus on gathering information, followed by other sections of the Guides in turn. When the Guides are used for in-the-moment teaching in veterinary practice settings, veterinarians and those they are teaching can choose to focus on various sets of tasks rather than all of the skills at once.

Relating specific issues to core communication skills

The skills collated in the Guides provide the foundations for effective communication in a variety of different veterinary contexts. There are many challenging situations for veterinarians when they communicate with clients, such as in breaking bad news, dealing with animal mortality or euthanasia, responding to gender and cultural issues, communicating with older clients or children, communicating with families or multiple employees on farms, or discussing financial matters. These issues clearly deserve special attention. However, we stress that the skills delineated in the guides are the *core* communication skills required in all these circumstances, providing a secure platform for tackling these specific communication issues. Some may perceive cross-cultural or interdisciplinary contexts in local, national or global veterinary medicine to require special communication skills. Gaining a deeper understanding of different cultures and contexts is important. However, here again we contend that cross-cultural or interdisciplinary sensitivity or just plain ordinary sensitivity to anyone with views different from our own requires the same communication process skills as those used to ensure accuracy, efficiency and supportiveness with clients (Kurtz and Adams 2009). Although the context of the interaction changes and the content of the communication varies, the process skills themselves remain the same. The challenge is to deepen our understanding of these core skills and the level of mastery with which we apply them.

The research and theoretical basis that validates the inclusion of each individual skill

In a recent Best Evidence Medical Education systematic review, communication skills were the only professional competency that met the criteria of having strong stakeholder consensus and strong outcome-based empirical evidence in support of success in veterinary practice (Cake et al. 2016). It is no longer appropriate to consider communication skills teaching and learning as simply raising awareness of the importance of communication in the consultation. Nor is it just a matter of sharing various approaches, of increasing the range of possibilities available, of treating all suggestions as equally valid. Certain skills and methods have now been shown to make a substantial difference to veterinarian–client communication and to ensuring patient health outcomes.

We are fortunate that over the last 45 years an extensive canon of theoretical and research evidence has accumulated which enables us to define the skills that enhance communication in veterinary and human medicine between veterinarian and client, physician and patient. Research clearly demonstrates how the use of specific skills can lead to improvements in client and veterinary satisfaction, follow-through and adherence, and other outcomes of care. We can now promote these skills as worth teaching, learning, and using with intention in clinical practice. We are able to confidently answer the question "where's the validity?" and effectively counter the suggestion that communication skills are purely subjective.

The curriculum of communication skills is not and should not be static. Research will continue to accumulate to challenge our preconceptions and move the goalposts of communication skills teaching and learning (Griffin et al. 2004; de Haes and Bensing 2009; Street et al. 2009; von Fragstein et al. 2008; Williams and Jewell 2012; Artemiou et al. 2013; Artemiou et al. 2014).

In this chapter, we have simply delineated a curriculum for communication skills teaching and learning, whether for formal communication programs or self-directed learning, by listing and briefly defining each skill. In the following six chapters, we describe the skills more fully and examine in depth the concepts, principles and research evidence that validate each skill.

Summary

In this chapter, we have defined the types of skills that constitute clinical communication. We have delineated the individual skills to be included in communication curricula for learners at all levels and introduced the conceptual and research bases that validate the choice of these particular skills. We have presented the curriculum of skills in the form of the enhanced Calgary–Cambridge Guides that not only list the skills but also provide a structure or conceptual framework that enables practitioners, facilitators and learners to make sense of the individual skills and how they relate to the consultation as a whole.

In the next six chapters we explore the individual skills on the Calgary–Cambridge Guides in depth. What is the rationale for using each skill in veterinary contexts, what is the research and theoretical evidence that validates each skill and how is each skill used in practice? Each of the chapters describes the individual communication skills that pertain to one task of the basic framework, presents the research evidence and conceptual underpinnings for each skill or skill set, and offers practical examples of the skills in action in a variety of veterinary contexts. We start by looking at the skills required for initiating the interview.

CHAPTER 2

Initiating the session

The beginning of the consultation is a particularly rich area to explore. In the opening minutes of any interaction we make our first impressions, begin to establish rapport, attempt to identify the problems or issues that the client wishes to discuss about their animal and start to plan a course for the consultation. The scene is set for the rest of the consultation. Clinicians tend to underestimate the potential difficulties and opportunities of these brief first minutes. Yet we know from research that many problems in communication occur in this initial phase of the interview. Of particular note is the tendency for clinicians to cut the initiation short by frequently interrupting the client or patient, which then contributes to problems later in the consultation.

At the beginning of almost every communication course or workshop no one says they want to focus on the initiation. Yet so often it becomes apparent as the course proceeds that it is the beginning of the consultation that is the root cause for many of their perceived difficulties later on.

Consultations occur in widely differing contexts: from new to review or follow-up appointments, from general to specialty practice, from the examination room to the stall or field, from the intensive care unit to the home. Although at first sight there are many differences between the beginnings of interviews in these very diverse settings, the overall objectives and individual skills required are remarkably consistent. Wherever they meet, the problems veterinarians and clients face in the initial stages of an interview are very similar.

The specific communication skills that clinicians choose to demonstrate at the beginning of the consultation are not merely social niceties: these skills have an important impact on the accuracy and efficiency of the interview and on the nature of the relationship with the client or patient. We therefore set initiation apart as a separate task, devoting a whole chapter to discussing what will take at most only a few minutes to achieve in real time.

Problems in communication

One of the aims at the beginning of the consultation is to identify what the individual seeking assistance wishes to discuss. Here the research evidence reveals some particularly salutary lessons:

- Dysart et al. (2011), in a study of small animal veterinarians in Canada, showed that veterinarians solicited concerns at the beginning of the interview in just over a third of appointments. The average length of time clients spoke before interruption when solicitations were offered was 15.3 seconds. The odds of a new concern arising during the closing segment of an appointment were four times greater when the veterinarian did not solicit the client's concerns at the beginning of the interview.

- In human primary care in Canada, Stewart et al. (1979) showed that 54% of patients' complaints and 45% of their concerns were not elicited.
- Starfield et al. (1981) found that in 50% of primary care visits the patient and the physician did not agree on the nature of the main presenting problem by the end of the consultation.
- Burack and Carpenter (1983) found that patients and physicians agreed on the chief complaint in only 76% of somatic problems and in only 6% of psychosocial problems in primary care visits in the USA.
- Beckman and Frankel (1984) showed that primary care physicians in the USA frequently interrupted patients so soon after they began their opening statement – after a mean time of only 18 seconds – that patients failed to disclose other equally significant concerns.
- Byrne and Long (1976) identified that physician–patient interviews in British general practice were particularly likely to become dysfunctional if there were shortcomings in that part of the consultation relating to "discovering the reason for the patient's attendance."
- Rhodes et al. (2004) in a study in a emergency department in the USA demonstrated that residents introduced themselves in only two-thirds of encounters, rarely indicating their training status (8%). Despite a tendency for physicians to start with an open-ended question (63%), only 20% of patients completed their presenting complaint without interruption. The average time to interruption was 12 seconds.

Clearly, there is little point in being an excellent diagnostician or possessing great factual knowledge if you are not dealing with the client's particular concerns or the patient's most significant problems!

An additional potential problem in veterinary medicine is that the client may consist of multiple people. For example, on dairy farms a team of many individuals may be responsible for the animals or in small animal medicine various family members may be involved. That may make it difficult to know with whom to talk.

Objectives

We begin our exploration of what to focus on in this first section of the interview by looking at our objectives, at what needs to be achieved. One of the principles of effective communication that we outlined in Chapter 1 is that *communication requires planning and thinking in terms of outcomes*. Objectives make us think about "Where do we want to get to?"; work on individual skills provides strategies for "How do we get there?"

Objectives during initiation include the following:

- establishing a supportive environment and initial rapport
- developing an awareness of the patient's well-being and the client's state of mind

- identifying as far as possible all the problems or issues that the client has come to discuss
- establishing with the client a mutually agreed agenda or plan for the consultation, including both the client's perspectives and the veterinarian's
- developing a partnership with the client, enabling the client to become part of a collaborative process.

These objectives encompass many of the tasks and checkpoints mentioned in other guides to the consultation. Here we provide a list of such guides and the tasks and checkpoints on them that are related to initiation; we have edited "patient" to "client" where appropriate. Appendix C contains the lists of these guides and the tasks and checkpoints on them that relate to Chapters 3 to 7 so you can see how other guides have recognized skills associated with those components of the consultation.

- Pendleton et al. (1984, 2003)
  - to understand the reasons for the client's attendance
  - to establish or maintain a relationship with the client that helps to achieve the other tasks.
- Neighbour (1987)
  - connecting: establishing rapport with the client
  - summarizing: "Have I sufficiently understood why the patient and client have come to see me?"
- AAPP 3-Function Model (Cohen-Cole 1991)
  - gathering data to understand a patient's problems
  - developing rapport and responding to the client's emotions.
- (Bayer) Institute for Health Care Communication E4 model (Keller and Carroll 1994)
  - engaging the client.
- The Four Habits Model (Frankel and Stein 1999; Krupat et al. 2006)
  - invest in the beginning.
- The SEGUE Framework for teaching and assessing communication skills (Makoul 2001)
  - set the stage.
- The Maastricht Maas Global (van Thiel and van Dalen 1995)
  - introduction
  - clarification.
- Essential Elements of Communication in Medical Encounters: Kalamazoo Consensus Statement (Participants in the Bayer-Fetzer Conference on Physician-Patient Communication in Medical Education 2001)
  - open the discussion
  - build a relationship.
- Patient-centered medicine (Stewart et al. 2003)
  - exploring both the disease and illness experience.
- The Model of the Macy Initiative in Health Communication (Kalet et al. 2004)
  - prepare

— open
— gather.
- The Six Function Model (de Haes and Bensing 2009)
  — fostering the relationship
  — gathering information.
- Institute for Healthcare Communication, Veterinary Communication Project (2004)
  — open the visit.

Skills

Having established the objectives of the initiation phase, the next step is to turn attention to the skills that help achieve these objectives. The following list of skills is taken from the Calgary–Cambridge Guides that were introduced in Chapter 1.

Preparation
- Puts aside last task, attends to personal needs and comfort
- Focuses attention and prepares for this consultation.

Establishing initial rapport
- Greets client(s) and patient(s) and obtains names as appropriate
- Introduces self; clarifies role and nature of interview; obtains consent if necessary
- Demonstrates interest and respect, attends to client's and patient's physical comfort.

Identifying the reason(s) for the consultation
- Identifies the patient's problems or the issues that the client wishes to address with appropriate opening question (e.g. *"What problems would you like to discuss today?"* or *"I know you've already spoken with my technician. It would be helpful if you would start by telling me the list of what you would like to discuss today."*)
- Listens attentively to the client's opening statement without interrupting or directing client's response
- Confirms list and screens for further problems (e.g. *"So that's updating vaccinations and Max seems more tired than usual; something else …?"* or *"What other things would you would like to discuss today?"*)
- Negotiates agenda, taking both client's and veterinarian's needs into account (e.g. *"We only have 20 minutes scheduled today. Let's make sure we get the ear infection evaluated, but delay discussing nutrition until your recheck appointment in a week. How would that work for you?"*)

What to teach and learn about initiating: the evidence for the skills

Preparation

As we have seen in Chapter 1, *unresolved uncertainties and anxieties can lead to lack of concentration which in turn can block effective communication.* In clinical practice, it is easy for your mind to still be on the last patient or client or telephone call, the growing queue of clients and patients still to be seen, the number of animals in the herd that still require your attention or your own personal needs. You may find yourself calling up records on the computer or completing a record as you greet the next client and patient. These thoughts, feelings and actions can easily get in the way of providing full concentration at the beginning of the consultation. The alternative is to prepare yourself so that you can give your full attention to the client and patient and are not distracted by other issues at this critical moment. Although this may be just one of many routine consultations of the day for you, for the client it may be a far more important and significant occasion. It is clearly helpful if you and the client approach the interaction with full attention.

Suggestions for preparation and achieving full concentration include:

- **putting aside the last task** – making sure that the last consultation will not impinge on the next, making arrangements to return to unresolved issues later
- **attending to our personal needs and comfort** – ensuring that hunger, heat, thirst, etc. do not disturb your concentration in the next interview
- **shifting focus to the consultation at hand** – preparing as necessary by reading the written or computerized records, searching for results or thinking about the animal's history
- **concluding these activities before greeting the client and patient** – being free to concentrate in as relaxed and focused a way as possible.

This kind of preparation and focus goes deeper than common courtesy and respect. A study looking at family physicians' perceptions of the causes of their self-admitted clinical errors (Ely et al. 1995) showed that hurrying and distraction were among the most common causes to which physicians attributed their mistakes.

Establishing initial rapport

There has been little research into the value of greetings in human or veterinary medical settings – presumably as it seems so obvious – but the following elements deserve consideration:

- greeting the client(s) and patient(s) where appropriate
- introducing yourself
- clarifying your role
- obtaining client's and patient's names and patient signalment as needed
- demonstrating interest and respect; attending to client's and patient's physical comfort.

Research colleague Elpida Artemiou (pers. comm 2016) conducted a pre-and post-training simulated oral assessment of 96 second-year veterinary students' communication skills. The preliminary findings reported here regarding initiation (as described on the Calgary–Cambridge Guides) represent a sample from the larger data set. In this sample there was an increase in time students spent initiating the session post training. This was due in part to an increase in students' use of an opening question and to an increase in efforts to develop a problem list with the client. Students missed explanation of their role and agenda setting consistently in both pre- and post-interactions.

Jansen (2010) audio-recorded and analyzed transcriptions of veterinary–farmer conversations occurring during dairy herd health visits. While veterinarians opened all visits informally (e.g. *How are you?*), only three out of seventeen used a formal opening which included agenda setting. During initiation and throughout the consultations Jansen found no instances of veterinarians following up on advice given in previous visits.

Establishing rapport with multiple people rather than an individual client may require particular attention, for example, when multiple family members or a variety of farm workers play a role in the care of the animal(s) and therefore might be considered to be clients (Williams and Jewell 2012). Individuals in these disparate groups may be present together or located in different places or on various schedules, so you may need to meet with them at different times. We encourage you to keep these permutations in mind throughout this chapter (actually throughout the book) even though, for convenience, we frequently refer to "client" in the singular just as we do in the Calgary–Cambridge Guides.

Greetings and introductions

Introductions are a fascinating insight into veterinarians' practices, particularly as they so often seem to be omitted. We have observed veterinarians or veterinary students forgetting to introduce themselves in clinics and heard clients comment that they were not sure who they were seeing or that they did not know the staff members interacting with their animal(s) or what roles those staff members played. In human medicine, patients frequently make similar comments about introductions.

If you have not met the client and patient before, it is relatively easy to welcome and introduce yourself using a combination of appropriate nonverbal approaches such as handshake, eye contact and smile plus a suitable verbal greeting:

"Good evening, I am Dr. Tammy Anderson, [pause] the doctor on emergency duty this evening. May I ask your name? And this is [gesturing to patient]?"

or

"Hello Ms. French. I am Dr. Pete Kennedy. I understand this is Kiki. And you have met my technician, Pam, already."

or

> "Hello, I'm Dr. Christine Jones, a veterinarian here at the clinic. Am I right that you are Indigo's owner, George Smith?"

In many situations veterinarians know their clients and patients well and do not need to introduce themselves every time. However, veterinary professionals sometimes assume that clients know who they are without any evidence that this is so and inappropriately omit a verbal introduction. They assume that if they have seen a client before, the client will remember who they are and therefore there will be no need to introduce themselves again. Veterinarians may also feel uncomfortable about introducing themselves to individuals such as family members or farm employees or even colleagues whom they may have met before but cannot now remember. We need to develop ways of overcoming such problems:

> "Hello, my name is Dr. Jones. Am I right in thinking we haven't met before?"
>
> or
>
> "You look familiar; have we worked together on past cases? I am the pathologist on duty, James Richardson."

Clarifying your role and the nature of the consultation

In large practices or practices where veterinary students come and go frequently, the uncertainty of not knowing who the clinician is or how they fit into the care of the patient can be unsettling for the client. In a study of 50 medical students, Maguire and Rutter (1976) reported that 80% failed to introduce themselves adequately and to explain their intentions. We have seen incomplete introductions in many veterinary settings. It would seem helpful for students, interns, residents, technicians and others to give their names and also explain their position within the team, the length of time they have to spend with the client, what they will do with the information obtained and how they will relate this information to their supervisor. Would it not be best to state from the outset that the interview is at least partly for the learner's benefit, if that is the case, or conversely, if this is the only opportunity the client will have to give their story and ask questions? Similarly, obtaining permission should be seen as an essential part of the introductory process for all members of the veterinary team:

> "Good morning, my name is Patty Newman and I am a third year veterinary student working with Dr. Mulligan. He has asked me to come get some information from you while he is finishing up with a phone call. Would you be willing to share with me what has been going on with your flock?"
>
> or

"Hi, I am Dr. Grant, an intern working at the emergency clinic. As an intern, I am a graduate veterinarian working under the guidance of the specialists here. That means you get multiple veterinarians working with you to care for Oscar the Grouch. I will be touching base with them at all the crucial points of your case. What are your thoughts about that plan?"

or

"Hello, I am Trish Anderson, one of the technicians here. I am working with Dr. Jones today. Do you mind if I ask you a few questions to get some information for the doctor before he joins us in 10 minutes?"

or

"Hello, my name is Catherine Singh. I am a second year veterinary student volunteering here at the clinic with Dr. Ko. I am here learning how to interview clients. I think Dr. Ko suggested to you that I might spend 15 minutes talking to you before he joins us to discuss your concerns with Oliver. Would that still be all right?"

It might be argued that this is superfluous for experienced veterinarians. But consider the situation in teaching hospitals or with field investigation units, advisory teams, group practices, interdisciplinary teams and emergency departments. Wherever different veterinarians or team members relate to individual patients and clients, you can prevent confusion by carefully explaining your role and the nature of the interview and obtaining consent rather than letting things go unsaid and be ripe for possible misinterpretation. These clarifications are also important when meeting new clients or patients or when circumstances dictate changing of roles.

"Hello Mr. Danners. I am the lead veterinarian with our field disease investigation unit. Dr. Harrington asked me to touch base with you related to your abortion storm. Do you have 15 minutes to talk?"

or

"Phillip, I would like to introduce you to Dr. Kate Miller. She is the internist that is going to take over Buster's care now that we got him through his colic surgery. She and I will work closely together so I will still be involved with his care, but she will be the primary person ensuring his care and keeping you updated on his progress."

or

"Hello, I'm Dr. Ko. May I sit here? I'm one of the surgeons here at the veterinary specialty hospital. Your regular veterinarian, Dr. Jones, has asked me to see you. May I spend 20 minutes with you now to discuss Oliver's problems and to perform a physical exam on him? I'll follow up with Dr. Jones so he knows what we've talked about."

Obtaining the client's and patient's names

In circumstances where you know the client or patient well, this is clearly an unnecessary step. But whenever there is a possibility of confusion, it is always advisable to check that you have the correct names and pronunciations and that the names match those in the medical record. Avoid making assumptions about marital status or preferred form of address.

Veterinarian: *"Hello James, Good to see you again. Am I correct in thinking this handsome creature is Foghorn Leghorn?"*

or

Veterinarian: *"Hello, I'm Dr. Jones. I'm one of the four veterinarians working at this veterinary clinic. Please have a seat if you wish. Can I just check – is it Mrs. Mary French? (pause) I don't think we've met before; what do you prefer that I call you?"*
Client: *"You're right; we haven't met before and please call me Mary."*
Veterinarian: *"Great, and this is Rex?"* (Pause)

Demonstrating interest and respect, attending to the client's and patient's physical comfort

Taking steps to build a relationship from the very beginning of the interview is particularly important. Demonstrating interest, concern and respect for the client and patient, including appropriate nonverbal behavior, is essential in laying the groundwork for productive and collaborative relationships. Findings in the study of Hamood et al. (2014) highlight the importance of balancing the communication between the animal and the client rather than focusing on one or the other.

The veterinarian's behavior and demeanor here are vital in enabling the client to feel welcomed, valued and respected. Taking steps to establish trust and develop the relationship early on will set the scene for efficient and accurate information exchange as the interview unfolds. In human medicine, Eide et al. (2003) demonstrated how very brief informal discussion helps build rapport very early on in the consultation and increases human patient satisfaction with very little investment of time. Beach et al. (2006) showed that when they had respect for particular patients, physicians showed positive affect and provided more information; patients were able to perceive this.

To build rapport you need to demonstrate respect and establish common ground. There are many ways to do this. You can talk about mutual personal interests that have little to do with the animal or you can make sure you both understand the same problem/issue list or you might just acknowledge out loud that you both have the animal's best interest in mind. Because this vital area requires attention throughout the whole interview and not just at the beginning, we discuss skills that contribute to building the relationship in every chapter and devote all of Chapter 5 to this topic.

Virtually everything that we describe about initiating the interview contributes to relationship building by encouraging the client's contributions and promoting a collaborative approach. However, before leaving our consideration of the skills associated with establishing initial rapport, we would like to comment on one particularly important item: attending to the client's and patient's physical comfort.

Environmental factors affect physical and psychological comfort. They influence position, posture and eye contact, our perception and attitudes and our ability to attend. If you are meeting at your clinic or hospital, are room temperatures appropriate? Is seating available for incapacitated or elderly clients? Are examining rooms equipped to accommodate a variety of veterinary patients safely? Have you taken into consideration the comfort of the client(s) and yourself? Is lighting neither glaring nor too dim? Are the client and you positioned so that no one must look into the glare of windows without shades or bright sunlight? In reception areas are materials available, such as magazines, aquariums, client education brochures, children's toys and the like? Whether at your clinic or a client's farm are you positioning people and animals to take into account the safety of all, including yourself?

If the client is seated, all the better if you are also seated as this puts everyone on a more equal footing, makes unobtrusive note-taking easier, and gives the impression that you are willing to take the time that is needed to give full attention to the patient and client. Interestingly, Swayden et al. (2012) showed in a randomized controlled study that postoperative surgical patients perceived physicians who sat rather than stood at their bedside as being present longer, even though the actual time the physician spent at the bedside did not change significantly. Patients with whom the physician sat reported a more positive interaction and a better understanding of their condition. We suspect these findings pertain to many veterinary contexts, too.

Where possible in clinic contexts, placing furniture so that you and the client can sit at a knee-to-knee angle rather than side by side or directly across from each other is helpful. People want easy eye contact, but not so direct that they cannot readily "escape." Wherever you are, to the extent possible, control extraneous sound levels so that everyone can hear. Whether the animal is on an exam table or not, take care to position everyone safely as well as conveniently for whatever interaction with the client and patient is needed.

As much as possible, when dealing with sensitive subject matter (e.g. giving bad news or euthanasia), close doors or if no privacy is possible, at least be aware of others who are nearby. Reassure the client and be aware that environment-induced uneasiness may inhibit or distract the client to the point of giving inaccurate or incomplete information. Finally, keep in mind that all these aspects of environment are as likely to influence you as much as they influence others.

Identifying the reason(s) for the consultation

Having exchanged introductions and established initial rapport, the next step is to determine what issues the client wishes to discuss. What is the client's agenda for the interview? Why are you seeing the client and patient today? In all contexts you need to clarify the list of problems or items that the client wishes to address, explain additional reasons of your own for seeing the patient, and take note of patient needs that the client may not have mentioned. This is an essential element of initiation even when a receptionist or technician has already spoken with the client and provided their perception of the problem list. This information guides the organization of the entire consultation and is also an important opportunity to begin establishing common ground and rapport with the client.

McKinley and Middleton (1999) have shown in a study in British general practice that almost all patients had specific pre-formed requests they wished to make of their physicians; almost half had specific questions they wished to ask; 55% wanted specific treatment; 60% had their own ideas about why they had developed their problems and 40% had specific concerns about their symptoms. Patients undoubtedly come to the physician with well thought out agendas that they want to have addressed. So do veterinary clients.

Perhaps this all seems so obvious as to be hardly worth mentioning, but in fact it's more complicated than we might think. Recall Dysart et al.'s (2011) findings reported earlier in the chapter showing that veterinarians often failed to solicit clients' concerns early in the interview and that they often have more than one concern. Also remember the evidence showing how often physicians fail to detect problems or issues patients wish to discuss and how frequently physicians and patients disagree after the interview about the nature of the main presenting problem. In a qualitative study in general medical practice in the UK, Barry et al. (2000) discovered that only 4 of 35 patients voiced all the concerns they wanted to discuss in the consultation. In all of the 14 consultations with problem outcomes, at least one of the problems was related to an unvoiced agenda item.

The veterinarian's behavior and approach in the initiation phase can have profound effects on the rest of the consultation, causing differences not only in the structure and timing of what occurs in the consultation but indeed in the very problems that are discussed. It is interesting to consider evidence from research on initiation in human medicine in order to compare it with some of what happens at the beginning of veterinary consultations:

- Several investigators have shown that human patients often have more than one concern to discuss: in a variety of settings including primary care, pediatrics and internal medicine, the mean number of concerns ranged from 1.2 to 3.9 in both new and return visits (Starfield et al. 1981; Good and Good 1982; Wasserman et al. 1984; Greenfield et al. 1985). These studies warn of the danger of physicians engaging in premature and limited hypothesis testing before identifying a wider spectrum of concerns.
- In a study of internal medicine residents and physicians in primary care, Beckman and Frankel (1984) have shown that:
  - the serial order in which patients present their problems is not related to their clinical importance; the first concern presented is no more likely than the second or third to be the most important as judged by either the patient or the doctor
  - physicians very often assume erroneously that the first complaint mentioned is the only one that the patient has brought
  - in follow-up visits, doctors often assume that the consultation is a direct

continuation of the last interview and omit the opening solicitation entirely, proceeding directly to questions about concerns elicited in previous visits.

If the first complaint mentioned is not necessarily the most important, why do we behave as if it is the only one likely to be offered? We all can recall consultations that have suffered from this approach with the real problem concerning the human patient or client surfacing very late in the interview after our precious allotted time has been used on a less important topic (Robinson 2001; Dysart et al. 2011). Sometimes it's even worse: we may not discover the main reason for the consultation at all and the interview may end without the patient/client mentioning their more important agenda item. Even more fundamentally, why do we explore the first sign or symptom mentioned before discovering all the other signs or symptoms that the patient/client has noticed even when, as we shall see in Chapter 3, this can lead to significantly less effective clinical reasoning?

How can we overcome these problems? How do we make a route-plan of the consultation rather than blindly setting off down the first road that we come across? Here we discuss three related skills that can help the veterinarian to understand the client's complete agenda early on, during the initiation of the session:

- the opening question
- listening
- screening
- agenda setting

The opening question
New consultations

Near the beginning of the interview, it is important to ask the client an open question such as *"What would you like to discuss today?"* We all tend to have a favorite stock question that we use repeatedly. Here are some examples of phrases we have heard veterinarians use:

"How can I help?"
"Tell me what you have come to see me about."
"What would you like to talk about today?"
"What can I do for you?"
"How are you doing?"
"How are things?"
"What's up?"
"What is going on with your herd/flock?"
"I understand you've called me here today to perform a lameness exam …?"
Nothing said (all implied in body language with appropriate pause).

The opening question of an inexperienced student may need to be different from that of the veterinarian responsible for the patient. Given a client whose animal was admitted to the tertiary care hospital some time ago and is therefore already in the system, the student's task may be to discover, primarily for their own benefit, what the client understands and what their concerns are at this point. On the other hand, veterinarians more often are working in a diagnostic capacity and need to use phrases such as *"Tell me what problems Riley has been having," "How can I help you and Riley?"* or *"I have a helpful letter from your veterinarian, Dr. Patel, but please start by telling me what the problems are from your perspective."*

The exact words that we use can become a mantra that we repeat without thought. But in fact the phrasing of this simple task can make a considerable difference to the nature of the rest of the interview. The format of this opening question can subtly change the type of response the client provides.

More general inquiries such as *"How are things?"* allow the client to comment in broad terms about how the new puppy is settling in or how the kids' soccer team is doing but might not discover the actual problem that they have come about. On the other hand, it may open up a useful conversation with a producer who is worried about feed prices and is considering switching rations, which may impact your nutritional plan.

"Tell me what you have come to see me about" is less medical, more open and might signal your willingness to listen to a wider agenda.

"What's on your agenda today?" or *"What's on your problem list today?"* certainly implies that you would like to encourage the client to make a list of all the problems that they would like to discuss, but might not be understood by all clients unless you explain, at least the first time you ask.

"The technician told me you were here for vaccines and a weight check – is that the complete list or is there something else you wanted to talk about today?" This acknowledges that someone else has already spoken to the client and invites the client to repeat themselves or add new information without it seeming awkward. When you expect to see clients anytime again we encourage you to tell them directly that it is very helpful if they prepare a complete list beforehand of everything they hope to discuss with you and that you will routinely ask for this list.

We are not suggesting that there is one correct opening method to be used on all occasions. However, there is a need for clinicians to raise their awareness and think more carefully about the consequences of how they start each consultation (Robinson 2001; Gafaranga and Britten 2003).

Heritage and Robinson (2006) used conversation analysis to explore the effect of various opening questions in primary, acute and outpatient visits. Compared to confirmatory questions in which the physician asks whether the patient has come for a particular reason (e.g. *"I understand you have some sinus problems today"*), general open-ended inquiries were associated with significantly longer problem presentations that included more discrete symptoms. In another human study, open-ended inquiries were positively associated with patients' evaluation of physicians' listening and relational communication (Robinson and Heritage 2006). Heritage (2011) has also looked at the evidence from conversation analysis in everyday non-medical conversations and explains how normal conversation differs from medical consultations. He explores why physicians have to put aside their normal conversational approach of assuming pre-existing shared understanding with the patient, based solely on information from the record or from another health practitioner (such as the triage nurse in primary care) and instead use highly open general inquiries as above at the beginning of the interview.

In veterinary medicine, Dysart et al. (2011) showed that an opening solicitation was categorized as either an open-ended question, which is a broad inquiry into a client's concerns that does not shape or direct the content of the response (e.g. *"What can I do for you today?"*) or a closed-ended question. Closed-ended questions (e.g. *"Any concerns?"* or *"Is Rory in today for his vaccinations?"*) are structured to elicit a specific and often one-word response (e.g. yes or no). In the study the use of open-ended solicitations resulted in significantly more client concerns being elicited than the use of closed-ended solicitations.

When the veterinarian is speaking with multiple clients involved in the care of the animals at different times or when someone other than the veterinarian has already talked with the client, a few additions to the opening solicitation are helpful. These additions clarify for the client what you already know and what you are now inviting the client to tell you. For example:

"I understand from Tammy [the technician], that Banjo has been having diarrhea and vomiting. Is that correct? [pause] What other concerns do you have?"

or

"I have been speaking to your herd manager about your increased incidence of mastitis. We are here to help you look into this problem. What other concerns do you have before we get started with a plan to investigate the mastitis?"

or

"The receptionist told me you were here for vaccines and a weight check – what else is on your list for today?"

Consider also the differences in the opening solicitation when referring and referral veterinarians are talking with the client. White et al. (2013) undertook a small study involving conversation analysis to look at the impact of the referral process during the initiation phase of human surgeon–patient consultations in New Zealand. In these referred consultations a central task of the opening activities was "… for the participants to establish a shared understanding of the reason for the visit incorporating not only their own understanding but also that of the referring doctor." Here the researchers suggest that overt recognition of the referral process by the surgeon (for instance, by explicitly mentioning the referring doctor and/or the referral letter) and the discussion that followed is important for accurately determining the agenda and organizing the surgical consultation, providing patients with the opportunity to participate in the opening activities of the visit, helping patients to overcome concerns about telling the surgeon something they already know, and progressing to appropriate exploration of the problem. In this study, problems arose when there was no recognition of the referral process (although this occurred in only one consultation), when the referral letter was unclear or when the surgeon's understanding of the referral (e.g. regarding the presenting problem or the goal of the consultation) did not align with the patient's and/or the referring physician's understanding.

We suggest that some of these same issues arise in veterinary medicine not only between referring and referral veterinarians but also during the initiation of the visit in primary care, emergency departments/clinics, teaching hospitals, or other settings where someone other than the veterinarian handles an intake interview or triage, be it a veterinary technician or receptionist (as in the examples above) or a veterinary student or intern. Or in settings like tertiary care hospitals where patients are moved from one service to another or group practices where, for example, different veterinarians may see chronic care patients on different occasions. Even though in these contexts the time elapsed may be only minutes or hours, the issues (e.g. inaccuracy or incompleteness in the "handover," incomplete or unclear records, unchecked assumptions, and clients' uncertainty or reluctance to repeat some important fact or sequence of events that they think their veterinarian already knows) may be similar.

When handovers are involved it is, of course, not only the way clinicians interact with clients or patients, but also the quality of communication between the various clinicians that makes a difference. In her research on equine referring veterinarians' expectations of equine specialists and veterinary referral centers, Best (2015) reported that effective and timely communication was the most important component of the referral process. Lack of communication, delayed communication, and incorrect information contributed to referring veterinarians' negative experience. For a more detailed look at this important aspect of interaction between veterinarians and its implications for communication with clients and outcomes of patient care, see Best's complete dissertation.

Another valuable resource on communication in handovers is a recent book reporting on a 3-year multidisciplinary research project that focused on nursing, medical and interprofessional handovers in a wide range of hospital contexts in human medicine. Edited by Eggins et al. (2016,), the book presents extensive empirical data and practical communication tools that emanated from that comprehensive project.

Follow-up visits

Follow-up visits have much more in common with new consultations than is often believed. The key here is not to make the assumption that you know the reason for the visit until you have actually asked the client and checked the patient. It is so easy to assume that the purpose of the consultation is a routine check of the animal and to move straight into *"How are you getting along with the new medication regime?"* when in fact the patient has a more pressing problem or the client has a different agenda item to discuss. Yet it can sound as if you do not remember the patient and client at all if you start as in a new appointment with *"What would you like to discuss today?"* Perhaps instead you might start with your understanding of the reason for the visit as in *"Am I right in thinking that you have come primarily for the follow-up visit to Max's surgery?"* and then ask the client to confirm if that is the only thing they want to discuss by adding *"I'd appreciate knowing if there is something else you would like to talk about today …"*

Listening to the client's opening statement
Learning how to listen at the beginning of the consultation is the first step to an efficient and accurate consultation

It seems at first glance that giving the client time, space and encouragement to have the floor while the veterinarian deliberately sits back and listens might not be the most efficient way of beginning an interview. In their discussion of time and physician–patient interaction, Levinson and Pizzo (2011) maintain that clinicians can be under so much pressure from time constraints that they feel the need to force the pace by quickly moving into questioning mode and taking the initiative. Similarly in veterinary medicine, this same time factor often leads veterinarians to explore the first item the client offers which, as we have seen, can be counterproductive. How do we address this problem? How do we establish that being fully present in order to be able to listen to the client from the very beginning of the consultation is rewarded by a far more efficient and accurate interview overall?

Listening rather than questioning allows veterinarians and clients to achieve more of their objectives for this part of the consultation

Reviewing the objectives for this first part of the consultation is helpful. The objectives fall into three broad categories. The first is to understand what the client wants to discuss today, to then add in anything else that you as the veterinarian wish to discuss, and to plan with the client how to approach the rest of the consultation. The second is to establish initial rapport and make the client feel an important part of the process. The third is to gauge how the client and the patient are doing given the circumstances.

How do veterinary professionals achieve all of these objectives with the greatest ease and efficiency? As you will see in Chapter 3, as soon as the veterinarian moves into detailed questioning, the client tends to become a passive contributor. The veterinarian then has to follow each closed question with another, their mind is forced away from the client's responses into diagnostic reasoning and the interview prematurely focuses onto one particular area. In contrast, following an open-ended initial statement or question with attentive listening allows the veterinarian to discover more of the client's agenda, to hear the story from the client's perspective, to appear supportive and interested and, by concentrating on both patient and client, to pick up cues that could otherwise be missed.

What is the evidence to support listening?

The importance of demonstrating listening skills from the very beginning of the consultation and throughout has been demonstrated by a number of researchers in both human and veterinary medicine.

In a Canadian focus group study, Coe et al. (2008) found participating pet owners identified the veterinarian taking the time to listen as a key factor in the positive experiences described by the pet owners. Participants indicated that this did not necessarily mean the veterinarian had to take more physical time; rather that the participants valued the veterinarian focusing complete attention on them and their animal(s) during the scheduled appointment time.

We have known for a long time from Byrne and Long's work in human primary care (1976) that many dysfunctional consultations arise because of difficulties in discovering why the patient has come. One of the problems here lies with the patient's tendency to withhold important concerns until later in the visit, when they have tested the water and gained confidence in the doctor. Anxiety or embarrassment about a particular problem or a serious worry might prevent mention of it until late in the day. These late announcements have been termed "hidden agendas" (Barsky 1981), a difficulty with which veterinary medicine is also familiar.

The term "hidden agenda" tends to focus attention on the client's apparent decision to withhold, delay or share information. However, an alternative interpretation of what is happening when clients bring in a new agenda item late in the consultation emphasizes the role that the clinician plays, and the influence that clinicians' behavior can have on the placement and flow of information provided by clients or human patients. The clinicians' own words and actions have a startling effect on whether (or when) they discover the full reasons for the consultation – the clinicians' behavior may well be more influential here than the clients'.

Byrne and Long (1976) showed that many physicians were not good listeners and had fixed routines of interviewing patients that demonstrate little capacity for variation to meet an individual's needs. In their ground-breaking research, Beckman and Frankel (1984) have taken this further by analyzing exactly how physicians' use of words and questions can so easily and inadvertently direct the patient away from disclosing their reasons for wishing to see the doctor. Their research revealed a host of thought-provoking facts:

- physicians frequently interrupted patients before they had completed their opening statement – after a mean time of only 18 seconds
- only 23% of patients completed their opening statement
- in only 1 out of 51 interrupted statements was the patient allowed to complete their opening statement later
- 94% of all interruptions concluded with the physician obtaining the floor
- the longer the physician waited before interruption, the more complaints were elicited
- allowing the patient to complete the opening statement led to a significant reduction in late arising problems
- clarifying or closed questions were the most frequent cause of interruption but any utterance by the doctor that specifically encouraged the patient to give further information about any one problem could also cause disruption: this perhaps surprisingly included echoing of the patient's words

- in 34 out of 51 visits, the doctor interrupted the patient after the initial concern, apparently assuming that the first complaint was the chief one
- the serial order in which the patients presented their problems was not related to their clinical importance
- patients who were allowed to complete their opening statement without interruption mostly took less than 60 seconds and none took longer than 150 seconds, even when encouraged to continue.

Does any of this happen in veterinary medicine? In a cross-sectional study of 334 veterinarian–client–patient interactions that was based on Beckman and Frankel's work, Dysart et al. (2011) asked many of the same questions but in small animal veterinary medicine. They found that:

- in 63% (n=211) of the consultations, the veterinarian made no solicitations (i.e. questions that probed the reasons for the visit or for the client's concerns)
- in the 37% (n=123) of the consultations where veterinarians did make solicitations, they used open questions 76% of the time and closed 24%.

In the 123 consultations where veterinarians made solicitations:

- the veterinarian interrupted the client 55% (n=68) of the time
- the mean length of time clients spoke before interruption was 15.3 seconds
- odds of a client's opening statement being completed before interruption in a wellness appointment were six times higher than in a problem appointment
- the most common reason for incompletion of a client's response was the veterinarian interrupting by using a closed-ended question
- most often interruptions occurred after the client had expressed at least one concern – the longer a client was allowed to speak, the more concerns arose or, said another way, the more complete the list of concerns and problems was
- when veterinarians used an open-ended question, the client spoke a mean of 13.2 seconds. The use of a closed-ended question resulted in the client speaking for a mean of 5 seconds
- the use of open-ended solicitations resulted in significantly more client concerns being elicited than the use of closed questions.

Beckman and Frankel and Dysart et al. have shown us that in human and veterinary medicine it is the early pursuit by closed questioning of the first problem mentioned that prevents clinicians from discovering all the issues that a patient or client wishes to discuss. The emphasis quickly shifts from a patient/client-centered to a clinician-centered format. Once this is done, the patient/client tends to remain in a more passive role, trying to comply by giving short answers, perhaps assuming that if the competent clinician needs to know something they will ask. Inefficient and inaccurate information gathering ensues. Not only does the interview steam ahead before the main concerns have been discovered but hypothesis testing proceeds without clients having a chance to tell their story or to provide information which closed questioning may well never discover.

Dysart et al. (2011) offer examples of several kinds of interruptions veterinarians use as clients are trying to describe their concerns:

- *"Which leg was she limping on?"* (closed question)
- *"It sounds like she could have ear mites."* (noninterrogative statement)
- *"So she is favoring her left leg more than her right one."* (recompleter)
- *"Tell me more about the scratching."* (elaborator)
- The veterinarian interrupts the client by speaking to the patient.

These could be useful approaches to history taking, but not when they interrupt the client who is trying to tell you their agenda.

The research in veterinary and human medicine clearly demonstrates that even minimal interruptions to clients' or patients' initial statements can actually prevent other concerns from appearing at all or can make important complaints arise late in the consultation. By asking individuals to start telling you more about any one problem, you restrict their options, preventing them from expanding on other information that they would like to tell you. The individual is faced with a practical problem when the clinician moves in with an interruption. Several additional studies from human medicine underscore the need to change our approach to this part of the interview.

In their study, Marvel et al. (1999) found that physicians interrupted 72% of their patients, and although physicians may well intend to return later to let the patient finish, this happened in only 8% of interviews. They discovered that an alternative approach to encouraging patients to disclose their full agenda was to follow each solicitation with a focused open-ended question such as *"Tell me more about the leg pain"* before reverting to another open-ended solicitation such as *"Is there anything else we need to take care of today?"* An example in veterinary medicine might be *"Tell me more about the limping"* followed by *"Is there something else we need to take care of today?"*

Ruiz Moral et al. (2006) in a study of third year family physician residents in Spain showed that patients mentioned new problems at closure (*"Oh, by the way ..."*) more frequently when physicians redirected the focus of the interview before patients completed an initial statement of concerns in the early moments of the visit. More than half of the trainees directed the focus of the interview before the patient had completed an initial statement of concerns. Early redirection did not save overall consultation time but made closures longer and more dysfunctional as patients raised new problems at the end of the interview.

Langewitz et al. (2002) conducted their study in the internal medicine outpatient clinic of a Swiss tertiary referral centre, a setting characterized by "difficult patients with complex histories." Suggesting that physicians may interrupt so frequently because they assume that patients will interfere with the time schedule if allowed to talk as long as they wish, Langewitz et al. wanted to know if this in fact would happen. The sample consisted of 335 patients who were making first contact with this clinic and 14 experienced internists who were trained to listen actively without interrupting until the patient indicated that their list of complaints was complete. Despite the complexities inherent in this tertiary referral setting, patients' mean spontaneous talking time was only 92 seconds and 78% of all patients finished within 2 minutes. Seven patients talked longer than 5 minutes, but their doctors felt the information they were giving was important and should not be interrupted.

Wissow et al. (1994) have shown that pediatricians' use of attentive listening is positively associated with parents' disclosure of psychosocial problems. Might this be similarly useful in veterinary medicine where, for example, spousal or animal abuse is an issue or with potentially suicidal clients?

Putnam et al. (1988) have shown that it is possible to teach residents in human medicine the skills of attentive listening and that such teaching leads to a significant increase in patient exposition without any associated increase in the length of the interview.

What are the specific skills of attentive listening?

Listening is often equated with "sitting and doing nothing", a passive rather than active approach. Yet as Egan (1990) says in *The Skilled Helper*:

> How many times have you heard someone exclaim, "You're not listening to what I'm saying!" When the person accused of not listening answers, "I am too; I can repeat everything you've said," the accuser is not comforted. What people look for in attending and listening is not the other person's ability to repeat their words. A tape recorder would do that perfectly. People want more than physical presence in human communication; they want the other person to be present psychologically, socially and emotionally.

In fact attentive listening is both active and highly skilled. It is needed during initiation and throughout the consultation. There are four specific skill areas that can help us to develop our ability to listen attentively:

- wait time
- facilitative response
- nonverbal skills
- picking up verbal and nonverbal cues.

1. WAIT TIME

Making the shift from speaking to listening at appropriate moments in the consultation is not easy. Inadvertently, we often find ourselves preparing our next question rather than focusing attention on what the client is saying. We may become so involved in formulating our next question that we divert our own attention from hearing the client's message and, by interrupting, fail to give the client adequate time to respond. Or we finish the client's sentence for them, perhaps trying to hurry them along or to anticipate what they are about to say even though we actually quite often do not know. Evidence from the world of education rather than medicine helps to illuminate the value to both veterinarian and client of allowing the client more space to think before answering or to go on after pausing.

Over 20 years, Rowe (1986) studied non-medical teachers in a wide variety of classroom settings. She found that when teachers asked questions, they waited 1 second or less for a reply. Similarly, they only waited 1 second after a student stopped speaking before they responded. However, if the teachers were trained to increase their pauses at each of these key points to 3 seconds, remarkable changes occurred in the student's behavior in class. The students contributed more often, spoke for longer, asked more questions, provided more evidence for their thinking and failed to respond less often. Difficult or "invisible" students started to contribute successfully. In turn, teachers asked their students less questions but of a more flexible nature and they increased their expectations of their students.

In the veterinary interview, using wait time effectively allows the client time to think and to contribute more without interruption and the veterinarian to have time to listen, think and respond more flexibly.

2. FACILITATIVE RESPONSE

Some veterinarians clearly are more able than others to encourage their clients to say more about a topic, to indicate to clients that they are interested in what their clients are saying and would like them to continue. This is often achieved very efficiently with minimal or no interruption. It is worth considering exactly what these minimal clues are that seem to be such powerful indicators to the client that we are listening.

We will look in more detail at facilitation skills in Chapter 3 but at this point we would like to consider which specific facilitative responses are of value in this opening phase of the consultation. Research has clearly shown that the skills employed in attentive listening are different at different stages in the consultation and that facilitation skills known to be helpful later on in the consultation are in fact counterproductive when used early on in the interview.

Beckman and Frankel's (1984) work provides clear guidance here again. They showed that repetition (echoing), paraphrasing and interpretation, which are all valuable facilitative skills later on in the interview, potentially act as interrupters at the beginning of the interview whereas other more neutral facilitative phrases such as "uh-huh," "go on," "yes," "um," "I see" serve to encourage the patient to continue along their own path.

3. NONVERBAL SKILLS

We provide a more detailed exploration of nonverbal skills when we look at "Building the Relationship" in Chapter 5. Here, however, we would like to flag some issues about nonverbal communication which are particularly relevant to the beginning of the consultation.

Much of our willingness to listen is signaled through our nonverbal behavior which immediately gives the client strong clues as to our level of interest in them, their questions or issues, and their animal's problems. Many individual components are involved in nonverbal communication including posture, movement, proximity, direction of gaze, eye contact, gestures, affect, vocal cues (tone, rate, volume of speech), facial expression, touch, physical appearance, and environmental cues (placement of furniture, lighting, warmth). All these skills can assist in demonstrating attentiveness to clients and facilitate the formation of a supportive relationship; ineffective attending behavior in contrast both closes off the interaction and prohibits relationship building (Gazda et al. 1995).

Among the most important of all the nonverbal skills is eye contact. We can easily be distracted from providing this by notes or computer or the animal as we try to listen to and understand our client. Yet poor clinician eye contact can be readily misinterpreted as lack of interest and can inhibit open communication (Goodwin 1981; Ruusuvuori 2001; Nordman et al. 2010). First impressions are very important here.

Communication research has shown that nonverbal messages tend to override verbal messages when the two are inconsistent or contradictory (Koch 1971; McCroskey et al. 1971). Perhaps this is because nonverbal communication is so much more elemental to us as a species – we had nonverbal communication long before we had the spoken word. If you provide the verbal message that you want the client to tell you all about their problem while at the same time you speak quickly, look harassed and avoid eye contact, your nonverbal message will usually win out. The client will correctly construe that time is at a premium today and may not tell you about the problem in sufficient detail.

The importance of both verbal and nonverbal facilitation skills lies in the message that they impart to the client. Two of the principles of communication that we outlined in Chapter 1 concerned reducing uncertainty and establishing mutually understood common ground. Facilitation skills are effective in encouraging clients to tell us their story because they directly signal to our clients something about our attitude to them, our interest in them and their story, and our helpful intentions. In the absence of these skills, the client remains uncertain about our interest in what they are saying and our need for them to continue with their account: we might be clear in our own minds that we wish the interview to proceed in a certain way but is our verbal and nonverbal behavior skillful enough for the client to share that understanding?

4. PICKING UP VERBAL AND NONVERBAL CUES

Another important listening skill is that of picking up clients' verbal and nonverbal cues. This requires listening and observation of both the client and the animal. Tuckett et al. (1985) found that human patients' ideas, concerns and expectations are often provided in nonverbal cues and indirect comments rather than overt statements. These cues often feature very early in the patient's exposition of their problems and the physician needs to look out specifically for them from the very beginning of the interview. The danger lies in either missing these messages altogether or assuming we know what they mean without checking them out with the client now or later in the interview. We take up this aspect of attentive listening in greater detail in Chapter 3.

What are the advantages of attentive listening?

Full attention through active listening allows you to:

- signal your interest to the client
- hear their story
- prevent yourself from making premature hypotheses and chasing down blind allies
- reduce late arising complaints
- hear both biomedical and client perspectives, as discussed in Chapter 3
- not have to think of the next question (which blocks your listening and renders the client passive)
- calibrate how the client is doing, including their emotional state
- observe more carefully and pick up verbal and nonverbal cues.

Listening attentively without interruption is also extremely helpful to the client whose ideas and concerns about their animal's health may be relatively undefined. Giving space to such clients allows them time to clarify what it is that they wish to discuss with the veterinarian. Not all clients have clear-cut agendas.

With so much to hear and see at the beginning of the interview, why not consciously set aside the first minute or two for the client and concentrate on listening and facilitating rather than questioning? Listening attentively instead of moving immediately to a series of questions about the history allows us to achieve more of our objectives. Although it requires very little time, using these early moments of the consultation wisely (however hard that may be) pays off handsomely.

In apparent veterinary emergency situations, we can hear objections to this approach to initiation. Yet consider a few examples. In an emergency situation where a dog has been rushed to the veterinary clinic immediately after being hit by a car, the veterinarian or a member of the veterinary team may check in with the client while the animal is being transported to the treatment room for assessment: *"I'm glad you were able to get her here so quickly. How are you holding up?"* This offers the opportunity for the client to share what is at the forefront of their mind and allows the veterinarian to assess the client's current state and feelings. Similarly, when called to attend to a uterine prolapse in a beef cow, the veterinarian can ask, while removing equipment from their vehicle: *"How has the rest of the calving season been going for you?"* This gives the veterinarian an opportunity to assess the broader situation on the farm while at the same time allowing the producer to share their thinking and feelings on that broader situation as the emergency proceeds.

Confirming and screening

The discussion above demonstrates how using an appropriate opening question combined with attentive listening and specific facilitation skills allows the veterinarian to discover more of the client's agenda in the early part of the consultation. Next we explore how making a further deliberate attempt to discover all of the client's concerns and issues *before* actively exploring any one of them can further increase the accuracy and efficiency of consultations.

Screening is the process of deliberately checking with the client that you have discovered all that they wish to discuss by asking further open-ended questions. Rather than assuming that the client has mentioned all their difficulties, double-check:

> Veterinarian: *"Susie, our technician, mentioned that you are here for Piper's routine vaccinations. What else did you hope we could help with today?"*

If the client continues, perhaps in this example mentioning a problem with Piper's ears, resume listening until the client stops again; then repeat the screening process, perhaps adding that it is helpful to have the client's full list right at the beginning of the interview, until eventually the client says that they have finished:

> Veterinarian: *"This is an important observation. In addition to updating the vaccinations, let's make sure we check her out to see what is going on with her ears. Was there something else on your list today?"*

At the end of this process when the client says, *"No, that's about it,"* it is useful to confirm your understanding out loud, thereby giving the client an opportunity to know what you have heard:

> Veterinarian: *"Let's make sure we're on the same page. Along with vaccinating Piper we want to check her ears to see if there is something causing her to shake her head a lot lately. And we'll check her to see if there is a reason she is scooting on the carpet. Does that hit on all your concerns and goals for this visit?"*

Often this method of checking reveals signs and concerns relating to the initial problem, but the client might not yet have revealed a totally separate problem:

> Client: *"Well, we've been thinking about getting a kitten. Do you have any advice for us about that?"*

A large animal example of screening and confirming the problem list might look like this:

> Veterinarian: *"You have the list of cows to preg check and I also noticed there are a couple of cows we should discuss that have SCCs [somatic cell counts] creeping up in your Dairy Comp record. What other things are on your list for today?"*

Resume listening until the client stops talking. Perhaps the client says there is a cow off feed. Then repeat the screening process.

> Veterinarian: *"No problem, we'll check the cow off feed as well. What else?"*

One last check:

> Veterinarian: *"So let me recap to make sure I have everything straight before we move on. We have the six cows on your list to preg check, the two cows with high SCC to check out, and then the one cow off feed. We have our list of cows to look at. Have we got your entire list or is there something more you were hoping we might be able to look at today as well?"*
> Client: *"If you have time I wouldn't mind you taking a quick look at the ventilation in the new calf barn and let me know your thoughts."*
> Or the client might raise a personal issue that affects the agenda:
> Client: *"Well, I've got a lot of hay down that needs to be wrapped and so I really don't have the time today for that cow to have a DA [displaced abomasum]."*

Interestingly, work by Heritage et al. (2007) in the USA demonstrated that using the phrase *"Is there something else you want to address in the visit today?"* was more effective in screening than the phrase *"Is there anything else you want to address in the visit today?"* Using "something" or "some other concern" strongly reduced the incidence of patients' unmet concerns without significantly increasing visit length. In contrast, using "anything" or "any other" was relatively ineffective in eliciting additional concerns and in reducing unmet concerns. This is as predicted by the field of linguistics which suggests that the word "any" is negatively polarized (with a subtle communication of an expectation of a "no" response) and the word "some" is positively polarized. It is not clear whether this result is generalizable outside of the USA and how much effect nonverbal communication has in ameliorating the differences between these words.

Confirming and screening are the last two steps in a four part approach to determining the client's complete problem list. Including:

1. opening question
2. listening

3. screening
4. confirming

offers many advantages to the veterinarian and the client over the alternative of:

1. asking
2. assuming
3. proceeding.

For the veterinarian, there is a better chance of discovering the client's full agenda, negotiating how best to use the time available and pacing the interview appropriately. Screening and confirming also provides a way for veterinarians to check out their expectations and assumptions about the client's reason for the visit, thereby helping the veterinarian to keep an open mind. For the client, screening establishes mutually understood common ground and provides the reassurance that you are really interested in their problems and thoughts. Both in turn enhance trust and disclosure. Helping the person reveal their most important concerns early on helps the client focus attention on how and when to introduce their unstated concern rather than on the agenda in progress (Korsch et al. 1968; Mehrabian and Ksionsky 1974). Screening and confirming help prevent uncertainty in the client's mind leading to distraction and blocking effective communication.

Clients may of course still reveal an underlying problem, a "hidden agenda," later in the interview when they have tested the water and gained confidence in the relationship. Screening encourages but does not guarantee early problem identification and we must still remain open to late arising complaints and be sensitive to the reasons that the client might have for delaying. In human medicine, Peltenburg et al. (2004) have demonstrated that some agenda items that emerge as the consultation proceeds were not anticipated by either physician or patient prior to the interview; this emerging agenda appeared to relate to the ability of the clinician to pick up affective cues.

Several North American texts propose the following sequence for the early part of the consultation (Riccardi and Kurtz 1983; Lipkin 1987; Cohen-Cole 1991; Baker et al. 2005):

- encouraging the client or patient to discuss their main concerns by attentive listening without interruption or premature closure
- confirming the list identified so far by summarizing or repeating the list out loud
- checking repeatedly for additional concerns, *"Is there something else you wish to discuss today?"*, until the client or patient indicates that there is nothing else to add
- negotiating an agenda for the consultation.

We shall look more closely at the skills of checking and summarizing in Chapter 3.

The balance between listening and screening

Having discovered the importance of screening for the full range of problems, learners often identify a dilemma about when exactly to screen and when to listen. A balance has to be achieved in the use of these two complementary skills that will be determined in part by the context of each interview.

In certain interviews, it is possible and beneficial to be quite up front about screening and to explain your plan to the client straightaway. So, as an example, the client referred to a specialist might receive the following introduction:

> *"Hello, I'm Dr. Smith. I've got a letter from your veterinarian so I've got some idea of why you've come today, but I'd like to hear the story from you first hand and then try to help as best I can. I'd like to start, if you agree, with us making a list of all the problems Dexter's been having and your concerns. Then we can explore them together in more detail."*

This approach makes the structure very clear to the client: it makes it apparent that the veterinarian wants to understand the whole of their agenda from the start and will then attend to all of their problems and concerns. Otherwise, the client may not know if they are expected to go ahead with explaining one problem in detail or to mention them all briefly.

At the other extreme is a client who immediately breaks into a story that they clearly need to tell. For example, a client who is worried she has done something wrong by not bringing her cat in sooner and feels guilty because she was preoccupied with final exams and may have ignored some important signs. Or a client who on sitting down starts to cry perhaps because he has reached a point of decision to euthanize his much-loved hunting dog. These times deserve our full attention now: here listening takes priority over screening. It would be inappropriate to interrupt and say, *"We'll come back to that. Is there something else that you would like to discuss today?"*!

Some clients come with their pre-written list (perhaps including ideas they got from the Internet, breeder, pet store, farrier, trainer, neighbor or animal psychic), thereby giving the veterinarian a perfect opportunity to screen the agenda and negotiate what is possible in the time today. Some veterinarians "teach" their clients to do just that and explain why such an opening list is so helpful. Other clients come with a well-rehearsed speech that they have prepared: the telling of it is essential for the client's peace of mind before the veterinarian and client can settle down to work together. Often this opening statement can be so rich in feelings, thoughts, ideas, concerns and expectations and give such clues to the patient's and client's situation that it would be a mistake not to give the client the floor to express their story. If you do not listen first, you might well miss clues that could be important in helping the client with their problem.

This dilemma can be resolved by another of the principles of communication that we have already discussed – *dynamism*. What is appropriate for one situation is inappropriate for another and we need to be able to adapt our approach to each individual and each situation as it progresses. To do this, we have to continually monitor how best to approach the consultation as we proceed. What is essential is, first, understanding that it is helpful to both listen and screen and then being flexible enough to use both skills appropriately in differing situations.

Agenda setting

Working in human health, Kaplan et al. (1997), Manning and Ray (2002) and Robins et al. (2011) indicate that screening naturally leads on to negotiating and setting an agenda which takes both the patient's and the physician's needs into account. With respect to veterinary medicine, Atkinson (2010a) emphasizes that a good consultation starts with the establishment of an agenda that includes the farmer's goals and is generally characterized by open questioning and listening. In keeping with our emphasis on developing a collaborative partnership between client and veterinarian, setting an agenda is an overt approach to clarifying how the interview should proceed that involves the client directly. For the client, the potential structure of the interview is made overt and an opportunity is provided for more involvement in deciding the agenda and more responsibility in what is taking place.

Like the rest of the initiation, agenda setting in veterinary medicine can be complicated by the fact that there may be multiple family members present or, in production animal or equine settings, multiple people responsible for the care of the animal who may have different valid perspectives on the problem list and agenda for the meeting with the veterinarian. Deciding whom to talk with as the client can be an issue not only here but throughout the consultation.

Agenda setting is an example of structuring early in the consultation. Priorities can be established and negotiated:

> *"Based on what you just told me, we should consider starting with a good physical examination and get some blood work. That will help us decide if these are new problems or if they are related to Ranger's previous diagnosis. Was there something else you had hoped we would do today?"*
>
> or
>
> *"Shall we start with Rex's recent hair loss and scratching, and then move onto revisiting his fear of lightning? That's the list of concerns that you've mentioned so far. What else is on your agenda today?"*

Additional items the veterinarian has for the agenda can also be included:

> *"After finishing Bangs vaccinations on these heifers, would you mind if we ran that bull we did surgery on a month ago in to take a look? I would like to see how he is healing up."*
>
> or
>
> *"Before I focus on Star's lame leg, I would also like to do a full physical, starting at her head in order to get a better picture of how she is doing, if that's all right."*

Problems with time can be acknowledged and negotiated:

> *"That's quite a list for us to get through and I'm not sure that we are going to have enough time to do it all justice; how about …?"*
>
> or
>
> *"We have three hours for this farm call. Based on the number of things you'd like to work on with me today, I think we should start by drawing blood for the coggins from the horses that need to travel, then evaluate the two lamenesses, see if we can get to one of the dentals, and then take a look at the new horse with the snotty nose before I leave, just in case it strangles. Will that work for today? What else were you hoping we'd do in today's visit?"*

In negotiating priorities, a balance may need to be struck between the client's personal hierarchy of concerns and the veterinarian's medical understanding of which problems might be more immediately important:

> *"I can see that you are worried and want to address Shad's scratching. If you don't mind, I'd rather we started by exploring the increased water intake and peeing you mentioned."*
>
> or
>
> *"Would you mind if we reordered the events for today? Based on a couple of the things you said about the calves, I would like to review your colostrum protocol and talk to Janet about how well that protocol is working for the crew first before we prescribe another antibiotic."*

Interestingly, Levinson et al. (1997) showed that primary care physicians who educated the patient about what to expect and the flow of the visit were less likely to have suffered malpractice claims.

Notice that in agenda setting and negotiating, you are not just telling the client what to do but are inviting the client to participate in making an agreed plan. One of the principles of communication that we discussed in Chapter 1 was that *effective communication promotes an interaction rather than a process of direct transmission.* Cassata (1978) explained how crystallizing agendas at the beginning of the consultation promotes just such an interaction, a two-way communication that encourages the patient to be a more active, responsible and autonomous participant throughout the consultation. Another of our five principles concerned *reducing uncertainty* – the combination of confirming the problem list, screening and overt agenda setting does just that by establishing mutually understood common ground. Joos et al. (1996) provide research validation of this approach. They taught internal medicine residents and physicians the skills of eliciting the patient's full concerns and negotiating an agreed agenda. They then demonstrated that physicians who received this training not only subsequently discovered more of their patients' concerns but equally importantly achieved this without any increase in the length of the visit. Mauksch et al. (2008) undertook a literature review to explore the determinants of efficiency in the medical interview. Three domains emerged from their review that can enhance communication efficiency: rapport building, upfront agenda setting and picking up emotional cues.

Rodriguez et al. (2008) taught practicing physicians the skill of "agenda-setting," eliciting the full set of concerns from the patient's perspective and using that information to prioritize and negotiate which clinical issues should most appropriately be dealt with and which should be deferred to a subsequent visit. The intervention resulted in statistically significant improvement in physicians' ability to explain things in a way that was easy to understand and marginal but significant improvement in the overall quality of physician–patient interactions compared to control group physicians.

We look in more detail at how to structure the entire consultation in Chapter 4 when we consider summary and signposting. We will describe how these methods encourage the veterinarian to consider where they have got to so far in the interview, what exactly they are trying to achieve next and how to verbalize these thoughts to the client. There are many advantages to this over simply moving forward without explaining the process to the client. For the veterinarian, organization of thought prevents aimless or unnecessary questioning and incomplete data gathering.

Summary

In this chapter, we have examined the skills of initiating the consultation, one of the most important parts of any consultation. The skills involved in establishing initial rapport, identifying the reasons for the client scheduling the appointment, and agreeing an agenda set the scene for the rest of the interview. These skills directly influence whether three important goals of medical communication – *accuracy, efficiency and supportiveness* – are achieved throughout the consultation as a whole.

As we have shown in the Calgary–Cambridge Guides, the skills of initiation are different from the skills of gathering information. Yet so often we do not separate out these tasks in our minds and they merge together with deleterious results. Clearly, having in mind a structure for the consultation as we progress through the interview is of vital importance. Before going on to explore the client's problems in detail, it is helpful to ask, *"Have I achieved my objectives for this first part of the interview: have I established a supportive environment and initial rapport; have I discovered the list of all the problems that the patient(s) has and that the client has come to discuss; have I established mutually understood common ground regarding the problem list and developed a mutually agreed plan for the consultation; have I enabled the client to become part of a collaborative process?"* Once these tasks have been completed, the veterinarian can then move on to gathering information about each problem.

CHAPTER 3

Gathering information

Having seen how vital the beginning of the interview is to successful communication in veterinary and human medicine, we now turn our attention to the next section of the interview – gathering information.

For many years, we have known of the overriding importance of history taking to diagnosis. Clinical studies from human medicine have shown repeatedly that the history contributes 60–80% of the data for diagnosis (Sandler 1980; Kassirer 1983; Peterson et al. 1992). In Hampton's study in medical outpatients, the history alone was sufficient to make the diagnosis in 66 out of 80 patients (Hampton et al. 1975). While we are unaware of such percentages in veterinary medicine, data gathering is most definitely important to diagnosis and working collaboratively with the client.

Fortunately, developments in communication theory and research have greatly improved our understanding of the *process* of gathering information. They have also opened up a whole new *content* area of history taking, namely, the client's perspective, including the client's concerns or issues, expectations, ideas about what is going on with their animal(s), etc. Interviewing in the healthcare professions has concentrated on pathological disease at the expense of understanding the highly individual perspectives and needs of each client in veterinary medicine and, in human medicine, each patient. As a consequence much of the information required to understand the client's perspective, and sometimes even the animal's problem(s), remains hidden. In veterinary and human medicine, studies of satisfaction, adherence, recall and physiological outcome all validate the need for a broader view of history taking that encompasses both the clinician's and the other person's perspectives.

Both the content and process skills of gathering information are central to effective consultations in veterinary and human medicine. Here we shall explore each of these areas in turn. Throughout this chapter we again rely on concepts, frameworks and research from both fields.

Problems in communication

There is considerable evidence of communication problems in the gathering information phase of the consultation.

- Shaw et al. (2004a) observed and video-recorded 300 veterinary consultations in small animal practices and found that clients asked on average only five questions per appointment. A subsequent study using the same database (Shaw et al. 2006) showed that veterinarians were verbally dominant in all of the consultations.
- Platt and McMath (1979) observed 300 encounters in hospital internal medicine

in the USA and showed that both a "high control style" (process) and premature focus on medical problems (content) lead to an over-narrow approach to hypothesis generation (perceptual) and to limitation of the patients' ability to communicate their concerns (content). These in turn lead to inaccurate consultations.

- Roshier and McBride (2013) recorded and analyzed 17 consultations across six veterinarians in the UK and administered a questionnaire to clients immediately following each consultation. Although on the questionnaire clients reported a total of 58 behavior concerns regarding their dogs, only 10 of these behavior concerns were actually mentioned during the consultation and none were fully explored or managed beyond the consultation. This issue may be compounded since clients may feel that it is inappropriate to mention behavioral concerns in veterinary appointments (Bergman et al. 2002). We wonder if another aspect of this problem is that for a variety of reasons veterinarians may feel unprepared or ill equipped to deal with some topics. Unfortunately this may affect a veterinarian's willingness to respond to cues or to collect important information.

- Maguire and Rutter (1976) showed serious deficiencies in senior medical students' information-gathering skills: few students managed to discover the patient's main problem, to clarify the exact nature of the problem and explore ambiguous statements, to clarify with precision, to elicit the impact of the problem on daily life, to respond to verbal cues, to cover more personal topics or to use facilitation. Most used closed, lengthy, multiple and repetitive questions.

- Gates and Nolan (2010) conducted a retrospective study between 1999 and 2006 that included fourth year veterinary students interviewing teaching hospital clients who had brought in 2679 dogs and 238 cats. The researchers found that students who had been assigned the task of taking a complete history that included heartworm, flea or tick preventatives' use did so with only 13% to 23% (percentages were based on amalgamated data regarding use of all three preventives). Clients whose pets were younger or presented with prior history of parasites or cardiac disease were no more likely to be questioned about preventive measures than those with healthy animals.

- In a qualitative study Agledahl et al. (2011) observed a consistent pattern in the consultations of hospital clinicians in Norway. The physicians were primarily concerned with their patients' biomedical health. This medical focus often overrode other important aspects of the consultations and physicians actively directed the focus away from their patients' concerns, rarely addressing the personal aspects of a patient's condition. Although physicians incorporated a polite and friendly approach, they did not pick up and explore the patients' cues to their underlying concerns and feelings.

- Research suggests that veterinarians may tend to make the least use of opportunities in the information-gathering segment of the interview. Shaw et al. (2004a) showed that veterinarians spend far less time gathering information from the client (9% of the statements per appointment – this excludes time spent gathering information via physical examination) compared to providing information (48%).

- Almost a decade later, in an Australian study of 64 visits, McArthur and Fitzgerald

(2013) also showed that veterinarians spend the least amount of time gathering information from their clients (6% of statements per appointment vs. 41% on client education and counseling).

- These findings notwithstanding, in McDermott et al.'s (2015) study using a questionnaire to which 1774 UK and US veterinarians responded, 73.2% said that obtaining a medical history was extremely important (1 = not at all important, 5 = extremely important).

Current trends in which veterinary technicians and sometimes receptionists are charged with obtaining problem lists, taking initial histories, and obtaining consent (Macdonald and Gray 2014) may be one reason veterinarians spend limited time gathering information. A second trend – namely the reliance on diagnostic tests and procedures – may also be contributing to the tendency to short change history taking, including the physical examination. A third potential explanation for this limited time spent on gathering information may be that veterinarians rely heavily on physical examination partly because the client may have limited understanding of animal disease or physiology. Veterinarians are looking for signs and indications from the animal to inform them of what is going on which then needs to be shared with the client to help them understand. Sometimes spending limited time gathering information is, of course, appropriate. However, it is worth asking whether the tendency for veterinarians to give part of this responsibility over to other members of the team or to technology or tests and physical examination, and to spend so little time on gathering information from the client, represents the best approach. The question is especially germane considering the effect this might be having on the detail and accuracy of information needed from the client and on aspects of the veterinarian's clinical reasoning process and relationship building that occur during information gathering.

Given time pressures, another possible problem for both veterinarians and physicians is moving too quickly down the clinical reasoning path before gathering sufficient information upon which to base that reasoning. This tends to limit what clinicians focus on during history taking and potentially results in missing important detail and/or arriving at wrong diagnoses. Sackett (2000) and Haynes et al. (2005) have written about this in human medicine and veterinary educators often refer to their work when teaching how to practice evidence-based medicine. Sackett defines evidence-based medicine as the integration of the best research evidence with clinical expertise and patient/client values.

And there is another issue. For many reasons perhaps related to time pressure or perceptions of clients' concerns over money, veterinarians can move prematurely to what Stivers (1998) refers to as "prediagnostic commentary" – premature because it occurs before we have gathered sufficient information. Stivers' study using conversation analysis to assess six video-recorded consultations is informative. She reported that veterinarians frequently engaged in prediagnostic commentary, that is, commentary typically delivered during physical examination that involves diagnostically relevant statements describing what the veterinarian is seeing or feeling and that anticipate or speculate on diagnoses and/or treatments that are being considered.

They used prediagnostic commentary to forecast to the client whether the diagnosis will be good news or bad so the client had some idea of what to expect and to allow the client to bring in their perspectives regarding diagnosis and negotiate diagnostic tests, treatments, costs and in some instances euthanasia. In this study, the veterinarians' out loud commentaries regarding speculations on diagnoses and suggestions of possible diagnostic tests and treatments were highly flexible, with the veterinarians frequently changing their point of view. Stivers points out that prediagnostic commentary can function as a helpful resource through which the veterinarian can explore the client's preparedness to allow and pay for treatments. On the other hand, the study showed that this commentary can happen too early in the interview, before veterinarians and clients have enough information to work with. Apparently because of the nature of what was said and when the prediagnostic commentary occurred, some clients heard such commentary as an invitation to negotiate the treatment and diagnosis before such participation was appropriate. Some veterinarians then adjusted their prediagnostic commentary, typically revising their position to fit with the client's point of view. In addition, when the veterinarian forecasted non-serious diagnostic options very early on and then the diagnosis turned out to be something more serious, the client had difficulty switching gears from non-serious to serious and the veterinarian was faced with making a marked revision of their earlier position. Whether on the serious or less serious side, the client's certainty regarding what was really going on appeared to be compromised and subsequently some clients did not agree with or show acceptance of the diagnosis and did not take it up. Prediagnostic commentary itself is not a problem – the problem is engaging in this commentary prematurely. Osborne et al.'s (2013) contention that we need to distinguish more carefully between listening to respond and listening to understand adds further insight into Stivers' findings.

A final issue with history taking in large and small animal veterinary medicine is that gathering information can become more complicated when multiple people are responsible for the health of the animal(s). Just finding out who does what and knowing whom to seek information from can be challenging, particularly since all parties may or may not be present during the consultation and since different individuals may have different takes on the information you are trying to gather. For example, Sischo et al. (2016, research in progress) found that management structures on large US dairies are evolving from an owner-operated to a distributed model where tasks and responsibilities are given to managers and workers. Many critical decisions are made by middle management and workers rather than by owners, and the communication between owners and these others is likely to be indirect (i.e. they do not talk directly to each other). In this study antibiotic use in calves depended on who was administering the antibiotics and the veterinarian may or may not have talked to that person. The veterinarian needs to understand the dynamics of information exchange on any given dairy and to know who is doing what in order to know whom to gather information from and whom to engage in subsequent explanation and planning.

Objectives

When gathering information the veterinarian's objectives go beyond obtaining physical examination findings and doing diagnostic tests on the animal while the client sits by passively. Even as you work with the patient, you need to ask questions of the client, make them feel listened to and valued, ensure mutual understanding between you and the client, and continue to develop a collaborative relationship. Objectives for this part of the visit therefore include:

- exploring the patient's problems or issues, including wellness and preventive care, to discover the biomedical history of the current problem, the client's perspective and background information
- ensuring that information gathered is accurate, complete and mutually understood by both veterinarian and client (establishing common ground)
- ensuring that the veterinarian not only hears but develops a way to remember the information gathered for use as appropriate throughout the interaction
- ensuring that clients feel listened to, that their information and views are welcomed and valued (confirmation, acknowledgment)
- continuing to develop a safe and accommodating environment for the patient and a supportive and collaborative relationship with the client
- structuring the consultation to ensure efficient information gathering and to enable the client to understand and be overtly involved in where the interaction is going and why.

As was the case for initiating the session, these objectives encompass many of the tasks and checkpoints mentioned in other well-known guides to the consultation – *see* Appendix C.

These objectives, like those of several other models, make it clear that both content and process skills are significant elements of information gathering. We would like first to explore the content related to this part of the veterinary consultation and then to look closely at the process skills for gathering information. Toward the end of this chapter, we discuss the influence of clinical reasoning on the process of information gathering and vice versa.

The content of information gathering in veterinary visits

So what information is it that veterinarians need to discover by the end of the visit? What information should they include in patients' records? To answer these questions it is useful to start by exploring two different approaches to information gathering: the more traditional approach to history taking and the integrated clinical method model. The latter is adapted from the work of Ian McWhinney and colleagues who called it the transformed clinical method model or the disease-illness model and, later, patient-centered care.

The more traditional veterinary medical history

The more traditional method of history taking is so firmly established in veterinary and human medical practice that it is easy to assume that it is the correct approach. Yet often in both contexts we make such assumptions without considering the origins of what we do and their relevance to modern-day practice.

Origins of the more traditional method

McWhinney (1989) has eloquently traced the origins, strengths and weaknesses of the traditional clinical method. Veterinary historian Brian Derbyshire (pers. comm. 2015) indicates that the evolution of the clinical method in veterinary medicine and human medicine emerged concurrently, perhaps because in the past veterinarians and physicians were often educated together. At the beginning of the nineteenth century, a new method of clinical medicine began to emerge, pioneered in post-revolutionary France. Schools of veterinary medicine began to appear in the preceding years, first in Lyon, France (1761) and then in London, England (1791), Mexico City, Mexico (1853), Guelph, Ontario (1862) and Ames, Iowa (1879). Prior to the nineteenth century medicine had lacked any scientific basis – patients' symptoms and signs had been the focus of clinicians' attention and there had been little understanding of underlying disease processes. Innovations such as the stethoscope now revealed a whole new range of clinical information. At the same time, physicians and veterinarians began to examine the internal organs after death and tried to correlate physical signs in life to post-mortem findings in death. From here on, the physical expression of the disease in humans and animals became central: it became the aim of the diagnostician to interpret the animal or human patient's signs or symptoms in terms of specific diseases and to provide a scientific explanation. This change was to herald the incredible advances in diagnosis and treatment of the twentieth century. The clinical method in both professions progressed in a parallel fashion.

By 1880, a fully defined clinical method had become established in human medicine that very likely influenced the veterinary profession as well, given the timing. In human medicine this is apparent from clinical records where the structured method of recording the history and examination that is so familiar today had already taken root (Tait 1979; Roter 2000). The history of chief complaint, history of past illness, medication and allergies, and a review of systems became the standard method of recording clinical inquiries in human medicine and forged an ordered approach to history taking. Veterinary medicine has followed a similar path (*see* Chapter 1, Box 1.2).

This method still dominates both human and veterinary medicine today and has been consolidated by the incorporation of powerful new methods of investigation that have further enhanced our ability to interpret the patient's problems in terms of underlying physical pathology. Imaging, microbiology, biochemistry and hematology are the essentials of both professions – they have taken our understanding of the disease process to the cellular level and beyond.

Strengths

It is the scientific approach to the patient that is the traditional clinical method's greatest strength. There is no doubt that the development of a method of classification of the underlying cause of disease paved the way for the advances in medical science that have followed. It provided the first real possibility of precise clinical audit with the pathologist giving clinicians feedback on their diagnostic skills. It gave a common language to unify the "medical approach."

This approach also provided clinicians with a clear method of taking and recording the clinical history, supplying a carefully structured template with which to arrive at a diagnosis or to exclude physical disease. It simplified and unified a very complex process, prevented the omission of key points and enabled the data extracted from the patient and, in veterinary medicine, the client to appear in a standard assimilable form.

Weaknesses

The strength of the traditional clinical method is also its weakness. As the professions have embraced the objectivity required to diagnose disease in terms of underlying pathology, they have increasingly concentrated on the individual parts of the body that are malfunctioning and have honed this process down to a cellular and now molecular level. Yet this biomedical focus so easily misses other issues as well as the client's perspective. The scientific method does not aim to understand the entire nature of the animal's problems or the impact on the animal, the client or others who may be affected. Subjective matters such as the client's beliefs, anxieties and concerns are not the remit of the more traditional approach. Science deals with the objective, that which can be measured, whereas the effect on the animal's or client's life, and the client's feelings, thoughts and concerns are unquantifiable and subjective, and therefore may be deemed less worthy of consideration.

Medical and veterinary students have been traditionally brought up in this world of the objective and the technological: they have been taught to concentrate on the underlying disease mechanism and thereby to avoid the patient's/client's perceptions and feelings as well as the impact of the problems on those involved.

An integrated clinical method

Over the past several years a number of ways for reconceptualizing how we think about interaction and relationships in healthcare have evolved. McWhinney (1989) and his colleagues in human medicine at the University of Western Ontario proposed their "transformed clinical method" to replace the traditional content of medical history taking. This approach, which requires physicians to understand their patients as well as their patients' diseases, has also been called "patient-centered clinical interviewing" to differentiate it from the "doctor-centered" approach that attempts to interpret the patient's illness only from the traditional perspective of disease and pathology (Stewart et al. 1995, 2003; Stewart 2001). Nogueira Borden et al. (2010) have applied the patient-centered model to veterinary medicine in their research. Similarly, in an article encouraging holistic health in veterinary medicine, Williams and Jewell (2012) expand the concept of patient-centered. They assert that health is more than the absence of disease and more than biomedicine. Whether in large or small animal contexts, holistic health in veterinary medicine is about looking after the biopsychosocial aspects of the animal's or herd's well-being and about the veterinarian's unique position in attending to aspects of the well-being of the people associated with the animals. Turning to family-centered pediatric care in human health as a model, Williams and Jewell propose the term "family-centered veterinary medicine." As applied to veterinary medicine, they suggest that family-centered veterinary care could literally include not only the patient(s) and the client, but also the family members or, in large animal practices, others who are responsible for the well-being and treatment of the animals.

Tresolini et al. (1994) suggested a somewhat different conceptualization of the healthcare process, namely, relationship-centered care. Based in human medicine, their intent was to recognize that the nature and quality of relationships are central to individual healthcare, the broader healthcare delivery system, and the well-being of both patient and physician. Taking this paradigm further, Beach et al. (2006) identified four principles of relationship-centered care that we have taken the liberty of adapting for veterinary medicine:

- Relationships in veterinary medicine ought to include dimensions of personhood, with veterinarians and clients bringing their authentic and whole person to the encounter. This principle also pertains to members of the family, employees in the veterinary practice and production animal contexts, veterinary colleagues, etc.
- Affect and emotion are important components of these relationships for all of the participants. Support is provided through the emotional presence of the veterinarian – this challenges the notion of detached concern.
- All healthcare relationships occur in the context of reciprocal influence (i.e. all of the participants have an influence on each other). While not precluding that the client's goals for the patient and the animal itself take priority, this acknowledges that veterinarians also benefit from serving clients and patients.
- Relationship-centered care has a moral foundation – people are morally committed to those with whom they are in relationship. The formation and maintenance of genuine relationships in healthcare is morally valuable.

Clearly these principles and the relationship-centered care approach apply to veterinary medicine. Relationship-centered care emphasizes the full range of relationships that impact veterinary practice and its outcomes, including:

- central relationships between veterinarian, client and patient
- relationship with self (i.e. the intrapersonal dimensions related to clinical reasoning, self-awareness, emotional intelligence, self-reflection, etc.)
- relationships between colleagues (i.e. other veterinarians within and beyond an immediate practice, staff, etc.)
- relationships with the community (i.e. immediate practice, hospital, industry partners, non-profit organizations, geographical communities [local and global], governing bodies, agencies, professional organizations, etc.).

Relationship-centered and patient- or client-centered care are complementary paradigms that have also been described as foundations for communication research and education in veterinary medicine (Adams and Kurtz 2006; Shaw et al. 2006; Kurtz

2006; Adams and Kurtz 2016, in press). Kristensen and Enevoldsen's (2008) concepts of "whole farm management" and attention to the "overall well-being of the farmer's household" fit into the relationship-centered care paradigm. So do Williams and Jewell's (2012) holistic veterinary medicine and family-centered veterinary care. Shaw et al. (2004b), Frankel (2006), Shaw et al. (2010), Shaw et al. (2012b), and Kanji (2012) have described relationship-centered care in the context of communication in small animal care. Relationship-centered care is a useful way to think about how we work, an important paradigm for veterinary medicine. Relationship-centered care takes the importance of patient-centered and client-centered care into account and adds a focus on the centrality of relationship, not only between veterinarian and client but between all the players involved.

Veterinary educators and researchers also draw on relational coordination – a model related to relationship-centered care – that refers to the coordination of work through relationships of shared goals, shared knowledge and mutual respect (Gittell et al. 2000, 2008a, 2009). Moore et al. (pers. comm. 2016), for example, looks at how relational coordination affects job satisfaction, intent to stay on the job, and burnout in veterinary practice. We discuss relationship-centered care and relational coordination further in Chapter 5.

Returning to McWhinney's "transformed clinical method," patient-centered medicine encourages physicians to consider both their own and the patient's agendas in

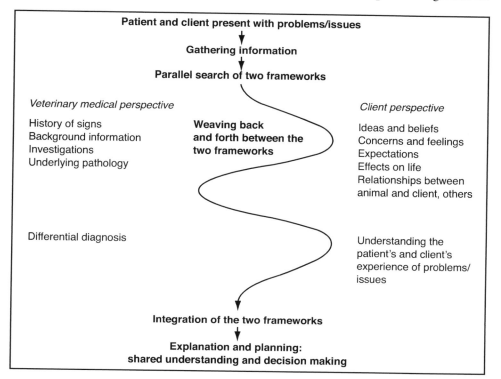

FIGURE 3.1 The integrated clinical method model. After Levenstein et al. (1989), and Stewart et al. (2003), which was adapted by Silverman et al. (1998)

each interview (Mischler 1984; Campion et al. 1992; Epstein 2000; Barry et al. 2001). In veterinary medicine, Williams and Jewell (2012), Nogueira Borden et al. (2010) and others have adapted the patient-centered approach to include the veterinarian's agenda, client's agenda, and patient's needs. We have therefore labeled this adaptation for veterinary medicine the "integrated clinical method model." Depicted in Figure 3.1, the integrated clinical method model attempts to provide a practical way of using McWhinney's concepts in everyday veterinary practice. For the sake of simplicity we refer only to the individual client in the model, using this term to include family members, employees and others – anyone who is involved with the well-being, management and treatment of the animals.

Definition of biomedical and client perspectives

The beauty of this analysis is the clarity with which it demonstrates how veterinarians need to explore two frameworks to fulfill their unique role as practitioners: the biomedical perspective and the client's perspective. Clearly it is the veterinarian's role to search for signs of underlying *biomedical* problems and the cause of disease in terms of pathophysiology. Discovering a diagnosis for the patient's problem(s) is the veterinarian's traditional and central agenda. The *client's perspective* in contrast refers to the client's unique experience of the patient's problems or issues or the client's point of view regarding issues related to the operating systems and management of animal facilities. The client's perspective is not as narrow as the biomedical perspective and includes the ideas and beliefs, concerns, expectations and effects-on-life that any animal-related concern raises for the client.

The client's perspective represents the client's response to events, understanding of what is happening, and expectations of help. Using different terms, the American College of Veterinary Nutrition (2012) recognized the importance of client perspective when they include "personal preferences, lifestyle and abilities of the owner" among the factors that need to be evaluated when conducting a nutritional history and prescribing a feeding protocol. The client's view of how a particular disease or issue affects an animal's quality of life or utility can vary from one animal or context to the next. For example, the client's and veterinarian's response to lameness in a horse that is used lightly or kept as a "pet" may be different from their response to lameness in a high-level dressage horse. The variation in clients' reactions to common diagnoses can be substantial. Their ideas, beliefs, feelings, concerns, expectations, support systems, previous life experiences and sense of what is practical influence clients' ability to make decisions and cope and even the information they give.

The importance of exploring both perspectives

In the past, some veterinarians have overlooked the client's perspectives as subjective and potentially confounding variables that get in the way of discovering the patient's underlying diagnosis. On one hand, a client's point of view about cause, their concerns over finances, their sense of anxiety or guilt or their reluctance to treat can interfere with the veterinarian's focus on the animal. On the other hand, not overtly attending to the client's perspectives can compromise the client's ability to provide information accurately, understand explanations, participate in decision making, and follow through with treatment plans. In their Canadian study analyzing small animal consultations, Shaw et al. (2008) showed that veterinarians focus on biomedical content during problem patient visits to the neglect of communication with the client about lifestyle and social concerns that could have an impact on the biomedical problems and their management. Nogueira Borden et al. (2010) analyzed 60 audiotaped visits pertaining to end of life decision making and/or euthanasia and showed that veterinarians in the study did little to explore the client's feelings, ideas and expectations, and the effect of the illness on the animal's function. Given such limited information in these areas, the researchers suggest that it would be difficult for the veterinarian to make recommendations and formulate a treatment plan that was in the best interests of the client and the patient or for the client to be meaningfully involved in decision making about the end of their pet's life.

Mischler (1984) has explained how the physician in his desperation to make a diagnosis selectively listens to patients' comments that help him interpret their problems from the technological perspective. He does not hear or pursue comments that give him insight into their world. Mischler described this as "two parallel monologues" in which patient and doctor talk at cross purposes in different languages.

Clinicians in fact have a *unique responsibility* to do both, to listen to both frameworks and not discard either (Smith and Hoppe 1991). The integrated clinical method model does not in any way negate the scientific disease approach but adds a client-centered arm as well. Veterinarians are not psychologists or counselors and they do have the responsibility and burden of diagnosing and treating disease or other problems. But if veterinarians consider their role as purely that of discovering and treating disease or recommending preventive care, they will not fully help their patients and clients with individual needs or set clients up to follow through with treatment plans and next steps.

In a survey of 378 Dutch dairy farmers regarding their mastitis control practices, Kuiper et al. (2005) found that farmers' beliefs and perceived self-efficacy were key factors affecting their practices. This speaks to the importance of asking about farmers' beliefs and other perspectives. The survey also found that veterinarians were the most important source of information affecting farmers' practices, followed by farm journals. External triggers such as sanctions, problems and incentives also influenced farmers' practices.

In a Canadian study of six client and four veterinarian focus groups, Coe et al. (2008) looked specifically at small animal clients' expectations regarding communication with their veterinarians. The findings reinforce those from human medicine and provide insight into what pet owners expect from veterinarians, namely:

- two-way conversation where veterinarians use language the clients understand, listen to what they have to say, and ask the appropriate questions so that the client can relate information that the client feels is important; clients expected veterinarians to ask the "right" questions so the client could give the right information back
- information up front, before the client makes a final decision about the care of their animal
- information provided in various forms (handouts, discharge instructions)

- information regarding the range of options for their animal's treatment
- respect for decisions clients make
- partnership with the veterinarian in the care of their animals that includes informed and shared decision making
- inquiry about the perspectives of other members of the client's family who will play a role in decision making about the animal.

These insights are very useful and underscore the need to ask individual clients what they need and expect from each visit. Veterinarians in this study recognized this fact but said they found this to be quite challenging to do – they had difficulty assessing individual clients' expectations and needs.

Working from a business perspective, Gabay et al. (2013) conducted a study of 109 small animal owners from one US veterinary practice to determine what these clients wanted from the practice. Focusing on what services to offer veterinary clients and how to position the practice from a marketing and advertising perspective, the study also offered insight on how to relate to clients during consultations. The researchers reported that these clients could be divided into three mindsets: a) responds to elements that convey warmth and reassurance, b) responds to technology, c) responds to treatment that is similar in nature to that given to people.

Veterinarians need to take into account both the traditional approach to gathering information and the client's particular perspectives. When a dog who has been hit by a car presents with a leg that needs to be amputated, the veterinarian may see their role in terms of treatment of the animal and its injured leg. That, of course, is appropriate. But the client's main concerns may be whether the dog can cope with three legs, and whether she can handle a dog with a missing leg – her agenda may concern discussing prognosis more than diagnosis. These two agendas overlap but both need to be addressed in order to fully serve the patient and the client.

The advantages of taking a history that includes both biomedical and client's perspectives are numerous:

1. **Supporting, understanding and building a relationship**

   Taking only a problem-oriented history on an obese dog case may only lead to an understanding of the food intake of the animal and exercise history without clarifying the client's abilities and inabilities. Failure to understand the client's work schedule and physical limitations easily leads to the veterinarian making seemingly reasonable medical recommendations that will be impossible for the client to adhere to, thereby resulting in frustration for both the client and veterinarian and ineffective treatment of the animal's obesity.

   Taking only a traditional disease-centered history relating to the destructive behavior of a 2-year-old golden retriever may well allow you to diagnose separation anxiety and plan management. While this is an absolutely necessary task, failing also to understand the impact of the behavior on the animal's relationship with the client or with other members of their family may well limit your effectiveness as a veterinarian. The client may become agitated at the mention of behavioral counseling as he and his wife may have already attempted this without success and his wife has indicated that if they do not resolve the behavior issue immediately the dog will need to leave their home. Or the client's wife may be ill and he might not want the ongoing stresses associated with the dog's behavioral problems. Managing this case effectively depends on your ability not only to diagnose effectively but also to understand the clients' perspectives and support them through their decisions for managing their dog's separation anxiety.

2. **The biomedical model does not provide all the information veterinarians need**
   There may not be a disease in traditional medical model terms to explain a client's request to euthanize an animal that appears to be in good general health. The request may have roots in the client's own personal unhappiness, in stress at home or at work, or in anxiety about their own health. Although it is clearly our responsibility to exclude physical disease, we will not find a disease in all our patients. Even if we do, we may personally struggle to justify the request of the client. For example, a young cat diagnosed with a first-time ear infection may appear relatively straightforward in terms of selecting a first line of treatment but because of financial concerns the client may feel the situation is unmanageable. Using just the biomedical approach, the client's request to euthanize their otherwise healthy cat may appear unreasonable. Until you explore the client's perspective you may also not find out about his current marital difficulties and his concern of losing his much-loved companion animal to his wife during the divorce. Another example that could be delicate to approach has to do with performance issues in equine athletes. Rider discomfort, imbalance or lack of fitness may be factors adversely affecting a sensitive horse's performance. The veterinarian needs to be astute and diplomatic in asking questions about the rider as well as about the working relationship between the rider and the horse to determine if there are both horse and rider factors contributing to poor performance. And there is another side to this: sometimes as a veterinarian you also have an ethical responsibility to look out for the client. For example, clients who are undergoing chemotherapy for cancer or who may be immunocompromised for other reasons may require particular kinds of information since contact with animals and some aspects of taking care of them are potential health threats for these people. You need to ask about the client's circumstances and tailor your care accordingly. Searching both biomedical and client frameworks can make the consultation more accurate, efficient and supportive.

   In human medicine, there is considerable research evidence to support the lack of organic disease to explain much about patients' problems. In 50% of patients presenting to general practitioners with chest pain, the cause was unproven after 6 months follow-up (Blacklock 1977). Similar statistics are available for tiredness, abdominal pain and headache. But it would be a mistake to think that this problem is restricted to human medicine – what about the dog that excessively licks the inside of its front paw, out of boredom, resulting in a granuloma or the horse with cribbing behavior that seems to subside with increased turnout. All veterinarians see patients whose problems are not necessarily caused by disease.

3. **Discovering the client's perspective can aid diagnosis and make for more effective and efficient interviews**
   Asking for the client's ideas can aid diagnosis. For example, consider the couple who bring in a dog with severe diarrhea who answer your question about what

they think might be going on by telling you that they went hiking a week or so ago and, even though they had bottled water for the dog, they wonder if the dog might have drunk water from a stream.

4. **Developing groundwork for explanation and planning**

When we explore explanation and planning in Chapter 6, we look at the research that demonstrates the central importance of eliciting and understanding the client's unique perspectives. We shall see that when veterinarians' explanations do not address their clients' individual ideas, expectations and concerns, the client's recall, understanding, satisfaction and compliance are all likely to suffer.

Tuckett et al. (1985) have shown that consultations go wrong where there is an incongruity between the patient and the physician's explanatory frameworks. Our client presenting with the young cat that has a first-time ear infection might well think that the costs will be ongoing due to the expensive experience of a friend whose dog has had chronic ear problems. The client might be perfectly happy to learn that the costs typically are not ongoing in these circumstances and you are open to working with him on staying within his financial boundaries. Unless you have discovered your clients' ideas and explained information in a manner that takes these ideas into account, clients may leave the consultation unconvinced that you really understand the problem or that the treatment plan you suggest is the best option. This belief may block the client's understanding and commitment to your explanations and undermine his acceptance of your treatment plan. A woman with an elderly cat showing signs of arthritis may not wish to use nonsteroidal anti-inflammatories because of personal experience with nonsteroidal anti-inflammatories in managing her own arthritis. Her concern may be increased due to her own online learning, where a website she found discussed the risks associated with the long-term use of these drugs in cats. Without understanding her experience and thoughts about risk, the veterinarian might prescribe a nonsteroidal anti-inflammatory drug that the client might not give to her cat.

So, after splitting the two arms of biomedical perspective and client perspective apart, the veterinarian has to put the two back together again. This is the stage labeled *integration* in the integrated clinical method model. Without this step it is impossible to achieve a shared understanding with the client about the nature of the problem and its management and difficult to enable the client to participate in shared decision making.

Basing negotiation regarding management plans on an open understanding of both veterinarian and client perspectives and reaching mutually understood common ground is the final aim. But as we shall see later in this chapter and in Chapter 6, understanding the client's perspective does not mean abrogating our responsibility as veterinarians and promoting an entirely consumerist approach. Consider the dairy producer who has a show calf exhibiting a dry cough with no temperature that you think requires no antibiotics. Discovering the producer's expectations before deciding on a treatment plan is helpful. A treatment plan can then be negotiated that is based on an accurate understanding of the producer's position. Finding out that the producer would prefer not to have antibiotics used in the show calf if at all possible, assures a more comfortable negotiation from the outset. If the client would prefer antibiotics, eliciting and addressing that expectation and explaining your position in relation to that point of view is vital. Only then can the producer understand your rationale and feel their position has at least been taken into consideration. For a small animal example, consider a situation where a 7-month old puppy intended to be a working dog comes up acutely lame for a short period of time and then the lameness resolves. Radiographs of the elbows are inconclusive. The veterinarian recommends a recheck and possibly repeat radiographs in 6 weeks. The client asks instead for an immediate referral for a CT (computerized tomography) scan of the elbows. By asking the client to explain this request, the veterinarian learns that another dog this client owned from this line had small fragments that were difficult to see on radiographs and once they were found, the damage to the joint was such that it limited that dog's athletic ability. As a study by Steihaugh et al. (2012) in human medicine demonstrates, overtly recognizing the client's perspectives makes it easier to tolerate disagreement; conflict and dissatisfaction can be anticipated and defused.

Working with an alternative template for the content of information gathering

The integrated clinical method model provides the basis for an alternative template for the content of information gathering in veterinary medicine. Introduced in Chapter 1 (Figure 1.4), this alternative template retains all the elements normally found in veterinary medical records and in addition includes the "new" content of the client's perspective. Explicitly demonstrating how the discrete elements of the traditional medical history and the components of the integrated clinical method model can seamlessly work together in clinical practice, this alternative content template

---

Content to be discovered

Biomedical perspective	*Client perspective*
Sequence of events	Ideas and beliefs
Analysis of signs	Concerns and feelings
Relevant systems review	Expectations
	Effects on life
	Relationship between animal and client, other

Background information – context

Environment and lifestyle
Past medical history
Current medications, adverse drug reactions, allergies
Genetic and familial history
Behavioral/social history
Review of systems

FIGURE 3.2 An alternative template for the content of information gathering. Adapted from Kurtz et al. (2003)

for veterinary medicine is an adaptation of a content template originally developed for human medicine (Kurtz et al. 2003).

This template makes intuitive sense to veterinarians. They readily see how the new and more traditional content fit together and also how this content model relates to the process skills of information gathering that we shall discuss shortly. The content template we provide here fits what happens in real-life clinical practice. Importantly, veterinary students having difficulty with structuring and taking good histories find the template immediately useful. As described in Chapter 1 (*see* Figure 1.4), veterinarians may also find this template a useful way to record information in the medical record and relate their findings to others.

The biomedical perspective

The information that the veterinarian needs to discover about the animal's disease or other problem(s) is identical to that of the traditional medical history. We have divided this into three equally important parts:

1. SEQUENCE OF EVENTS – TIMELINE

Before analyzing the clinical signs in depth, it is useful for the veterinarian to discover the exact sequence of events over time in relation to the problem areas that the client has identified. We discuss the process skills that enable this to be achieved in the most effective fashion in the next section of this chapter.

2. ANALYSIS OF SIGNS

The veterinarian also needs to analyze each clinical sign in depth, an approach that the traditional methodology of history taking has always stressed. Physical examination is of course a part of this investigation. WWQQAA+B is an example of an aide-memoire that clinicians in both human and veterinary medicine use when gathering information needed to investigate a sign or symptom.

WWQQAA plus B

1. **Where** – the location and radiation of signs or symptoms
2. **When** – when it began, frequency and fluctuation over time, duration, times of occurrence
3. **Quality** – client's characterization of the problem
4. **Quantity** – intensity, extent, degree of disability
5. **Aggravating and alleviating** factors
6. **Associated manifestations** – other signs or symptoms
7. **Beliefs** – the client's beliefs about the signs or symptoms.

At the end of this chapter we discuss DAMN-IT, another commonly used acronym that assists with clinical reasoning rather than information gathering. There we also consider the interdependence between information gathering and clinical reasoning.

3. RELEVANT SYSTEMS REVIEW

A further essential element consists of the components of the systems review that are relevant to the particular part of the medical history that is being discussed. For example, a client has explained that their cat seems to be having pain in and around their stomach and you have determined the sequence of events and assessed this particular sign. The most appropriate next step in exploring the biomedical perspective is to work through the review of the gastrointestinal system, including relevant negatives; physical examination is a critical part of this investigation. It is equally important to review with the client how other relevant systems have been working, including those that might not have come up on physical examination. Perhaps this patient has had previous bouts of loose stool over the past year and has been using the litter box more frequently, indicating a longer duration of the problem or suggesting what part of the GI tract may be of greatest concern. It is important to bring this part of the systems review forward rather than leaving it to near the end of the interview as part of the full systems review. Doing so fits better with the clinical reasoning process. Since veterinarians start to problem-solve early on in the interview, they need information about relevant systems at this point rather than later in the interview.

The client's perspective

The veterinarian needs to gain information and understanding about the client's perspective, the "new" content of the veterinary medical history, including:

- **ideas and beliefs** – the client's beliefs, theories or thoughts about causation of their animal's problem(s) or about health and what influences or contributes to it
- **concerns and feelings** – the client's concerns about cost, feelings of guilt, worries about what the signs mean, the animal's behavior
- **expectations** – the client's hopes of how the veterinarian might help, outcomes that the client wants from the visit
- **effects on life** – the effect the problem or issue has on day-to-day living for the animal or client or both
- **relationship between animal, client and others** – the client's view of their relationship with and responsibilities toward the animal and the direct or indirect effect they perceive this to have on the animal or decisions about the animal.

Background information: context

Of course, the veterinarian also needs to discover the background information. This information provides insights into the context within which current problems or symptoms are occurring. Such information is necessary to make a fully informed interpretation of current events. The level of detail required here depends on how complete the history needs to be. Background information includes:

- environment and lifestyle (e.g. living quarters and conditions, diet, exercise, daily routines, other animals, use of animal, health of contact animals or humans, travel history, relationship between animal and client, family members or others such as farm employees)

- past medical history (e.g. illnesses, surgeries, reproductive history, trauma, preventive care)
- current medications, adverse drug reactions and allergies (e.g. drug and other)
- genetic and familial background
- behavioral/social history
- review of systems that were not covered above.

For species specific details regarding content, see the historical investigation pyramids in Chapter 1 and Appendix B.

The process skills of information gathering

We now turn our attention to the communication process skills of gathering information. How do we go about gathering all the information from the client and about the patient that we have discussed above? What impact do communication process skills have on the content that is gathered? What communication skills can we employ to be most effective in this phase of the veterinary interview?

Box 3.1 delineates the communication process skills needed for gathering information effectively. We would like to stress that used appropriately these process skills apply equally to taking a more complete or focused history and in all settings, whether in hospital, clinic, barn, feed lot, zoo, etc. As indicated earlier, "client" refers to whoever is present representing the animal.

Box 3.1 Gathering information

Exploration of the patient's problems and client's issues
- **Client's narrative:** encourages client to tell the story of the problem(s) from when first started to the present in own words (clarifying reason for presenting now)
- **Questioning techniques:** uses *open and closed questioning techniques*, appropriately moving from open to closed
- **Listening:** listens attentively, allowing client to complete statements without interruption; leaves space for client to think before answering or go on after pausing
- **Facilitative response:** facilitates client's responses verbally and nonverbally (e.g. use of encouragement, silence, repetition, paraphrasing, interpretation)
- **Cues:** picks up client's verbal and nonverbal cues (body language, vocal cues, facial expression, affect); checks them out and acknowledges as appropriate. Observes patient behavior carefully
- **Clarification:** checks out statements that are vague or need amplification (e.g. *"Could you explain what you mean by seems to be in pain"*)
- **Time-framing:** establishes dates and sequence of events
- **Internal summary:** periodically summarizes to verify own understanding of what the client has said; invites client to correct interpretation and provide further information

- **Language:** uses concise, easily understood questions and comments; avoids or adequately explains jargon.

Additional skills for understanding the client's perspective
- **Actively determines and appropriately explores:**
  — **client's ideas** (i.e. beliefs, theories re cause)
  — **client's concerns** regarding each problem (e.g. worries, financial issues)
  — **client's expectations** (i.e. goals, what help the client expects/wants for each problem)
  — **effects of** each problem on the patient's and the client's life
  — **relationship between animal, client and others**
- **Encourages expression of feelings.**

Exploration of patient's problems and client's concerns/issues

In Chapter 2 we examined the beginning of the interview and saw the advantages of initiating the consultation carefully and making a plan of the consultation in conjunction with the client rather than blindly setting off down the first road that appears. This chapter examines each skill separately and then puts them together into a practical approach that veterinarians can use in everyday practice.

We start by exploring the central importance of questioning techniques to information gathering. Readers will note our recommendation in Box 3.1 that asking the client to relate chronologically what is going on is the first approach to consider after initiation. However, the skill of discovering the client's narrative is a specific application of the use of open questioning techniques and is easiest to consider after we have discussed questioning in more depth.

Questioning techniques

It is easy to assume at this point in the consultation that the veterinarian's influence on events is limited, that the client will tell their story efficiently or inefficiently, whatever the veterinarian does or says. But in fact veterinarians' actions and utterances profoundly influence clients' replies and the type of responses they provide. How we ask questions plays a central role in the quality and quantity of information that we obtain.

Veterinarians exert considerable control over the interview. We direct the client to an area for further exploration and by the nature of our questions and responses impose certain limits to the client's freedom to elaborate. Yet very often we are not consciously aware of the effect that we are having. The way that many veterinarians have been taught to take a history can lead to inaccuracy and inefficiency. Traditional questioning methods may not encourage appropriately comprehensive history taking or effective hypothesis generation. How can we make this process more intentional so that we can more adeptly choose to use different questioning approaches as and when required? A few definitions are helpful.

What are open and closed questions?

Closed (or closed-ended) questions[10] are questions for which a specific and often one word answer, such as yes or no, is expected. They limit the response to a narrow field set by the questioner. The client usually provides a response of one or two words without elaboration.

Open (or open-ended) questioning techniques in contrast are designed to introduce an area of inquiry without unduly shaping or focusing the content of the response. They still direct the client to a specific area but allow the client more latitude in how they answer, suggesting to the client that elaboration is both appropriate and welcome.

Here are some simple examples of these questioning styles:

Open: *"Tell me about the lameness."*
More directive but still open: *"What seems to make it better or worse?"*
Closed: *"Have you checked her temperature?"*

Because asking questions is not the only way to gather information, the term "question" is something of a misnomer here. More accurate would be the broader open and closed "questioning techniques." Many open techniques are in fact not questions at all but directive statements:

"Start at the beginning and take me through what has been happening ..."
"Tell me more about that ..."
"Tell me how he's been doing since the surgery last week ..."
"I've read the referral letter from Skippy's veterinarian, but it would be very helpful if you can tell me in your own words how this progressed from when you first noticed a problem right up until now."

---

rather than actual questions:

"What has been going on from when you first noticed her favoring the leg until now?"
"How has she been feeling since the operation?"
"What were your thoughts about how this fits in with your financial concerns?"

The examples in both boxes are equally useful open approaches to gathering information.

---

10   We use the terms closed and closed-ended as well as open and open-ended interchangeably in this book, as does the literautre.

We would like to emphasize that both open and closed questioning techniques are valuable. Yet McArthur and Fitzgerald (2013) reported that small animal veterinarians used no open questioning techniques in 15% of visits. Jansen (2010) found that 6 out of 10 dairy veterinarians in her study used no open-ended questions during herd health conversations that varied in length from 54 to 166 minutes. Dysart et al. (2011) showed that even when open questioning techniques were used, small animal veterinarians interrupted clients' responses midstream with a closed question 55% of the time. In our efforts to demonstrate that veterinarians tend to use closed questions too often, at the wrong time and at the expense of open questions, we do not mean to imply that veterinarians should not use closed questions at all. Both are essential but achieve very different ends. Their use at different times in the interview needs to be chosen with care.

When should we use open and closed methods: the open-to-closed cone

Understanding how to intentionally choose between open and closed questioning styles at different points in the interview is of key importance. Starting with open questions and later moving to closed questions is called the *"open-to-closed cone"* (Goldberg et al. 1983). The veterinarian uses open questioning techniques first to obtain a picture of the problem from the client's perspective. Later, the approach becomes more focused with increasingly specific though still open questions and eventually closed questions to elicit additional details that the client may have omitted. The use of open questioning techniques is critical at the beginning of the exploration of any problem – their power as an information-gathering tool here cannot be overemphasized. Two common mistakes are to interrupt the client before they have finished responding to a good open-ended question or to move to closed questioning too quickly. A third mistake is to use open techniques only at the beginning of the consultation. Using multiple open-to-closed cones throughout the interview, for example whenever you begin exploration of a new issue or topic, is more appropriate. A fourth potential mistake is to use such a broad open-ended question initially that clients are unsure how to respond. For example: *"Tell me about a day in the life of Cleo?"* You know you have asked too broad a question when the client responds with: *"Well, what do you want to know?"*

What are the advantages of open questioning techniques?

Why does staying open before moving to closed questions provide maximum efficiency in information gathering? Look at what might happen if we were to use two very different approaches to the same scenario.

A consultation relying on closed methods might go like this:

Veterinarian: *"Now what about the nasal drainage, what color is it?"*
Client: *"Yellowish."*
Veterinarian: *"Is the drainage milky or clear?"*
Client: *"Milky I guess."*

Veterinarian: *"Does it get worse with exercise?"*
Client: *"Maybe, I am not sure I can tell."*

or

Veterinarian: *"Now about this lump – how long has she had it?"*
Client: *"Well, I first noticed it three weeks ago."*
Veterinarian: *"Has it gotten any bigger?"*
Client: *"Yes."*
Veterinarian: *"How much?"*
Client: *"I'd say from about the size of a grape when I first noticed it to the size of a plum now."*
Veterinarian: *"Have you noticed lumps anywhere else?"*
Client: *"No, just there."*

An initially more open-ended questioning style might reveal very different information:

Veterinarian: *"Tell me about the nasal discharge."*
Client: *"Well, it started about two weeks ago. I thought it was just his allergies at first, but then it did not go away. It is really stinky and seems to come and go through the day. I am really worried it is something bad."*
Veterinarian: *"That is an understandable concern with what you have been telling me."*
Client: *"This horse's mother had a terrible sinus infection that ended up being a bad tooth. It took us forever to get her healed up and back into training."*

or

Veterinarian: *"Tell me about the lump you mentioned finding on her."*
Client: *"Well, I first noticed it three weeks ago and really didn't think much of it. I was just running my hand under her neck and noticed it. My last dog, Jake, had lots of fat lumps as he grew older and I figured that was what it was with her as well. But I was brushing Abby this week and noticed the lump again; it seemed to have grown a lot in the past couple of weeks. I thought I should bring her in and have it looked at just in case. It doesn't seem to bother her, though."*
Veterinarian: *"I see, tell me more about it."*
Client: *"Well, when I first noticed it I'd say it was about the size of a grape and now it is about the size of a plum. With Jake I was always able to move the fat lumps around; whereas with this one it seems more attached to her. I haven't noticed any other lumps on her, though. To be honest, I'm thinking we should probably just take it off to be safe."*

Why is there such a difference in the information obtained with open questioning? The advantages of open questioning methods are that they:

- encourage the client to tell their story in a more complete fashion
- prevent the stab in the dark approach of closed questioning
- allow the veterinarian time and space to listen and think and not just ask the next question
- contribute to more effective diagnostic reasoning
- help in the exploration of both the biomedical and the client perspectives
- set a pattern of client participation rather than veterinarian domination.

1. ENCOURAGING THE CLIENT TO TELL THEIR STORY IN A MORE COMPLETE FASHION

Closed questions give the veterinarian more control over the client's responses but limit the possible information that can be obtained. Open questions in contrast encourage the client to answer in an inclusive way and may well provide much of the information that is being sought. By asking an open question, information about a problem can be obtained quickly and efficiently. In the above examples, more useful information about the lump and the client's thoughts was discovered with two open questions than with four closed questions.

2. PREVENTING THE STAB IN THE DARK APPROACH OF CLOSED QUESTIONING

In the closed approach, all the responsibility rests on the veterinarian. They have to consider which areas might be worth enquiring about and then frame appropriate questions to ask. Clearly, the information obtained will only relate to those very areas that the veterinarian thinks are likely to be relevant and the veterinarian may well forget to ask about key areas of importance. Each question is like a stab in the dark, potentially a very inefficient process. In the open method, the client can mention areas that the veterinarian might not have considered – in the above example of closed questioning the veterinarian may not have thought to ask about the client's prior experience with their previous dog and would have missed the important information gained regarding the client's current thinking. This does not decry the value of closed questioning later on in the interview process. Closed questions are essential to clarify points or screen for areas not yet mentioned, but this is more efficiently achieved after first eliciting a wider view of the problem and hearing more of the client's story.

3. ALLOWING THE VETERINARIAN TIME AND SPACE TO LISTEN AND THINK AND NOT JUST ASK THE NEXT QUESTION

In the closed method, the veterinarian has to follow each closed question with another. Instead of listening and thinking about the client's responses, the veterinarian is formulating the next question to keep the flow of the interview going which in turn can interfere with listening and hearing important information. The open method allows the veterinarian time to more carefully consider what the client is saying and pick up cues as they emerge.

4. CONTRIBUTING TO MORE EFFECTIVE DIAGNOSTIC REASONING

Unless veterinarians use open questioning techniques at the beginning of their information gathering, it is all too easy to restrict diagnostic reasoning to an over-narrow field of inquiry. Bonnett (pers. comm. 2015) has observed that veterinarians start the process of problem solving very early on in the consultation. They quickly attempt to match the initial information presented by the client and patient to their underlying knowledge of individual diseases and to organizational frameworks that they have previously developed to aid problem solving. They then direct their further questioning to confirm or disprove their initial thoughts. This has been called "anchoring," which is a cognitive bias describing the common human tendency to rely too heavily on the first piece of information offered (the "anchor") when making decisions (Groopman 2007). A number of researchers have shown that physicians take this same approach (Kassirer and Gorry 1978; Barrows and Tamblyn 1980; Gick 1986; Mandin et al. 1997; Groopman 2007). Open methods allow clinicians more time to generate their problem-solving approach and provide them with more information on which to base their theories and hypotheses. Closed questioning in contrast too often quickly leads to premature closure, to the exploration of one particular avenue that may well prove inappropriate and lead inexorably to a dead end. The clinician may have to start again and generate a different problem-solving strategy – inefficient and inaccurate information gathering ensues. In our examples above, listening to the client's story with the use of open questions has allowed the clinician to avoid the trap of early closed questioning about the possibility of a particular problem and has enabled the discussion and exploration of additional signs, symptoms or concerns that will help to form a more accurate working hypothesis.

5. HELPING IN THE EXPLORATION OF BOTH THE BIOMEDICAL AND CLIENT PERSPECTIVES

Closed questions as explained above are not an efficient initial method of exploring the biomedical aspects of a problem. They are even less helpful in discovering the client's perspective. Because closed questions by their nature follow the veterinarian's agenda, they will tend to concentrate on the clinical aspects of the problem and omit the client's ideas. Open questions in contrast encourage clients to talk about their unique point of view, to tell their story in their own way using their own vocabulary. Clients can choose what is important from their own perspective and the veterinarian can better understand the client's personal experience and input regarding the animal's problems or issues. Most importantly, open questions allow the client time to organize their stories into a more logical framework and make them more understandable, not only to the veterinarian but to the client.

6. SETTING A PATTERN OF CLIENT PARTICIPATION RATHER THAN VETERINARIAN DOMINATION

Dysart et al. (2011) found that when veterinarians did not solicit the client's concerns at the beginning of an interaction the client was four times more likely to bring up concerns late in the visit resulting in the veterinarian having to extend the length of the appointment, ignore the concern or defer it to another visit. As discussed in Chapter 2,

Beckman and Frankel (1984) found that 94% of all interruptions in human medicine concluded with the physician obtaining the floor. In veterinary medicine, Dysart et al. (2011), found that following an interruption by the veterinarian the client was provided the opportunity to return to what they were saying only 28% of the time. The early pursuit of one problem by closed questioning shifts the whole emphasis from a client-centered to a veterinarian-centered format and once this is done, the client tends to remain in a more passive role. Once you begin closed questioning, clients will often not volunteer anything that is not explicitly asked – most clients defer to your lead. Open questions allow the client to participate more actively, signal that it is appropriate to elaborate, and make the veterinarian's willingness to listen apparent.

Why is it important to move from open to closed questioning techniques?

As the consultation proceeds it is important for the veterinarian to become gradually more focused. The veterinarian needs to use increasingly specific open questions and eventually move to closed questions to elicit important details. They then use closed questions to investigate specific areas that do not emerge from the client's account, to analyze a problem in detail, and to do a relevant review of systems (though even this can begin openly, e.g. *"Tell me about any problems or differences you have noticed with his breathing ..."*).

In Chapter 4, we explore how to move from open to closed questioning with the use of clear and explanatory transitional statements and shall see how summary and signposting can help overcome the perceived loss of control and potentially more disordered information gathering inherent in the use of open questioning. In Chapter 5, we will also look at the importance of nonverbal communication to the success of question asking and see how even closed questions asked in a facilitating manner can encourage the client to tell more of their story.

What is the evidence for the value of open and closed questioning techniques?

In an observational study of 284 video-recorded visits, MacMartin et al. (2015) found that 172 had nutrition discussions. Of these, 98 visits contained veterinary-initiated nutrition discussions. Looking at transcriptions of these 98 visits, the researchers studied the effect of question design on dietary information veterinarians collected and found that 75% of the time the veterinarian used a simple *what* question to initiate the topic of patient diet (e.g. *What kind of food does she eat? What food are you feeding him?*). Sixty-one percent of the time clients provided only one food item and 28% of the time only two. Seventy-five percent of the time the client was not asked about any other food item. The researchers indicate that these findings deviate considerably from Abood's (2008) suggestions for best practice whereby nutritional history taking should commence with open-ended questions inviting a broad range of nutrition-relevant information from clients.

In her commentary on dietary histories and nutritional assessment, Abood (2008) lists a number of communication skills critical to these tasks that are required in daily interactions among practice staff, veterinarians and their clients, including the ability to:

- ask open-ended questions
- evaluate the owner's knowledge and understanding of the situation
- listen actively to client responses
- interpret verbal cues and silence accurately
- recognize the client's nonverbal cues
- assess the emotional state of the client because it can influence the client's ability to provide information about their pet or to understand instructions.

Roter and Hall (1987) investigated the association between primary care physicians' interviewing styles and the medical information that they obtained during consultations with simulated patients. They found that physicians on average elicited only 50% of the medical information considered important by expert consensus, with a worrying range of 9–85%. They found that the amount of information elicited was related to the use of both appropriate open and closed questions. However, open questions prompted the revelation of substantially more relevant information than closed questions.

Shaw et al. (2004a) found that veterinarians primarily used closed questioning. In general 13 closed questions (range 0 to 42) were used per appointment compared with 2 open-ended questions (range 0 to 11). In 25% of the visits the veterinarian did not use any open-ended question.

Stiles et al. (1979) have shown that human patients at a hospital-based medical walk-in clinic were more satisfied with the information-gathering phase of the interview if they were allowed to express themselves in their own words rather than provide yes/no or one-word answers to closed questions.

Takemura et al. (2007) found significant positive relationships between three particular interview behaviors and the amount of information obtained in real family medicine interviews: the open-to-closed cone, facilitation, and summarization.

Evidence of the relative value of open and closed questioning comes from the detailed studies of Cox et al. (1981a, 1981b, Rutter and Cox 1981, Cox 1989). Their research showed that the number of topics raised by the interviewer, often via closed questions, was significantly associated with a larger number of symptoms being discovered to be definitely absent, which can be very important information.

Open-ended questioning techniques are, of course, not foolproof. Sometimes in spite of asking a good open-ended question, you may not get much information. Several realities can be at play here.

- The person who brought the animal in may not know the animal well or may not have much information to give.
- Clients may have limited experience with being asked an open-ended question and are caught off-guard.
- You may have asked a few closed questions in a row and the client perceives that you want short answers even to open-ended questions.
- You may have left too little time for them to think and respond before you interrupted with another question.

Eliciting the client's story

Listening is just as important in information gathering as it is during initiation of the consultation. But before you can start to listen, how do you set the client off in the right direction, how do you ask the client to give you further information about each of the patient's problems or about the problems in the herd?

From the discussion above, it is clear that open rather than closed questioning techniques at the beginning of problem exploration will pay dividends.

> "Tell me what has been going on with your flock."
>
> or
>
> "Tell me about Star's hind-end lameness."

will be far more advantageous than

> "So I understand you have been having high death loss in the flock. When did that start?"
>
> or
>
> "You mentioned Star was lame in the hind end. Which leg is it exactly?"

One particularly useful way to begin gathering information in an open way is to encourage the client to tell the story of their animal's problem from when it first started up to the present in their own words.

> "Please walk me through what has happened from the beginning, from the first case you noticed to now?"
>
> or
>
> "So, tell me from the beginning."

This is a natural way to find out about the client's perspective and to gather much of the information that you need in an orderly fashion. It allows the client to tell their story to you chronologically in the same way that they have experienced the problem and in much the same way as they would to a friend or colleague. From a biomedical standpoint, it provides the veterinarian early in the interview with a clear picture of the sequence of events. This important component of the biomedical perspective enhances accuracy. Asking the client to tell their story chronologically also provides you with an organizational framework that contributes to clinical reasoning and helps you as well as the client keep details of the history in mind more easily. In contrast, consider how difficult it is to elicit the sequence of events using closed questioning, which may explain why this valuable aspect of the history is sometimes overlooked.

This approach offers all the advantages of open questioning while providing the client with a simple way to tell their story chronologically. It is an excellent way to understand the client's perspective and it helps prevent what Mishler (1984) has called "two parallel monologues" in which patient and physician talk at cross purposes. The role of the veterinarian is to listen carefully and, if necessary, guide the client through their storytelling, possibly seeking brief clarification but quickly returning to *"then what happened?"*. The device of the client's narrative allows you to make some interruptions without necessarily taking the floor from the client; you can return control to the client by asking them to continue their story. However, this should be done sparingly because once you have interrupted it is all too easy to hold onto control with closed questions and forget to re-establish the client's narrative.

Adams and Frankel (2007) suggest that the stories clients tell about their animals establish client and patient identity. These narratives may contain anecdotal and biographical information that is important to the clinical reasoning process and ultimately the diagnosis of the problem. Adams and Frankel conclude that veterinarians may have to encourage and allow space for clients to tell their stories to facilitate this important form of engagement.

Degeling (2012), a small animal veterinarian in Australia, reinforced these points, indicating that attention to the client's narrative can improve clinical reasoning and give the client's perspective a more prominent place within that process. He asserts that veterinarians must consider shaping space for the clients to tell their stories about the patient because storytelling can help the veterinarian to better understand the patient's behavior, the context within which the owners will make their decisions about their animal's care and the reason that the client has come to see the veterinarian. Equally important, storytelling and attentive listening on behalf of the veterinarian can help ensure shared knowledge going forward with the care of the patient.

Open questioning and the client's narrative are ideal ways to enter the arenas of the biomedical aspects of the patient's problems and the client's perspectives simultaneously. High quality information can be obtained about both.

Attentive listening

As the client tells their story, the veterinarian needs to listen attentively without interrupting. We have already covered the importance of attentive listening in depth in Chapter 2 when we looked at the beginning of the interview. As we have seen, attentive listening is a highly skilled process, requiring a combination of focus, facilitation skills, wait time and picking up cues. More recently this process has been referred to as "mindful listening."

If we look again at the advantages of attentive listening listed in Chapter 2, we can see how many features are shared with the advantages of open questions mentioned earlier in this chapter. This similarity is because attentive listening is a direct consequence of the use of open questions: it is almost impossible to employ active listening and closed questioning together.

Facilitative response

As well as listening, it is important to actively encourage clients to continue their storytelling. Closed questioning is so predominant that clients may well initially respond even to excellent open questions with only a word or two unless they are encouraged to continue. Any behavior that has the effect of inviting clients to say more about the area that they are already discussing is a facilitative response. When we began our discussion of facilitative responses in Chapter 2, we looked at the research evidence showing that certain skills such as echoing or repetition could be counterproductive when used too early in the interview. At the beginning of the interview, our objective is to obtain as wide as possible a view of the patient's problem(s) and the client's whole agenda before exploring any one problem or issue in detail. Now let's turn our attention to the use of facilitative responses in the information-gathering phase. What are the skills that are useful here when we are trying to encourage clients to talk about each problem and issue in greater depth?

The facilitative response involves both verbal and nonverbal communication skills. In this chapter we focus primarily on verbal communication and also discuss selected nonverbal skills. We explore nonverbal communication in greater depth in Chapter 5.

The following responses can be used to encourage the client to say more about a topic, indicating simultaneously that you are interested in what they are saying and that you are keen for them to continue:

- encouragement
- silence
- repetition (echoing)
- paraphrasing
- sharing your thoughts.

Encouragement

Along with nonverbal head nods and the use of facial expression, veterinarians practicing attentive listening use innumerable verbal encouragers that signal the client to continue their story. This is often achieved very efficiently with minimal or no interruption and yet provides the client with the necessary confidence to keep going. Such neutral facilitative comments include "uh-huh," "go on," "yes," "um," "I see" – we all have our own particular favorites. Although veterinarians and learners often use "OK", clients frequently interpret this response to mean "OK, fine, that's all I need" – a signal that the veterinarian wants the floor – and the clients stop talking. Beckman and Frankel (1984) have found that this interpretation of "OK" is especially likely early in the interview.

Use of silence

Most verbal facilitation is ineffective unless immediately followed by nonverbal attentive silence. In Chapter 2, we discussed the work of Rowe (1986) on wait time and how the use of brief silence or pause can very easily and naturally facilitate the client to contribute more. Longer periods of silence are also appropriate if clients are having difficulty expressing themselves or if it seems that they are about to be overwhelmed by emotion. The aim of providing a longer pause is to encourage clients to express out loud their thoughts or feelings. There is a delicate balance here between comfortable and uncomfortable silence, between encouraging communication and interfering with it by creating uncertainty or anxiety – the veterinarian must attend carefully to the client's accompanying nonverbal behavior. However, remember that anxiety is more often felt by the veterinarian than the client; clients usually tolerate silence better than clinicians.

If you feel that a silence is producing anxiety or the client eventually needs further encouragement to speak, particular attention must be given to how the silence is broken. For instance:

> *"There is a lot going on here. Would you be willing to share your thoughts with me?"*

acts to allow the client to stay with their thoughts and further facilitates the process – as does repetition of the client's last words.

Repetition or echoing

Repeating the last few words that the client has said encourages the client to keep talking. Veterinarians often worry that this "echoing" will sound unnatural but it tends to be easily accepted by clients. Note how repetition encourages the client to continue with their last phrase and is therefore slightly more directive than encouragement or silence. In some research, echoing could act as a possible interrupter when used at the beginning of the interview (Beckman and Frankel 1984).

Following through the example used earlier, we see how the skills mentioned can be used to explore the biomedical and client's perspectives of a problem:

> Veterinarian: *"Tell me what has been going on with Diamond."* (open question)
> Client: *"Well, she has been coughing and has had a snotty nose since we brought her home from the trainer last week. She does not seem to be as rambunctious as her usual self and her appetite seems off."*
> Veterinarian: *"Yes, go on."* (encouragement)
> Client: *"It is just that she started so well and we really think she has a chance at making the futurity. With all the horses with strangles in the area, I am really worried that's what she has and that would put her out of training for this."*
> Veterinarian: (silence – accompanied by eye contact, slight head nod)
> Client: *"I have a lot of time tied up in her training and breeding and I really need to see some success this year."*
> Veterinarian: *"How are you going to cope … You have a lot tied up in her …"* (repetition)
> Client: *"Well, we really wanted a daughter out of this stallion and she seems to have so much promise."*
>
> or

Veterinarian: *"Tell me about the lump you mentioned finding on her."* (open question)

Client: *"Well, I first noticed it three weeks ago and really didn't think much of it. I was just running my hand under her neck and noticed it. My last dog, Jake, had lots of fat lumps as he grew older and I figured that was what it was with her as well. However, I was brushing her this week and noticed it again – it seemed to have grown a lot in the past couple of weeks. I thought I should bring her in and have it looked at just in case. It doesn't seem to bother her, though."*

Veterinarian: *"Yes, go on."* (encouragement)

Client: *"Well, when I first noticed it I'd say it was about the size of a grape and now it's the size of a plum. With Jake I was always able to move the fat lumps around; whereas with this one it seems more attached to her. I haven't noticed any other lumps on her, though. To be honest, I'm thinking we should probably just take it off to be safe."*

Veterinarian: (silence – accompanied by eye contact, slight head nod)

Client: *"I just can't have anything happen to her right now, I've spoken with my parents and they are willing to loan me the money to do whatever needs to be done, if it comes to that. They are the ones that told me to bring her in."*

Veterinarian: *"Your parents told you to bring her in …"* (repetition)

Client: *"Yes, I've recently lost my job and was hesitant to bring her in because I just don't have the money right now, but I'm also really worried about her. So, they told me they would help with whatever was needed and to just bring her in, to get her checked out."*

Paraphrasing (reflective listening)

Paraphrasing is restating in your own words the content or feelings behind the client's message. Not quite the same as checking or summarizing (see below), paraphrasing is intended to sharpen rather than just confirm understanding and therefore tends to be more specific than the original message. Paraphrasing is a way to check if your own *interpretation* of what the client actually means is correct. Continuing our examples:

Veterinarian: *"Are you thinking that you are going to be out the investment in her breeding and training because of this respiratory problem?"* (paraphrase of content)

Client: *"That is part of it. If she can't show or does not do well, I think our business will be sunk."*

Veterinarian: *"It sounds like you have a lot riding on this horse and you are worried about the pressure that is putting on you and your business."* (paraphrase of feeling)

or

Veterinarian: *"It sounds like you are in a very difficult financial position at the moment."* (paraphrase of content)

Client: *"Yeah, I mean my parents have offered to help, though I don't want to take advantage of them. I am really worried about the fact this lump is growing so quickly. I remember with Jake the veterinarian indicated that was something we should watch for."*

> Veterinarian: *"It sounds like you are very concerned about what this lump might mean for Abby."* (paraphrase of feeling)

Paraphrasing combines elements of facilitation, summarizing and clarification. It is particularly helpful if you think that you understand but are not quite certain, or you think that there might be hidden feelings or unstated information behind a seemingly simple message. Paraphrasing is a very good facilitative entry point into checking the client's perspective. It also gives clients clear opportunity to clarify or add to what they are saying or to correct your interpretation.

Sharing your thoughts

Sharing why you are asking questions is another excellent way to encourage the client to be more inclusive in their answer and acts as a very effective facilitative tool:

> *"Sometimes we can exacerbate respiratory disease by pushing youngsters too hard when they are not ready – do you think this could be a factor here?"*
>
> or
>
> *"Sometimes, when a cat starts urinating outside of the litter box it can be brought on by stress resulting from changes in their environment or their daily routine – I was wondering if you think that could be the case for Mokey."*

This is ostensibly a closed question but the fact that the client can understand the reasoning behind your request allows them to answer and then elaborate. The more direct *"Are you pushing the filly too hard this early in her training?"* is far more likely to produce a one word response containing little information (and perhaps a sense of defensiveness, in this case). We shall discuss the issue of sharing your thoughts with the client further in Chapter 5.

What is the theoretical and research evidence for facilitation?

The facilitative skills enumerated above are the key skills of non-directive counseling. They have been extensively discussed by Rogers (1980), Egan (1990) and others and are widely accepted as crucial elements of any communication in which the aim is to encourage the client to talk more about their concerns and issues without undue professional direction. Levinson et al. (1997) showed that primary care physicians who used more facilitation statements (soliciting patients' opinions, checking understanding, encouraging patients to talk, paraphrasing and interpretation) were less likely to have suffered malpractice claims.

Picking up verbal and nonverbal cues

Through attentive listening and verbal and nonverbal facilitation, we make clients feel comfortable and welcomed, indicate that we are interested in what they are saying and encourage them to continue and elaborate even further. But surprisingly, although we may be listening and give the impression that we are taking in everything that the clients are telling us, we may not have actually heard what clients are saying! We may be eliciting the information beautifully but failing to register it. This is akin to taking the heart rate of a patient but instantly realizing after removing the stethoscope that you did not register the rate mentally. It becomes even more complex in veterinary medicine because we also have to attend to a third party, namely, the animals: their behavior (including vocalizations), our own nonverbal behavior toward the animals, and how the clients and patients are interacting with each other. We do pick up and respond to animals' nonverbal behavior (MacMartin et al. 2014) and it is important. However, this large topic is beyond the scope of this book.

Certainly veterinarians are trained to recognize animals' behavioral cues, but are our clients really giving us these nonverbal opportunities? Research in human medicine confirms that patients in primary care, surgical and other hospital settings are indeed giving physicians numerous nonverbal cues (Levinson et al. 2000, Salmon et al. 2004, Mjaaland et al. 2011a). Since we are talking about human interaction, we suspect the same is true in veterinary medicine. Hearing what the client is saying is a vital ingredient in gathering information. This not only relates to what the client is telling us overtly but also what they are telling us indirectly or perhaps even unintentionally through verbal and nonverbal cues. Clients are generally eager to tell us about their own thoughts and feelings but often do so indirectly through verbal hints or changes in nonverbal behavior (body language, vocal cues such as hesitation or a change in volume, facial expression, affect). Picking up these cues is an essential skill for exploring both the biomedical (*"and he's had this … sort of … well, it doesn't really seem to be painful …"*) and client's perspectives (*"things haven't been easy …"* or *"I'm rarely at home …"*) (Tuckett et al. 1985; Branch and Malik 1993; Cegala 1997; Suchman et al. 1997; Lang et al. 2000).

And hearing the cue in itself is still not enough. We need to respond, to check out each cue with the client and acknowledge it as appropriate. Levinson et al. (2000) found that human patients gave cues throughout the interview from the opening to the closing minute, but that physicians only responded positively to patient cues in 38% of cases in surgery and 21% in primary care and in the remainder entirely missed the opportunity to respond to the patients' cues. Where the cue was missed, half of the patients brought up the same issue a second or third time and in all of these cases, the physician again missed these further opportunities to respond. In a follow-up study to their previous study, Mjaaland et al. (2011b) demonstrated that when patients expressed negative emotions or gave verbal or nonverbal cues to such emotions, physicians tended to move away from this communication without follow-up or exploration, particularly if the feeling was expressed as an explicit concern.

The danger therefore is twofold: either missing the message altogether or, having heard or seen it, assuming we know what it means without checking it out with the client. Clients' cues and the assumptions we make about them need to be explored and acknowledged throughout the interview. Although it can be appropriate to hear a cue and decide to leave your response to later, there is a danger to this course of action. First, there is a considerable chance that you will forget your mental note.

And, second, an immediate response and acknowledgment of the client's cue acts as confirmation to the client that you are interested and helps ensure an atmosphere conducive to even more disclosure.

The Levinson et al. (2000) study also showed that picking up and responding to cues *shortens* visits. Primary care visits that included at least one cue were longer when the physician missed the opportunity to respond than when physicians demonstrated a positive response (mean time 20.1 minutes vs. 17.6 minutes). Findings were similar in surgery (14.0 minutes vs. 12.5 minutes). Visits in which patients repeatedly brought up emotional issues after the physician missed an opportunity to respond were longer than visits where physicians made at least one positive response (18.4 vs. 17.6 in primary care and 15.5 vs. 12.5 in surgery visits). Levinson et al. concluded that these two aspects of the medical encounter – patient cues and physician response – were "a key to building a trusting patient-physician relationship, thus ultimately improving outcomes of care." Picking up cues and responding are also keys to efficient practice.

Kanji et al. (2012) found that in appointments where veterinarians and clients used a high sympathetic or empathetic tone and a low hurried and low rushed tone, clients subsequently adhered to recommendations, with low hurried and low rushed tone being the more influential factor. Reciprocity theory (Roter and Hall 2006) helps explain this – one person's positive action (in this case less hurried or rushed tone, something that is communicated via verbal and nonverbal cues) results in the other person reciprocating with a positive action. This is similar to the effect of nonverbal mirroring that we discuss in Chapter 5.

Later in this chapter, when we explore techniques for exploring the client's perspective, we shall look at some of the ways in which clients' cues can be picked up and responded to.

Clarification of the client's story

Clarifying statements that are vague or need further amplification is a vital information-gathering skill. After an initial response to an open-ended question, veterinarians may need to prompt clients for more precision, clarity or completeness. Often clients' statements can have two or more possible meanings: it is important to ascertain which meaning is intended.

Clarifying is often open in nature:

> *"Could you explain what you mean by Xena is not right?"*
>
> or
>
> *"Can you be more specific about what you meant when you said you don't think the heifers are gaining weight like you think they should?"*

but may also be closed:

"When you say not right, do you mean he appears to be straining to pee?"

or

"Have you been weighing each of the heifers to monitor their weight gain?"

If the client doesn't provide dates for important events in the animal's history, ask for them. Check that you understand the sequence of events correctly if you are uncertain. And to improve accuracy, learn to timeframe your own questions. Compare:

"Has she had any coughing?" (undated)
"Has she ever had any coughing?"
"Has she had any coughing in the last two weeks, since raising her hay off the ground?"

or

"Do you typically have a veterinarian involved with pregnancy diagnosis?" (undated)
"Is a veterinarian ever involved in preg checking?"
"Was there a veterinarian involved with the pregnancy diagnosis of the herd this fall?"

Too often we ask the first or second when we mean the third. When clients answer "occasionally," which question are they answering?

Internal summary

Summarizing is the deliberate step of making an explicit verbal summary to the client of the information gathered so far and is one of the most important of all information-gathering skills. Used periodically throughout the interview, internal summary helps the veterinarian with two significant tasks – ensuring accuracy in the consultation and facilitating the client's further responses.

Accuracy

With respect to accuracy, summarizing is a highly effective practical test of whether you have understood the client correctly, enabling the client to confirm that you have understood what they have said or to correct your misinterpretation. It is a means of ensuring that you and the client have attained *mutually understood common ground*. Platt and Platt (2003) liken the process to two authors passing drafts of a work back and forth until both are satisfied. Takemura et al. (2007) found a significant positive relationship between summarization and the amount of information obtained in family medicine interviews.

Remember to summarize both biomedical aspects and client perspective. Summarizing both helps to fulfill two of our previously stated objectives for this phase of the interview, namely:

- exploring and understanding the client's perspective so as to understand the meaning of the problems and issues for the patient and client
- exploring the biomedical perspective so as to obtain an adequate "medical" history.

Summarizing periodically tells you whether you have "got it right." If you have, the client will confirm your picture with both verbal and nonverbal signs of agreement. However, if your understanding is inaccurate or incomplete, the client will tell you or provide nonverbal signals of being unhappy. Without overt verbal summary, we rely on conjecture and assumption that we have understood our clients correctly.

Summary as facilitation

Internal summary also serves as an excellent facilitative opening. Followed by a pause and attentive listening, it is an important way to enable the client to continue their story without explicit direction from the veterinarian. It acts as a facilitative tool by inviting and making space for the client to go further in explaining problems and thoughts.

Veterinarian: *"Do you mind if I check my understanding of what has been going on? Three weeks ago there were two horses with snotty noses at the trainers. It does not sound like they were seen by a veterinarian but several clients voiced concern that it could be strangles. Last week when you brought her home from the trainers you noticed that your filly had a snotty nose and a cough and does not seem to have her normal energy level or appetite."* (Pause)

Client: *"Yes. We started her on antibiotics yesterday and they have not seemed to help so we called you."*

or

Veterinarian: *"Can I just see if I've got this right? You first noticed the lump on Abby three weeks ago and really didn't think much of it. While brushing her this week you noticed it again and it seems to have gotten larger. It has grown from the size of about a grape to a plum. However, it doesn't seem to bother her and you have not noticed any other lumps on her. You are worried because it seems more attached than the lumps you had experienced with Jake and so you're currently thinking it should come off. Is that right?"* (Pause)

Client: *"Yes, and I am concerned about the cost since I don't have a job at the moment."*

The advantages for clients are numerous – internal summary:

- clearly demonstrates that you have been listening
- demonstrates that you are interested and care about getting things right – it confirms the client

- offers a collaborative approach to problem solving
- allows the client to check your understanding and thoughts
- gives the client an opportunity to either confirm or correct your interpretation and add in missing areas
- invites and allows the client to go further in explaining their problems and thoughts by acting as a facilitative opening
- demonstrates the veterinarian's interest in the client's perspective as well as the biomedical aspects of the case.

The advantages for the veterinarian are also significant – internal summary:

- maximizes accurate information gathering by allowing you to check the accuracy of what you think the client has said and rectify any misconceptions; it promotes mutually understood common ground
- provides a space for you to review what you have already covered
- allows you to order your thoughts and clarify in your mind what you are not sure about and what aspect of the story you need to explore next
- helps you to recall information later
- allows you to distinguish between and consider both biomedical data and client perspective
- helps the process of clinical reasoning.

In Chapter 4 we explore summary as a way to structure the consultation and discuss the evidence for its use. We take up end summary in Chapter 7.

Language

The use of concise, easily understood questions and comments, without jargon, is important throughout the interview. We shall be concentrating on this aspect of communication when we take a close look at explanation and planning in Chapter 6.

Additional skills for understanding the client's perspective

The skills of problem exploration outlined here will enable the veterinarian to discover information about all three elements of the history: the biomedical perspective, the client's perspective and background information.

As the story unfolds, the client will relate information about both biomedical and client perspectives and the skilled interviewer will be able to weave between these two vital aspects of the case. However, the skills needed to ensure understanding of the client's perspective – namely, determining and acknowledging the client's ideas, concerns and expectations and encouraging the expression of feelings and thoughts – have a different intrinsic quality which requires additional expertise from the veterinarian.

What is the evidence to support exploring the client's perspective of the problems and issues?

Earlier in this chapter, we looked in detail at the integrated clinical method model and the importance of exploring both the veterinarian's and the client's perspectives in the consultation. Research undertaken in a variety of veterinary contexts validates the importance of understanding the client's perspective of their animal's problems and related issues.

As noted earlier in this chapter, the client's perspective includes:

- ideas and beliefs
- concerns and feelings
- expectations
- effects on life of client and animal
- relationship between animal, client, and others.

In a Canadian study of 44 clients across 8 veterinary clinics, Adams et al. (1999) looked at clients' grief following the death of their pets and found that there was great variability across clients in terms of their grief experiences and needs. Several factors contributed to these differences including the client's beliefs, life stage, past critical life events, the animal's attributes and the client's relationship with the animal. In a subsequent cross-sectional study involving 177 clients from 14 veterinary practices, Adams et al. (2000) found that different clients may have very different perspectives about the kind or amount of support they need regarding end of life issues or whether they need support at all. Thirty percent of clients whose pets had been euthanized experienced severe grief while 70% experienced sadness and may or may not have wanted any support from their veterinarians.

Looking at a very different aspect of client perspective, Kristensen and Enevoldsen (2008) investigated Danish dairy farmers' expectations regarding a herd health management program. They found substantial differences in the perspectives of veterinarians and farmers. While veterinarians believed that farmers' primary focus was on production and profit, farmers had other priorities that the veterinarians rarely explored, such as animal welfare and being part of a team with shared ambitions and goals. While veterinarians thought farmers were motivated to increase herd size primarily by a desire to improve financial performance, one farmer had no interest in increasing his herd size to improve profitability because he wanted to spend more time with his family and a second farmer was not so motivated because he wanted to take care of all his animals individually. The researchers concluded that instead of making assumptions about farmers' expectations and priorities, veterinarians need to check with their clients about what motivates them, including clients' perspectives on lifestyle, and social as well as biomedical and economic issues.

In a more recent study of veterinarians and dairy farmers in the Netherlands, Derks et al. (2013) found that veterinarians rarely asked farmers what their goals were for the farm or the herd and instead made assumptions about what the farmer was thinking. The researchers reported a mismatch between farmer and veterinarian perceptions about goals and objectives for the farm. Findings indicated that veterinarians should more actively seek information about farmers' needs regarding herd health, since farmers do not readily volunteer this information.

As part of a Dutch national mastitis control program, Jansen et al. (2010) asked eight veterinary practices to identify hard-to-reach farmers. Twenty-four farmers agreed to participate. In semi-structured interviews, the farmers indicated that their dairy veterinarians demonstrate limited active listening and pay little attention to fostering a balanced conversation with the farmer (i.e. letting farmers do their fair share of the talking).

For the following subsections we have included some research from veterinary medicine – additional veterinary studies related to these subjects are presented in Chapters 5 and 6, where they are more helpfully placed. Here we present several studies from human medicine that offer useful insights and reflect what we teach in our educational programs. These studies may also serve to stimulate future research in veterinary contexts.

Anthropological and cross-cultural studies

Many of the concepts that helped to formulate McWhinney's disease-illness model (and the integrated method model adapted from it) came originally from anthropological and cross-cultural studies. Kleinman et al.'s (1978) seminal review paper explored how patients' explanatory frameworks of their illness are culturally shaped. Our social, cultural and spiritual beliefs about health and illness influence our perception of symptoms, expectations and help-seeking behavior (from families, friends and professionals). Illness behavior is governed by cultural rules with marked cross-cultural variations in how disorders are both defined by society and dealt with by the individual. Kleinman et al. (1978) quote examples of the wide range of explanatory frameworks of illness in ethnic minorities living in the USA and point out that cultural minorities often will not respond to illness in the way expected by their professional advisors. In all our interactions there is potential for differences in explanatory models which can inhibit effective communication. These differences also exist within a culture across class and family boundaries.

Similarly, in veterinary medicine many of our social, cultural and spiritual beliefs about animals' health and illness influence our perspectives and impact the care of animals. For example, laminitis is a problem in Egypt, but owners there are often opposed to euthanasia, which sometimes means those horses die of complications from their laminitis. Owners in some cultures want to keep their animals intact. In some cultures obesity is a sign of affluence. Even within the same culture, ranching and farming families sometimes make medical decisions about their animals differently from how people who reside in urban settings might. Finding out about each individual's culturally influenced perspectives is important for thinking about alternative management options and making recommendations.

It is not only clients'/patients' beliefs that are culturally determined but veterinarians' and physicians' beliefs too. Even within modern Western medical practice itself, there are large cultural differences that determine what is perceived as "clinical reality." The biomedical viewpoint is "culture specific and value laden" rather than, as we so often think, "objective." In a study of health beliefs related to culture in a multicultural urban setting, Chugh et al. (1994) showed clearly that beliefs within a cultural group are often as diverse as beliefs between cultural groups. This research reminds us that understanding the diversity of health beliefs related to culture is important but that it is still essential to discover the health beliefs of each individual.

As Kleinman and his colleagues recommend, physicians should not only elicit their patients' explanatory model but also openly compare and discuss how their ideas conflict with their patients' ideas. This as an essential step to improving compliance with medical advice; compliance is likely to be poor if the physician has not explained their recommendations in relation to the patient's beliefs and if the physician's advice does not seem to help with the problem as the patient sees it. Clearly these recommendations and insights have application to veterinarians and their clients. Only by discovering the client's perspective can we explain and plan in terms the client can understand and accept. The client's ideas and beliefs, concerns and expectations need to be built into our explanation of the problem(s) so that we cover the questions that are most important from the client's perspective and together reach some degree of common ground. It is important to get to a position where our explanations and recommendations make sense in the client's world. This is the stage labeled "integration" in the integrated clinical method model (*see* Figure 3.1).

Exploring the client's beliefs involves a three-stage process:

- **identification** – discover and listen to the client's ideas, concerns and expectations
- **acceptance** – acknowledge the client's views and their right to hold them, without necessarily agreeing with them; then pause so as to make space for the client to say more if they wish
- **explanation** – explain your understanding of the problem in relation to the client's understanding and reach mutually understood common ground.

We discuss acceptance in greater depth in Chapter 5 and explore this three-stage model further in Chapter 6 when we look at the influence that eliciting the client's perspective has on clients' recall and understanding of our explanations.

Outcome studies

In human medicine, many studies confirm that eliciting and responding to patients' perspectives has a significant impact on outcomes of care (e.g. The Headache Study Group of the University of Western Ontario 1986; Orth et al. 1987; Brody and Miller 1986; Roter et al. 1995; Kinmonth et al. 1998; Roter 2000; Stewart et al. 2000a; Alamo et al. 2002; Croom et al. 2011 – if you are interested in more detail regarding findings from each of these studies, see pages 90–92 in Silverman et al. 2013).

As Street et al. (2009) indicate in their analysis of physician–patient interaction, the influence of communication skills on outcomes is important even though it may be an indirect pathway. In other words communication skills do not necessarily directly cure patients. Applied to veterinary medicine, the direct and indirect pathways Street et al. describe look like this: when clients' perspectives are taken into account, information exchange is likely to be more complete, honest and accurate; clients feel accepted and are in a better position to hear and accept veterinarians' diagnoses and recommendations, including those relating to preventive medicine; clients and veterinarians are more likely to feel satisfied and to develop relationships based on partnership; and because of all of these factors, compliance and follow-through are likely to be greater, which in turn impacts outcomes of care.

Satisfaction and compliance studies

This is a compelling topic for veterinary medicine because of its impact on animal and client-related outcomes as well as practice success. In Chapters 5 and 6 we explore in much greater detail the research showing how taking the client's perspective into account influences outcomes. For now we will reflect on just a sample of studies.

In both veterinary and human medicine understanding the clients'/patients' perspective is critical for satisfaction and compliance. Korsch et al. (1968) and Francis et al. (1969), in their seminal study of 800 visits to a pediatric walk-in outpatient clinic in Los Angeles, were among the first to tackle the physician–patient interaction, using rigorous methods. Satisfaction and compliance with the consultation was shown to be reduced if physicians demonstrated:

- lack of warmth and friendliness
- failure to take concerns and expectations into account
- use of jargon
- lack of clear explanations of diagnosis and causation.

This research showed that mothers' expectations were often not elicited by the pediatrician and that only 24% of mothers' main worries were mentioned. Lack of response to mothers' expressed worry or expectation led mothers to "click off" from the interview and give little further information. On the other hand when the needs that mothers perceived to be urgent were met, mothers appeared attentive and amenable to the physicians' ideas and plans. The highest incidence of dissatisfaction on follow-up occurred in those visits where neither expectations nor main concern received attention. No further time was taken when expectations were discovered.

Jansen et al. (2010) conducted a study to determine the factors that contributed to "hard to reach" farmers' reluctance to take up information that pertained to udder health. They concluded that veterinarians have ample opportunities to reach these farmers by tailoring communication to these farmers' specific needs and that such tailoring requires gathering information about farmers' needs and preferred approaches to working with the veterinarian.

Joos et al. (1993) and Kravitz et al. (1994) have shown that human patients were significantly more satisfied if their prior expectations of help were fulfilled in the interview. However, many patients' desires for further information or specific help remained unmet.

In a Canadian study of 90 consultations, Adams et al. (2005) found that dog owners were nine times more likely to comply with recommendations when medications were required once or twice a day versus three times a day. The researchers concluded that in order to enhance compliance, veterinarians must ask about the client's lifestyle and home situation to help in choosing a dosing regime that is manageable for the client.

Kanji et al. (2012) showed that clients who adhered to a dentistry and/or surgery recommendation were more satisfied with their office visit than those clients that did not adhere. Satisfaction had to do with how well the veterinarian understood the reason for the client's visit, how well the veterinarian involved the client in the entire appointment, the veterinarian's recognition of the role that the pet played in the client's life, etc.

Eisenthal and Lazare (Eisenthal and Lazare 1976; Eisenthal et al. 1979; Eisenthal et al. 1990; Lazare et al. 1975) studied human patients' expectations extensively by looking specifically at "how the patient hoped the doctor might help them" as well as at their presenting symptoms. They clearly demonstrated that patients' expectations are often not obvious from the chief complaint, that clinicians need to make a specific inquiry to discover their patients' expectations and that doctors do not routinely ask for patient's expectations. Their research showed that when physicians did ask for patient's expectations, patients were more likely to feel satisfied and helped and also to adhere to a negotiated plan. Most importantly, their research clearly demonstrated that this increased satisfaction was apparent regardless of whether or not the request was granted.

Britten et al. (2000) identified 14 categories of misunderstanding that included patient information unknown to the physician, physician information unknown to the patient, conflicting information, disagreement about attribution of side effects, failure of communication about physicians' decision, and relationship factors. All the misunderstandings were associated with lack of patients' participation in the consultation in terms of their voicing of expectations and preferences or their voicing of responses to physicians' decisions and actions. Misunderstandings were all associated with potential or actual adverse outcomes such as non-adherence to treatment.

Understanding and recall studies

Tuckett et al.'s research (1985) on information giving demonstrates the great importance of eliciting the patients' beliefs and views of their illness in enabling patients to understand and recall information provided by the physician. Their research efforts were hampered by the very few examples that they were able to find at all of physicians asking for patients to volunteer their ideas, or even of doctors asking the patient to elaborate on their ideas if they were spontaneously brought up. Physicians often evaded their patients' ideas and positively inhibited their expression. This behavior led to a considerably increased likelihood of client failure to understand and recall.

Physicians' understanding is also enhanced by patient-centered interviewing. Peppiatt (1992) showed in a study of 1000 interviews undertaken by one family physician that 77% of patients either spontaneously offered or responded to requests to express a cause for their condition and that 20% of patients' ideas of causation helped the doctor decide on a cause with 9% enabling the doctor to actually make a diagnosis.

Are client/patient-centered interviews longer?

Stewart (1985) looked at 133 interviews in primary care and compared their "patient-centeredness" score with the length of the consultation. Low scores for patient centeredness produced interviews of on average 7.8 minutes, intermediate scores 10.9 minutes and high scores 8.5 minutes. Her conclusion was that physicians could expect to take longer while they are learning the skills. But physicians in this study who had *mastered* the patient-centered approach took little extra time compared with physicians who did not employ these techniques. Roter et al. (1995) also found no increase in the length of interviews in primary care following training in the skills of "problem-defining and emotion-handling."

Roter et al. (1997) found five distinct communication patterns in primary care visits in the USA:

1. "narrowly biomedical," characterized by closed-ended medical questions and bio-medical talk
2. "expanded biomedical," like the restricted pattern but with moderate levels of psychosocial discussion
3. "bio-psychosocial," reflecting a balance of psychosocial and biomedical topics
4. "psychosocial," characterized by psychosocial exchange, and
5. "consumerist," characterized primarily by patient questions and physician infor-mation giving.

They found no evidence that patient-centered consultations took any longer than strictly biomedical interviews.

Using Roter's same system of analysis, Shaw et al. (2006) found that veterinarians used two communication patterns. In 58% of the 300 consultations in the study they used a biomedical pattern (characterized by a high degree of biomedical talk) and in 42% a biolifestyle-social pattern (characterized by shared biomedical and lifestyle-social talk). Appointments oriented to biomedical communication were significantly longer than those oriented to biolifestyle-social communication. Relationship-centered care scores (defined as the ratio of client-centered to veterinary-centered talk) were significantly higher for the biolifestyle-social appointments.

Levinson et al. (2000) showed that primary care and surgical office visits where physicians missed opportunities to pick up patients' emotional cues tended to be longer than visits with a positive response.

In Abdel-Tawab and Roter (2002)'s study patient-centered consultations were only 1 minute longer than physician-centered consultations despite markedly improved patient satisfaction and adherence.

Recall the Mauksch et al. (2008) literature review regarding determinants of effi-ciency in human medical interviews. That review found three skill sets or domains that could enhance communication efficiency: rapport building, upfront agenda set-ting and picking up emotional cues.

How to discover the client's perspective

Earlier in this chapter we presented the literature establishing how important it is for veterinarians to get the client's perspective. There are two alternative ways of exploring the client's point of view. The first is by directly asking for the client's ideas, concerns, expectations and feelings; the second is by picking up cues (i.e. verbal and nonverbal hints) provided by the client during the course of the consultation.

Del Piccolo et al. (2007) concluded that listening, together with supporting and emotion-centered expressions, activate cue emission by encouraging the patient to add new information or to direct the physician's attention to issues of importance, whereas physician closed questions tend to suppress cue expressions. On the other hand, soliciting human patients' expression of personal needs by open inquiry and active listening followed by acknowledging and sensitively handling patients' expressions of needs will satisfy those needs and lower cue offers.

Interestingly, Cegala and Post (2009) found that physicians engaged in significantly more exploration of patients' disease and illness when interacting with high participation patients than when interacting with low participation patients. Active participation in medical interviews by patients influenced physicians to adopt a more patient-centered style.

Picking up and checking out cues

The research in this area shows that clinicians tend not to pick up or at least not to respond to many of the verbal and nonverbal cues that people give, that they respond better to informational cues than to those regarding emotion, and that – contrary to what we tend to think – generally responding to cues takes less rather than more time. We have not found research on this topic done in veterinary medicine but have certainly observed these missed opportunities in both teaching and practice settings across the profession.

Patients are keen to tell healthcare providers about their own thoughts and feelings. In Tuckett' et al.'s research (1985), 26% of patients spontaneously offered an explanation of their symptoms to the physician. However, when patients did express their views, only 7% of doctors actively encouraged their patients to elaborate, 13% listened passively and 81% made no effort to listen or deliberately interrupted. Half of patients' views were expressed covertly rather than overtly with overt cues being picked up far more readily than covert cues. The conclusion here is that many patients provide cues which physicians unfortunately ignore. Zimmerman et al. (2007) undertook a systematic review, documenting 58 original quantitative and qualitative research articles demonstrating patient expressions of cues and/or concerns, all based on the analysis of audio or videotaped medical consultations. Yet again, their overall conclusion was that physicians missed most cues and concerns and adopted behaviors that discouraged disclosure. Communication training improved the detection of cues and concerns.

It should be emphasized that cues do not only appear as verbal comments. Nonverbal cues in body language, speech, facial expression and affect are also highly significant. To ensure accurate interpretation of such nonverbal behavior, it is important to observe the patient and client carefully and then sensitively verify your perceptions with the client.

Clients' cues are usually a short cut to important areas requiring our attention. So why do we often fail to respond to these cues? Perhaps it is in part due to issues of control. Veterinarians have traditionally controlled the interview via closed questions that limit clients' contributions and render them more passive (Shaw et al. 2004b, 2006). When veterinarians pick up client cues, perhaps they feel that responding will take them off their pre-planned flight path and are uncertain of where it might lead or how much time it may take. Some veterinarians may start to feel that they are losing control of the consultation or are concerned that they are opening up emotional territory which will make everyone uncomfortable. An awkward moment ensues that is all too easy for the veterinarian to side-step by ignoring the client cue and returning to safer ground.

In veterinary medicine we may also fail to pick up cues regarding the client's perspective because we are preferentially listening for cues about the patient's disease or problems. If the client says, *"It's been difficult at home and I know Spike is overweight but I just haven't been able to take him for his daily walks,"* it is so easy to preferentially pick up the weight issue rather than finding out what turns out to be highly relevant information affecting the client's ability to care for the animal. In this actual case the client's husband was in a serious accident and caring for him took up time that the client would otherwise have spent walking the dog.

Box 3.2 provides a variety of effective ways to pick up and respond to clients' cues.

Box 3.2 Examples of ways to pick up verbal and nonverbal cues

Repetition of cues
- *"frustrated …?"*
- *"excited about her potential …?"*
- *"worried …?"*
- *"worse than last time …?"*

Picking up and checking out verbal cues
- *"You said that you were worried that her lameness might be something serious; what theories did you have about what it might be?"*
- *"You mentioned that your previous horse had been diagnosed with navicular disease – are you thinking that's what she might be experiencing as well?"*
- *"You have noticed some real potential from the new bull you added last year. Are you thinking you want to move to more of this type of cross in the future?"*

Picking up and checking out nonverbal cues
- *"I noticed that you really light up when you talk about your new pair of alpacas."* (Pause)
- *"This is a diagnosis that often brings up a lot of emotion for people. I sense that you are feeling that right now. Do I have that right?"*
- *"You don't look very convinced with our plan for today's appointment – what are your thoughts?"*
- *"You appear to be very upset about what has happened here. Let's take some more time to discuss things. … What questions do you have at this point?"*

Asking specifically about the client's perspective

Picking up client's verbal and nonverbal cues is important. However, even if we do this well, asking specifically about the client's perspective rather than just making assumptions about what they mean is still a very necessary task (Platt et al. 2001). It is particularly helpful to find out about and acknowledge clients' ideas, hypotheses and even beliefs about what they think is going on, how serious they believe it is, what is likely to happen, how they think the animal's problem(s) might affect them, etc.

Box 3.3 Ways to find out about clients' ideas and beliefs

- *"Tell me what you're thinking."*
- *"What are your thoughts on what might be going on with her?"*
- *"Do you have any theories on how this might have happened?"*
- *"You've obviously given some thought to what is going on. It'd be helpful for me to know what you are thinking. Tell me about what you think is causing it."*
- *"What do you think might be happening?"*
- *"Have you any ideas about it yourself?"*
- *"You have a lot of experience in the industry. I would imagine you have some suspicion about what might be going on."*
- *"I know horse people like to talk about other horse people's issues. Do you have anything in mind based on what has been discussed at the barn?"*

Lang et al. (2002) in a family practice clinic setting showed that in response to sequenced questioning about the patient's perspective, 44% of patients revealed specific, significant concerns that had not been otherwise disclosed. Among patients without prior contact with their physicians, satisfaction with the encounter was significantly higher when such sequenced questions were used than when they were not.

Direct questions need careful timing, with good signposting of intent and attention to detail in wording (*see* Chapter 4). Bass and Cohen (1982) showed that when parents in a pediatric practice were asked *"What worries you about this problem?"*, the majority of parents responded with *"I'm not worried"* whereas the phrase *"What concerns you about the problem?"* produced previously unrecognized concerns in more than a third of parents. Linguist colleague Clare MacMartin (pers. comm. 2015) explains that when we use "worry" clients may edit out information, thinking that the issue is not at the level of "worry." Perceived to be less negative, "concern" seems to result in less defensiveness, increase the likelihood of obtaining more information, and connote a more actionable issue.

Box 3.4 Ways to ask about concerns

- *"What concerns do you have at this point?"*
- *"Is there anything particular or specific that you are concerned about …?"*
- *"What are you concerned that it might be?"*
- *"What was the worst thing you were thinking it might be?"*
- *"Is there a specific disease you are concerned about?"*

Many veterinarians find entering the realm of clients' feelings particularly difficult or inappropriate. It doesn't fit naturally with the objective approach of the traditional clinical method and is something that veterinarians may tend to avoid. Impassive objectivity can be appealing – feelings are often difficult to handle and may be painful to the veterinarian as well as the client. Veterinarians are reluctant to "open a Pandora's box" of their client's emotions and feelings and might consider dealing with feelings to be beyond their training or responsibility or that it will take too much time. Physicians appear to be similarly reluctant. Maguire et al. (1996) reported that when responding to patient emotion, physicians used a ratio of three inhibitory behaviors or responses for every facilitative response.

It is important to recognize that dealing with feelings and concerns in the veterinary context is not about fixing the problem but rather about eliciting and acknowledging the client's perspective so as to be able to use relevant insights gained to help guide further information gathering, relationship building, explanation and planning. Evidence from the neuroscience literature demonstrates that feeling understood is a powerful incentive for focusing and engaging in the interaction (Fogassi 2011; Zak 2011).

Box 3.5 Skills involved in discovering and responding to clients' feelings

Picking up and checking out verbal cues
- *"You mentioned you are not happy with her progress. Could you tell me more?"*
- *"I heard you mention that you have high hopes for this ram. It would be helpful for me to know more."*

Repeating verbal cues
- *"angry …?"*
- *"worried …"*

Picking up and reflecting nonverbal cues
- *"I sense that you're frustrated – would it help to talk about it?"*
- *"You are obviously attached to your lizard. I noticed you talking to him when I walked in the room."*

Asking direct questions
- *"How did that leave you feeling?"*
- *"Cancer is a scary term. Do you mind telling me what is going on for you?"*

Using acceptance, empathy, concern, understanding to allow the patient to feel that you are interested in their feelings (*see Chapter 5*)
- *"I don't think anyone ever wants to make this kind of decision. Deciding when the best time is to let our best friends go is tough."*
- *"I can see that this has been very difficult for you to talk about."*

Using feelings questions early on to establish your interest in the subject

Asking for particular examples
- *"How did you feel after Felix's last chemotherapy treatment?"*
- *"Can you remember a time when you felt like that – what actually happened?"*

Asking permission to enter the feelings realm
- *"Would you be open to sharing how you are feeling at this moment?"*

How to end the discussion of concerns or feelings without getting drawn into lengthy discussion
- *"I appreciate you telling me about your concerns. It helps me to understand the situation much better. Is there anything else you'd like to tell me about it?"*
- *"I think I understand now a little of what you have been feeling – let's look at the practical things that we can do together to help."*
- *"Understanding how you are feeling is very helpful to me; it'll assist us when it comes time to make decisions."*

Determining clients' expectations, whether realistic or not, is important. Clients' expectations include what they expect of the veterinarian or the veterinary team, what they want from the visit, their hopes for the animal as a result of treatment, their perceptions about how successful or good or reasonable outcomes will be for the animal and for themselves.

Box 3.6 Ways to ask about client expectations

- *"What are you hoping we can achieve for Harley today?"*
- *"Given the limited time you have for this morning's herd health, what would you like to accomplish?"*
- *"What options would you be open to considering for her?"*
- *"How best might I help you with this?"*
- *"You've obviously given some thought to how we might address this. What were you thinking would be the best way of tackling it?"*
- *"What were you hoping we might be able to do for this?"*
- *"What do you think might be the best plan of action …?"*
- *"Do you have a sense of how you think we should proceed?"*

EFFECTS ON LIFE
Open questions about how the animal's problem is affecting the animal or the client are excellent entries into the client's perspective of the problem and in particular often lead the client to talk openly about their thoughts and feelings.

RELATIONSHIP BETWEEN ANIMAL AND CLIENT, OTHERS
It helps the veterinarian to know whether the relationship between the animal and

the client is strong or indifferent, whether this is a hunting dog or a show horse rather than a pet, etc. – it influences how to work with a particular client. There are also many situations where multiple people are responsible for the animal and in the event that these relationships have some bearing on the patient's health, it is useful to discover the client's perception of these relationships. For example, consider situations where that other person's relationship with the animal contributes to excessive feeding or over exercise.

Putting the skills of information gathering together

We have now explored the individual process skills of information gathering. But how in practice can we best combine these skills to negotiate a path through this section of the interview? How can they be used most effectively to discover the content of:

- the biomedical perspective
- the client's perspective
- background information?

Exploration of both the biomedical and the client's perspectives

Sequence of events
Encourage the client to tell their story by using open questioning methods
Listen attentively
Facilitate
Use more focused open questions
Clarify and determine timeframe
Pick up and respond to verbal and nonverbal cues regarding both the biomedical problem and client perspective
Summarize both the biomedical perspective and client's perspective
Signpost to (i.e. overtly indicate to the client that you are moving to):

Further analysis of each symptom and the relevant systems review
Start with open questions and gradually move to closed
Signpost to:

Further exploration of the client's perspective
Use predominately open questions
Acknowledge client's views and feelings
Signpost to:

Finding out about background information:

Use increasingly focused questions, and eventually closed

This is one practical approach to combining the process skills that veterinarians can use in everyday practice once they have completed the initiation phase of the interview and identified the list of the patient's problems or issues and client's concerns. There are of course many ways to combine these skills. The key is to be flexible and dynamic, responding to the patient's needs and the client's cues and responses as you go.

The continuum of open to closed questioning techniques

In the approach suggested here, there is a continuum of open to closed questioning techniques: the interview gradually moves from open to closed questions as each specific component of the content of the history is explored.

Initially, open questioning techniques are used at the start of the exploration:

"Walk me through what has been going on from when you first noticed the problem until now."

or

"Tell me what has been going on from just before you first noticed Dexter's vomiting right up until now."

As the interview proceeds, you may need to become more directive, guiding the client to elaborate further on specific areas of both the biomedical and the client's perspective that have surfaced as they tell their narrative. You can do this by employing more focused verbal encouragement in the form of more directed open statements and questions:

"Tell me more about the vomiting and diarrhea."
"You mentioned he seems not right; tell me more about what you mean by that."
"You said you are worried about him. Can you tell me more about that?"
"Did you notice anything else while all this was going on?"
"What did you notice with the lameness?"
"To help me make optimal vaccination recommendations it would help to know what Fido's lifestyle is like."
"What is going on with the herd?"

As the exploration of the problem progresses, important facets of the biomedical perspective may well not emerge from the client's account and the gradual movement from open to closed questioning ensures that these areas are explored. Each issue needs to be explored thoroughly as we have described earlier in this chapter and more focused questions are essential here. Again, these more directive questions can be open at first and then increasingly closed if necessary:

> "Tell me about the travelling that Yin and Wally have done."
> "Have you been to Florida of late?"

You will also want to explore the client's perspective. As described earlier, open questions are most profitable here, although sometimes more closed questions can be useful:

> "Do you have specific ideas about what is going on?"
> "Are you thinking that there might be a resistance issue with the parasite?"
> "What are your thoughts on the cause of his vomiting?"
> "Do you think he might have gotten into something poisonous?"

As the interview proceeds, you will have started the process of clinical reasoning. Your perceptual skills will drive further focused questioning. For example, a client presenting their dog with vomiting and diarrhea might not consider recent environmental exposure as a contributing factor. After careful listening and the judicial use of open questions, you might ask the specific closed question:

> Veterinarian: "Is Bailey ever exposed to water that other animals, especially wildlife, have access to?"
> Client: "Well, we like to take him to the conservation area north of the city so we can let him off leash. There's wildlife there."

Be careful that your closed questioning is not too focused. It is easy to ask the client an inappropriate closed question: we think ahead too quickly, think of a possible answer to a question we have posed to ourselves and then test our own premature hypotheses. Instead, ask the question that was in your mind right from the start! Two examples that illustrate this problem would be:

> The veterinarian above wonders about his patient's exposure to wildlife and other animals in relation to a diagnosis of leptospirosis. Instead of asking a general question such as "Tell me about Bailey's exposure to areas where there is wildlife or other animals," he thinks ahead, about exposure to free-standing water accessed by wildlife and other animals, and asks, "Does Bailey ever drink from lakes, ponds or swampy areas?" The client says no and the veterinarian moves on without an answer to his original question.
>
> or
>
> The veterinarian is concerned that a modification of the treatment protocol may be to

blame for the increased incidence of a problem in the herd. Instead of asking a general question like *"Have there been any changes to the protocols lately?"* he assumes that maybe it is related to a new employee and asks, *"How are things going with the new calf manager?"* When the client answers fine, the veterinarian does not continue back to query any other changes in protocol.

Next you need to gather details about the relevant background information of the patient's environment and lifestyle, including animal use, past medical history, current medications, adverse drug reactions and allergies, genetic and familial background, behavioral/social history and review of systems. At this point in the process of information gathering, increasingly directed questions are used until you arrive at the review of systems which becomes almost a checklist of closed questions. Important information is lost if a systematic approach to the exclusion of associated signs and other physical examination findings is not employed. Although this may only discover which signs or findings are definitely absent, this is still highly useful diagnostic information that cannot otherwise be assumed. Negative findings can be as important as positive ones.

The more complete versus more focused history

It is worth emphasizing that both the process and content frameworks outlined here are equally applicable whether you are doing a more complete or more focused history. We recognize that time generally prevents doing a truly complete history or, for that matter, a complete physical examination. Nevertheless, with a new patient and client or a more complex situation, a more complete history and physical is generally needed than with a known patient. Then again, even with a known patient, things frequently change for patient and/or client and that requires gathering more complete information rather than simply making assumptions based on previous interactions. In more focused histories information obtained is not the same as in the complete history. While the problem list, biomedical history of the patient's problems and client's perspective are still vital and cannot be truncated, only certain relevant and actively selected parts of the background information are sought – the full systems review for instance is almost never completed. There is therefore a more selective and judicial approach to the background information. The only real difference between a more complete and more focused history is the level of detail collected regarding background information. As for the physical examination, however complete it may be, it clearly does not take the place of the information that must be obtained from talking with the client.

Why do communication process skills so frequently seem to be a casualty of the transition from the classroom to "real-life" practice? Part of the explanation may be that there is a mismatch between what we teach about history taking in clinical communication or professionalism courses and how we expect students, interns and residents to perform in classrooms or during clinical rotations and oral examinations elsewhere in the curriculum. This became clear yet again during a discussion we had with a recently graduated resident who at first insisted that the focused history had to be mostly directed toward biomedical information obtained through closed questions. As he talked, the following insight was reconfirmed: all too often when students and residents are asked to take a history in clinical rotations or during an oral examination, what they are really expected to demonstrate is their knowledge of content by saying it out loud in the form of the questions they ask. Almost inevitably that means using closed questions focused on the biomedical history throughout, especially if this is during a time-truncated oral examination. Looking again at the pyramids, teachers and learners have to be careful not to oversimplify history taking by translating the items in the pyramids into a checklist of closed questions.

All of us tend to focus on that with which we are familiar and comfortable. Artemiou et al. (2015) offer research that explores this notion further. They conducted a pre-post communication skills assessment of 96 second-year veterinary students which required 23 examiners, including 11 veterinary clinical sciences faculty and 12 from elsewhere (basic sciences, education, and communication faculty members, laboratory technicians, a hospital administrator). As part of the assessment checklist, examiners were asked to provide written feedback during and after each student's participation in an interaction that gave students opportunity to demonstrate their communication skills. Out of 403 written comments, 56 had to do with the student's clinical knowledge such as: *"failed to address diet"* (referring to the student), *"not realistic in the delivery of expectations to the client"* (referring to prognosis), *"missed the mark on diagnostics"* or *"failed to discuss a probable diagnosis like diabetes or hyperthyroidism"*. The veterinary clinical sciences faculty evaluators provided 91% of these comments. The researchers concluded that clinical sciences faculty scores were influenced by their clinical expectations of the students even though the examination checklist had only to do with communication process skills.

Unfortunately some learners (and probably some faculty and practitioners) also tend to associate history taking in real-life practice with closed questioning and a narrow emphasis on biomedical history. Seeing this, students too often perceive that in actual practice the veterinarian simply abandons the initial listening phase and moves quickly into closed questions and physical examination. Is it any wonder that as they move from their early training years to practice, many students seem to lose track of the process skills that we have advocated so far in this book such as listening, screening, agenda setting, facilitation, using the open to closed cone, summarizing, asking for the client's narrative and building relationship?

In veterinary medicine another potential challenge regarding completeness has to do with the shift from veterinarians taking full responsibility for the history to the increasingly common practice of receptionists finding out the reason(s) for the visit and veterinary technicians taking the initial history. Depending on their level of training, technicians generally are responsible for taking only partial histories such as those that are guided by checklists (eating, drinking, vomiting, diarrhea, etc.). When the veterinarian picks up the history a few potential difficulties can result. First, the veterinarian may rely too heavily on the information the receptionist has passed on and/or the technician's written or verbal recounting of the history, thereby missing important information that with their deeper knowledge base and judgment they would have gathered about the patient's condition or needs and the client's perspective. Distributing the tasks of history taking across staff members can be helpful. On the other hand, involving multiple team members in information gathering requires careful training and coordination so that this relationship augments rather than hinders the veterinarian's thought process and their interaction with the client. Even when staff members are carefully trained there may be gaps in the history, or other inaccuracies, and the time allotted for handovers between technician and veterinarian may be too brief to be thorough or may not happen at all. If clients are asked the same or seemingly similar questions by the technician and veterinarian, clients may get confused about what information to share or not or frustrated if they do not get to tell you important details of their story. Another issue may arise because people are hesitant to repeat information and so may not give you information they have already related. You can make this easier for clients by introducing the way the tag team is working and indicating how the client might participate:

> Veterinarian talking to client: *"I have gotten some idea of your concerns today from Jessica* [veterinary technician]. *I want to make sure I understand your perspective so I may ask you to repeat some of the information you have already told her. I do this to make sure I really understand what is going on. Will that work?"*

If something like this is not explicitly said, the veterinarian may short change both initiating and gathering information, thus potentially compromising accurate understanding and losing significant opportunities to build relationship with the client.

Gathering complete and accurate information is also complicated when the client is not a single individual, but rather multiple caregivers in a household or multiple team members on farms. Here, too, veterinarians can help with explicit comment:

> Veterinarian talking to producer: *"I stopped to say hi to Larry* [lead hand] *while I was driving in. He mentioned how busy you are taking the crops off the fields. This is good to know. Let's make sure we take the time pressure you're under into account as we decide how best to treat that injured cow – my receptionist said you thought she was pretty dire."*

In summary, the relational coordination issues that are part of either having someone other than the veterinarian take the history or having to take history from more than one person can impact diagnostic accuracy, client satisfaction, client's understanding of what they are supposed to tell each person and clarity about the role that each team member plays in the practice.

The effect of clinical reasoning on the process of gathering information

Just as with approaches to history taking, the effect of different approaches to clinical reasoning should not in any way influence the communication process skills required for information gathering – these process skills are important regardless of the clinical reasoning process the veterinarian is using. Yet the way that many veterinarians take a history can lead to inaccuracy and inefficiency which can affect clinical reasoning. Commonly used closed questioning methods do not encourage appropriately comprehensive history taking which in turn compromises effective pattern recognition and, in unfamiliar situations, hypothesis generation. Communication skills and clinical reasoning are closely connected to each other.

When learners start to see patients, they initially use a variation of *hypothetico-deductive reasoning* to attempt to solve clinical problems. In this approach, all the information is obtained from the physical examination and conversation with the client first. Then the student stands back to consider what the differential diagnosis might be. Students next "guess" at potential diagnoses and then consider how to rule them in and out. This is a very early approach to clinical reasoning that is generally not used by clinicians in real life unless they are well away from their area of subject expertise. As clinical reasoning at this stage of a student's development is often an after-event, it may not interfere with the interviewing process.

In both human and veterinary medicine, as clinicians develop subject expertise, they adopt increasingly more sophisticated approaches to clinical reasoning (Elstein and Schwarz 2002; Dornan and Carroll 2003; Maddison et al. 2015). The first is *more advanced hypothetico-deductive reasoning* in which, after eliciting the presenting problems, the clinician forms a number of diagnostic hypotheses (no more than five or six) in the early minutes of the interview and then validates or rejects these hypotheses by selective questioning ("rule in/rule out"), selective physical examination and selective investigations. Hypothesis generation occurs early and drives the questions that the clinician asks as the interview proceeds. One drawback to this approach is that it is tempting for practitioners to go for findings that support their "favored" hypotheses rather than those that could refute them, especially when they perceive a lack of time. As Osborne (2010) has pointed out in the veterinary context, taking short cuts in clinical reasoning and information gathering that result in a misdiagnosis ultimately may be more detrimental to patients than the illness itself. This, of course, can also happen when using the other approaches to clinical reasoning.

In the next variation, *schema driven clinical reasoning*, clinicians use pre-formed schema or mental flow diagrams to help solve the problem (Mandin et al. 1997). This approach is only possible with increased subject expertise and knowledge. Schema enable inductive reasoning to occur – highly selective and discriminating questioning can enable large diagnostic areas to be ruled in or out at a time and can allow fast navigation through a well-defined problem area.

Highly experienced clinicians use a method of clinical reasoning that is not available to students – *pattern recognition*. As their career progresses, clinicians continually accumulate details and key features about specific conditions as templates or memory structures known in human medicine as "illness scripts" (Schmidt et al. 1990; Elstein and Schwarz 2002; Norman 2005). These are often "pegged" to particular patients. When confronted with a specific problem, the clinician searches their "bank" of illness scripts to see if a pattern can be recognized. Initial impressions will then be tested for "goodness of fit" by further inquiry. Such pattern recognition is not a short cut but, rather, an essential skill that all clinicians use – it is predicated on having seen a large number of patients over many years.

It is useful here to consider an approach to ruling in or out various diagnoses that veterinarians frequently use during the clinical reasoning process. The approach is known by the acronym DAMN-IT (Osborne 1983, 2005, 2010):

- **Degenerative** or developmental
- **Anomalous** or autoimmune
- **Metabolic**, mechanical or mental
- **Nutritional** or neoplastic
- **Inflammatory**, infectious, ischemic, immune-mediated, inherited, iatrogenic, idiopathic
- **Traumatic** or toxic.

Potentially helpful at various points throughout the consultation, this approach to clinical reasoning and diagnosis influences the veterinarian's thought process and can serve to remind veterinarians of information they may still need to gather using the communication skills and strategies described throughout this chapter. Note that the DAMN-IT approach does not take the place of communication skills and strategies such as appropriately used questioning techniques, the content gathered through sign analysis or physical examination, exploration of client perspectives, effective use of summary, etc.

How do the different clinical reasoning approaches influence the process of information gathering?

All of the different approaches to clinical reasoning described above necessitate clinicians starting the process of problem solving early on as the interview proceeds. At first sight, this might suggest that clinicians employing such techniques should move more quickly to closed questioning as they test out hypotheses, schema and recognized patterns, thereby narrowing the field of potential diagnoses.

In fact, the opposite is true. All of these approaches are critically dependent on adopting the same approach to the process of information gathering that we have described earlier in this chapter. The potential danger of all the approaches is starting down a path of clinical reasoning prematurely. Early closed questioning can quickly lead to the exploration of one particular avenue that may well prove inappropriate and lead inexorably to a dead-end. The clinician may have to start again and generate a different problem-solving strategy: inefficient and inaccurate information gathering ensues. Consider here also how any of these clinical reasoning patterns may be affected when the initial problem list and history are collected by someone other than the veterinarian. Or when information is gathered from multiple people, often at different times and in different places.

All of these approaches to clinical reasoning in fact depend on a clear and careful questioning and listening phase through which clinicians can obtain enough of the picture first so that eventually they can apply the right schema or increase the chance of recognizing the right pattern and ruling various diagnoses in or out accurately. Wise use of the process skills of screening, open questioning, attentive listening and discovering the client's/patient's narrative in the opening minutes of the interview allow clinicians more time to generate their problem-solving strategies and provide clinicians with more information on which to base their theories and hypotheses. Here we see how perceptual, content and process skills in communication are inextricably linked and cannot be considered in isolation.

What is the relationship between clinical reasoning, clinical communication and medical problem solving?

It is helpful here to revisit the Clinical Method Map in Chapter 1 and then consider the interdependence of clinical reasoning and clinical communication as they impact medical problem solving (Kurtz 2016):

- *Clinical reasoning* involves the thought processes you engage in as you collect information and opinions from various sources (e.g. the patient, the client and others, physical examination, diagnostic tests, other veterinary staff and professionals, the medical record, etc.) and synthesize that information with your knowledge and experience to generate hypotheses, differentials, diagnoses and action/treatment plans – these perceptual skills occur at the intrapersonal level of communication (i.e. communication within the self).
- *Clinical communication skills and capacities* are what you employ to initiate interactions with those involved; develop the relationships with clients and their significant others, patients, referring veterinarians and other colleagues, nurses/ technicians, allied health professionals, etc. that are necessary to engage in effective (i.e. accurate, efficient, supportive) interactions; gather information from others accurately and efficiently; structure your interactions so all participants can engage in them at optimal levels; give explanations and participate in planning and decision making; close interactions; and follow up appropriately with those involved – communication content and process skills play major roles here, along with perceptual skills related to feelings, attitudes, values, biases, intentions and capacities.
- *Medical problem solving* is what you get when you have well developed clinical reasoning and clinical communication skills and capacities and are adept at integrating all of them.

Said another way, the evidence-based process and content skills that are important in clinical communication have the potential to influence clinical reasoning significantly. Conversely, clinical reasoning has a considerable influence on the particular process and content skills used during interactions.

Summary

In this chapter, we have looked at both the theory and the practice of gathering information. We have explored the content of information gathering and discussed the strengths and limitations of the more traditional method of history taking. We have examined the need for an integrated clinical method that takes into account both the clinician's and the client's perspectives of the problem being discussed. We have also examined the process of information gathering and demonstrated that accurate and efficient information gathering is not achieved simply by examining the patient and interrogating the client but, rather, that it requires the more effective initial techniques of using open questions and listening. And we have looked at the additional skills needed to explore the client's perspective.

Before moving on to the physical examination or to the explanation and planning phase of the interview, the veterinarian needs to think through the skills outlined in the Gathering Information section of the Calgary–Cambridge Guide and to consider: "Have I explored the biomedical aspects of the patient's problems or issues effectively? Have I explored the client's perspective and understood the meaning of the problems or issues from the client's point of view? Have I discovered the background information? Have I ensured that the information gathered is accurate and appropriately complete? Have I confirmed that I have understood the story correctly? Have I continued to develop a supportive relationship and collaborative environment?"

CHAPTER 4

Providing structure to the interview

In this chapter, we explore the communication skills that veterinarians can employ to structure the consultation to the benefit of veterinarian, client and patient. Providing structure is one of two tasks of the interview that we intentionally show in the Calgary–Cambridge Guides as continuous threads throughout the interview rather than as part of a sequential pattern. Providing structure, like relationship building, is a task that occurs throughout the interview. It is essential for the five sequential tasks to be achieved effectively.

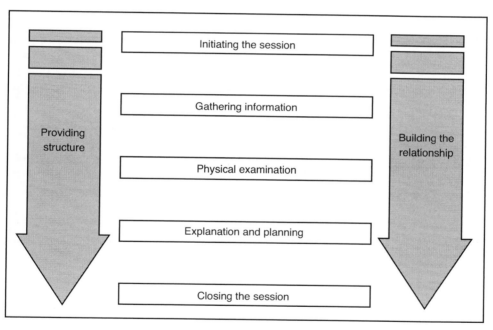

FIGURE 4.1 The basic framework

The consultation is not an aimless or chance meeting, a social chat between two equal friends. It is a highly choreographed discussion between a professional and a client in which both parties often behave in certain stereotypical patterns according to tacit traditions, rules and customs. The interview proceeds along set pathways that both parties may be subliminally aware of but rarely openly discuss.

How is the structure of the meeting determined? Although veterinarians can all recall interviews with clients in which they have felt completely out of control, the almost invariable pattern is that it is the professional who sets the parameters of the consultation and determines the structure of the interaction. The greater degree of power implicitly rests with the veterinarians – they can determine the time available for discussion, move the interview to new areas at whim, decide how many topics can be discussed today and terminate the interaction when they wish. Clinicians exert considerable control over the consultation. Their behavior imposes limits on another person's freedom whether they like it or not (Pilnick and Dingwall 2011).

Power of course leads to responsibilities. What are our responsibilities in directing the consultation? What do we want to achieve in structuring the consultation? The traditional approach to structure is via a series of closed questions in which the client is a mainly passive contributor to the consultation. In this book, we have taken a client/patient-centered or relationship-centered approach to the interview and the skills that we have identified promote a more collaborative partnership between client and veterinarian. This is not because of our own subjective opinion but because in most circumstances the skills that enable this approach have been shown in both practice and research to produce better outcomes for patients, clients *and* veterinarians.

The concept of a collaborative partnership implies a more equal relationship between client and veterinarian. However, as veterinarians control the shape of the interview, this shift in power will only occur if veterinarians structure the interview appropriately – it will not happen on its own. Veterinarians in effect determine the level of contribution of the client, their degree of involvement in the direction that the interview takes and the balance between veterinary-centeredness and relationship-centeredness (Coe 2008; Nogueira Borden et al. 2010; Robins et al. 2011; Shaw et al. 2004b; Shaw et al. 2006; Kanji et al. 2012; McArthur and Fitzgerald 2013).

An awareness of structure at all times throughout the interview provides the veterinarian with appropriate influence on the overall parameters of the encounter and of their working day. Used appropriately it also enables the client to become more involved in the consultation and to take part in a more balanced relationship.

Objectives

The task of providing structure involves the following objectives:

- Enabling a flexible but ordered interview
- Helping the client to understand and be overtly involved in where the consultation is going and why
- Encouraging the client to be part of the structuring process
- Encouraging client participation and collaboration
- Enabling accurate information gathering and giving
- Using time efficiently.

These objectives encompass some of the tasks and checkpoints mentioned in other well-known guides to the consultation: *see* Appendix C.

Skills

In his comments on structuring the interview, Cassata (1978) emphasizes the importance of two-way communication in every part of the consultation and in particular stresses the importance of making expectations and agendas overt at the very beginning of the interview. This encourages participation, ownership and collaboration on the part of everyone present. In Chapter 2, we explored how the following three skills can facilitate this collaborative approach and at the same time lead to more efficient consultations:

1. problem identification
2. screening and confirming
3. agenda setting.

Here we concentrate on four additional skills that are relevant throughout the interview and enable us to work with the client to orchestrate an overtly structured consultation:

Box 4.1 Additional structuring skills that are relevant throughout the interview

---

Making organization overt
- **internal summarizing:** summarizes at the end of a specific line of inquiry to confirm understanding before moving on to the next section
- **signposting:** progresses from one section to another using transitional statements, including rationale for next section; uses categorization and other forms of signposting.

Attending to flow
- **sequencing:** structures consultation in logical sequence
- **timing:** attends to timing and keeping interview on task.

What to teach and learn about providing structure: the evidence for the skills

Making organization overt

How can we help clients understand the structure of the interview and become more involved in the consultation? The key here is to make the organization overt. Robins et al. (2011) explore the concept of transparency in human medicine, of clear signaling to the patient about the process as well as the content of the interview, so that not only the physician but also the patient understands where the interview is going and why. They clarify how physicians providing statements about what they are working on or signaling that they are making a transition promotes relationship building, reduces uncertainty for the patient and enables a more collaborative consultation. Transparency involves making the organization of the interview overt to the other person throughout the interview. Robins et al. (2011) demonstrate in their study that physicians spent little time using such process-related transparency and in particular did not orient the patient to the progress of their interviews. In a Canadian veterinary study of 300 visits to 50 veterinarians (150 each of wellness and problem visits), the mean number of orientation statements (e.g. *"I would like to examine him now"*) was 11 in both wellness and problem visits, with a range of 0 to 60 (Shaw et al. 2008). These statements comprised 6% of the visit. In their Australian study, McArthur and Fitzgerald (2013) found that veterinarians used a mean of 17 orientations (range 2 to 51) and a mean of 14 transitions (range 2 to 47). The two veterinary studies show that veterinarians, like physicians, use orienting statements but with considerable variability across visits.

Summarizing
What is summarizing?
Summarizing is the deliberate step of providing an explicit verbal summary to the client. There are two kinds of summary:

- internal summary which focuses on a specific part of the interaction
- end summary which concisely pulls together the entire interaction.

We explore end summary in more detail in Chapter 7.

Why is internal summary a key skill in structuring the consultation?
In Chapter 3, we explored the role of internal summary as one of the most important of the information-gathering skills. Here we discuss its equally vital role in structuring the interview. Understanding how to structure a consultation via agenda setting, summarizing and signposting is a key area in communication skill teaching.

   Traditionally veterinarians have imposed structure on the consultation via closed questions which, as we have explained earlier, keep veterinarians "in control" at the expense of rendering the client passive. But, as we have seen, this approach can be highly inefficient, can lead to inaccuracy in obtaining quality information, and can feel unsupportive to the client. But if staying open and using attentive listening is so effective, why do we shy away from it? Perhaps it is because:

- it can feel like we have lost control of the consultation
- we worry we will not need or be able to remember all that we are being told
- information flows out in a less ordered form – we seem to be receiving a cloud of unprocessed information that is not in an order that we can easily assimilate
- we worry that the client will talk too long and about irrelevant issues or topics.

These are very genuine concerns – there is no doubt that open methods do seem to produce a less ordered consultation. However, there is a way out of this difficulty: *structuring the consultation via summary and signposting* provides an alternative method for the veterinarian to obtain order and appropriate control without sacrificing the benefits of openness.

Summarizing as a structuring tool allows you to:

- pull together and review what you have heard so far
- order the information into a coherent pattern
- realize what information you still need to obtain or clarify
- gain space to consider where the consultation should go next
- separate and consider both veterinarian's and client's perspectives.

Learners grappling with the techniques of open questions and attentive listening find summarizing especially useful – when unsure of what to ask next or what the client has already said, summarize and play for time! The very act of summarizing and the client's response will normally establish the most appropriate path forward without embarrassment or apparent loss of momentum.

Veterinarian: *"OK, she calved three days ago on her own; however, she has not had a great appetite. So, you have been drenching her with 4 ounces of glycol twice a day. And she is off her feed now."*
Client: *"Yeah and I could really use a boost in milk right now."*

or

Veterinarian: *"So you want to vaccinate the herd and make sure we evaluate the three new foals because you think that they are having more severe diarrhea than what makes sense for foal heat."*
Client: *"Yes, that's right. My neighbors just lost two foals at this age and I am really nervous about what is going on with ours. Thank you."*

What is the evidence for the value of summarizing in the consultation?

Here we present the evidence for the value of summarizing to both "gathering information" and "providing structure to the interview." We have identified five research papers that validate the importance of summarizing.

In their study of veterinarians and dairy farmers, Derks et al (2013) reported that veterinarians seldom summarize important points made during explanation and planning.

Cox et al. (1981a) demonstrated that checking by repetition led parents of children referred to a child psychiatric clinic to be more voluble.

Maguire et al. (1996) showed that summarizing is one of several skills (along with the use of open questions, focusing on and clarifying psychological aspects, empathic statements and making educated guesses) that facilitate cancer patients to disclose more of their significant concerns.

Takemura et al. (2007) found significant positive relationships between three particular interview behaviors and the amount of information obtained in family medicine interviews: the open-to-closed cone, facilitation, and summarization.

Quilligan and Silverman (2012) sounded a cautionary note that summary may not always be beneficial and is perhaps more complex than previously described. In a qualitative study with simulated patients, the use of summary did appear to improve accuracy in the consultation. However, if summary was not carefully introduced, inaccurate summaries could make the patient question whether or not they had been heard. Also, the overuse of summary, particularly when summarizing very small segments of the interaction, could lead the patient to question whether they had been clear, and potentially damage the rapport between patient and doctor. Summary therefore needs to be used flexibly to suit the client.

Despite limited direct research on summary in clinical settings in human and veterinary medicine, there is impressive theoretical evidence from the discipline of communication to underpin the value of summarizing. In Chapter 1, we describe five principles that characterize effective communication. One of these principles is that *effective communication is a helical rather than a linear process – reiteration and repetition are essential.* Summary is an efficient way to build this principle into information gathering and explanation and planning.

A second and related principle is that *effective communication ensures an interaction rather than a direct transmission process.* Just imparting information or just listening is not enough: giving and receiving feedback about how the receiver interprets what the sender is saying or doing and the impact of the message becomes crucial. Sender and receiver are interdependent. Establishing mutually understood common ground requires full participation from both (Dance and Larson 1972). Summarizing is the key skill in the information-gathering and structuring phases of the interview that enables this principle to be put into practice; it provides intentional feedback to the client about what you think you have heard when listening to their story. At the same time, it gives clients opportunity to add details they may have forgotten to say and to correct anything you may have misinterpreted or misunderstood. As we shall see later, additional skills are required in the explanation and planning phase to ensure a similar degree of interaction.

Let's look further at these critical pieces of theory in the context of history taking. Without feedback from the veterinarian, how does the client know whether they have made themselves understood? You might say that nonverbal cues are being transmitted by the veterinarian in attentive listening that allow the client to know that the veterinarian is concentrating on and interested in their story and has understood their message. But this is an assumption. We cannot assume that exemplary listening by itself leads to correct understanding – communication is complicated and many misinterpretations are possible. The key question to ask yourself as a veterinarian is: "How do I know that what I have understood from the client is an accurate representation of what they wanted to tell me?" From the client's perspective, the question becomes: "I know that the veterinarian seems to be listening but how do I know that they have understood me?" How do both client and veterinarian know that they have established mutually understood common ground?

There are many possible sources of distortion in communication as any message is sent between two parties. Consider a client giving their story to a veterinarian. Possible distortion can occur at the following points:

- what the client says might be ambiguous
- the client uses jargon with which the veterinarian is not familiar and the veterinarian does not check out their understanding
- the client may have simply forgotten to say something
- the client may have misunderstood the veterinarian's question
- having already told their story to one member of the veterinary team, the client may assume this new individual already knows it
- the client may have been led off topic and have never returned to complete the unfinished comment
- the client may have inadvertently made a verbal mistake that distorts their meaning
- the client may give a nonverbal cue such as a laugh which suggests something unintended to the veterinarian
- the client may have said exactly what they meant but distortion occurred in the circumstances of transmission of the message (e.g. a noisy barn prevents the veterinarian hearing fully what was said)
- the client may have an agenda that is not being addressed by the veterinarian and therefore may attempt to modify how they answer questions to bring in that agenda
- the veterinarian hears the correct message but misinterprets what was meant
- the veterinarian understands what was meant but makes an incorrect assumption about what lay behind the message
- the veterinarian may have personal biases and prejudices which affect accuracy (e.g. based on gender or race or age of the client, the veterinarian's medical training, the location of the interview, or previous experience with the client).

All these distortions can lead to inaccurate history taking. The only way to be sure that the message has been formulated properly, received correctly and interpreted and understood is through feedback. In the veterinarian–client interaction, it is unlikely that the client will feel confident enough to ask us to demonstrate our understanding of their story! Unless we as veterinarians take responsibility by giving feedback via summary as the interview proceeds, we will leave the client uncertain as to whether they have been understood and we ourselves will be unsure that we have obtained an accurate account. Importantly, all these distortions can also lead to inaccuracy and misunderstanding during the explanation and planning phase, especially if you switch the placement of "veterinarian" and "client" in each item listed above.

Signposting and making transitions
What is signposting?
Signposting is a statement that introduces and highlights or draws attention to what you are about to say. For example, you might say: *"Listen carefully, this is important,"* or *"It's really important to find out where Nanook might be getting food other than his food bowl, so please think carefully with me."* It can also serve to categorize information so that people will pay more attention or can remember something more readily. For example: *"There are three things you need remember. First ..., second ..., third ...."*

> Veterinarian: *"You mentioned two areas there that are obviously important, first the redness you have noticed in Tuffy's right ear and second his behavior around your grandkids. Let's think about these one at a time. First, let me take a look at his ear and ask you a few more questions about it. … Now let's talk about Tuffy's behavior around your grandkids …"*

It is helpful to use a signposting statement to introduce your first summary rather than just launching into it. This not only announces what you are going to do but also invites clients to think with you, to add in forgotten areas or correct your interpretation if you got something wrong. For example:

> Veterinarian: *"There is a lot going on here. Can I summarize to make sure I have it all straight in my mind before we go on and to check that we haven't missed anything?"*

Then the interactive process can continue, as the client says:

> Client: *"No, not quite, you missed the part about him getting into the trash two days ago. Oh, and I forgot to tell you that …."*

Like the other structuring skills, these various examples of signposting can be useful at any point in the consultation and will likely appear multiple times. It is one of a constellation of skills that help you and the client stay oriented throughout the interaction so that you can think together more effectively.

What are transitional statements?

Transitional statements can be thought of as a particular kind of signpost. These statements draw attention to the fact that the consultation is moving from one topic to another (e.g. from questions about diet to questions about activity) or from one section to another (e.g. from gathering information to explanation and planning). Transitional statements help to do two things:

- progress from one section or topic to another
- provide the rationale for the next section or question.

> Veterinarian: *"It is urgent that we take a look at Jester so we can gauge the extent of his injuries. I want to make sure we have enough information to make good decisions for you and him so let me ask you just a few questions about what happened and then I'll take a good look at his injuries."*

Use transitional statements so that:

- the client understands where the interview is going and why
- you can share your thoughts and needs with the client
- you can ask permission
- the consultation is structured overtly for you both.

Possible places to use transitional statements during consultation include when moving:

- from the introduction into the gathering-information stage
- from open to closed questions
- into specific questions about the client's ideas, concerns or expectations
- into different parts of the history
- into the physical examination
- into explanation and planning
- into closing.

Signposting, transitional statements and summarizing take on another role when you are talking to multiple people – often at different times – who are responsible for the care of the animal or the herd. They help to draw attention or alert each individual to what has been or will be communicated to other people. For example, each person may need to be oriented to where you are in the information-gathering or giving process.

> *"When your mother brought Max in yesterday we agreed that he needs to get more exercise and change his diet so he can lose some weight. Can you think of any ways that you might be able to help?"*
>
> or
>
> *"I've already talked with the farm's nutritionist about what you are feeding. Now I'd like your input about the feeding schedule and how the animals are faring."*

Here again, summarizing and signposting (including transitional statements) together provide an overt structure apparent to each of the people – each of them can then understand more accurately and collaborate more appropriately with you and with each other. This is so much better than structuring via the use of closed questions where the clients are left in the dark about the process of the consultation.

Another of the five principles of effective communication we discuss in Chapter 1 is *reducing unnecessary uncertainty*. Unresolved uncertainties can lead to lack of concentration or anxiety which in turn can block effective communication. By knowing where the interview is going and why, much possible uncertainty and anxiety is reduced. This will let the client concentrate on what is going on in the interview without worrying that one of their main concerns might not be addressed. When multiple people are involved, this will help to clarify what you need from each of them and how they can better work with each other.

Levinson et al. (1997) showed that primary care physicians who used more signposting, which was described in this study as orientating statements, were less likely to have suffered malpractice claims.

Summarizing and signposting together therefore:

- are key skills promoting a collaborative and interactive interview
- make the structure overt and understood to the client
- allow you and the client to know where you are going and why
- allow the client to add information that they haven't yet told you
- allow you to signal a change in direction
- establish mutually understood common ground and reduce uncertainty for the client.

Signposting, transitional statements and summarizing are equally important during the explanation and planning, and closing phases of the interview. In Chapters 6 and 7, we discuss how to use these skills in these contexts and offer additional relevant evidence.

Attending to flow
Sequencing
After agenda setting and negotiation have established an overt and agreed plan for the interview, it is clearly the responsibility of the veterinarian to help carry out the agreed upon agenda and maintain a logical *sequence* that is apparent to the client as the interview unfolds. In a Dutch study analyzing 17 veterinarian–farmer conversations, Jansen (2010) showed that the majority of conversations lacked structure. In a UK study analyzing 48 recorded small animal consultations conducted by 13 small animal veterinarians, Everitt et al. (2013) found that consultations did not occur in a linear fashion but rather jumped around in an iterative fashion. The researchers identified the main reason for this to be the veterinarian responding (more or less immediately) to the client's concerns and agenda whenever the client raised them. As we discussed in Chapter 3, Stivers (1998) identified similar issues with respect to sequencing. For us, the solution goes back to the importance of getting and acknowledging out loud a problem *list* that includes the client's perspectives, and setting an agreed upon agenda during the initiation phase of the interview. This scaffold is the structure upon which the interview will unfold. If the client raises additional concerns or agenda later, agenda setting becomes a multi-step process – rather than simply responding to such items immediately, the veterinarian can acknowledge them as they arise, place those concerns within the existing scaffold or agenda, and return to deal with them efficiently in their appropriate place. In other words, the veterinarian still has responsibility for the structure but at the same time carefully incorporates the client's perspectives. A flexible but ordered approach to organization with clear transitions via signposting from one section of the interview to the

next – or even from one topic to the next – helps both veterinarian and client to be more efficient and accurate during data gathering.

One of the key ways to achieve this is for the veterinarian to have in their head at all times a clear structure to the interview, such as the Calgary–Cambridge content and process guides coupled with the species specific pyramids. The ability to take stock at points throughout the consultation and consider what has and what has not been achieved so far allows the veterinarian to regain control over what might otherwise become a meandering consultation, confusing to veterinarian and client alike. In fact a clear structure paradoxically enables flexibility. Knowing the steps and how to return to them provides you with the confidence to allow the interview free flow: "structure sets you free." All of these structuring processes enhance accuracy and are also likely to contribute to more effective clinical reasoning.

Timing

Another important skill for the veterinarian to use is timing. There is no doubt that time issues are a constant concern in modern medicine and that all veterinarians feel under pressure of time to complete interviews as efficiently as possible. Achieving all the different needs of veterinarian, client and patient is not easy in the time available. However, as we have shown in Chapter 3, patient-centered interviews in human medicine take little extra time compared with more traditional approaches. Shaw et al. (2006) showed that biomedically focused appointments in veterinary medicine were on average 1.5 minutes longer than biolifestyle-social appointments. This finding contradicts the notion that relationship-centered appointments that take into consideration the client's full spectrum of concerns, establishment of rapport and involvement of the client in decision making take too long.

A key skill is being able to manage time effectively in the consultation, to pace the session so that balanced amounts of time are taken over each section of the meeting. This is not just about pacing but also about the perception of time. Thorne et al. (2009) in Canada have explored the issue of time on the human patient's perspective in the cancer care context. They have elegantly shown that despite the omnipresence of time pressure, some clinicians pay considerable attention to the quality of the patient experience and find communication approaches that manipulate and manufacture time to optimal advantage. Patients reported how some physicians were able to utilize the small amount of time available more effectively by being "present" for the patient both verbally and nonverbally, negotiating time by offering future appointments or contact, and manufacturing a sense of time even when time was limited by encouraging questions or creating an impression that they were not rushed.

In a focus group study of veterinarians and pet owners done by Coe et al. (2008), veterinarians indicated that being pressed for time interfered with their ability to explain options for the care of the animal. Coe et al. (2009) found that appointments containing a cost discussion were significantly longer than those without cost. Veterinarians who scheduled appointments every 30 minutes were significantly more likely to have a cost discussion than those who scheduled 15-minute appointments. Shaw et al. (2012a) found that veterinary satisfaction was not related to length of appointment.

Veterinarians frequently question whether there is adequate time in veterinary visits for more information gathering and for client- or relationship-centered care. Shaw et al. (2010) showed that after being trained on skills from the Calgary–Cambridge Guides, veterinarians improved regarding the amount of information gathered and their rapport building. Importantly, veterinarians accomplished this with no increase in length of visit.

So how much time do veterinarians have? In small animal visits where research has been done, the mean length of visit and range, including physical exam in most cases, were as follows:

- 13 minutes (range of 2 to 49 minutes), n=300 – USA (Shaw et al. 2004b)
- 15.12 minutes (range 2 to 63 minutes), n=334 – Canada (Dysart et al. 2011)
- 24 minutes (range 11 to 43), n=48 – USA (Shaw et al. 2010)
- 11 minutes 45 seconds (range 4 to 28), n=48 – UK (Everitt et al. 2013).

Everitt et al. concluded that the standard 10 minutes frequently allotted to veterinary consultations in the UK may be inadequate to address the needs of the veterinary/patient/client consultation. They may well be right.

Summary

In this chapter, we have looked at the skills involved in providing structure to the interview and how they need to be utilized throughout the medical encounter. We have looked at issues of power, control and ordering within the interview and have seen how the veterinarian needs to explicitly consider the structure of the interaction that will take place and make this apparent to the client. We have explored the advantages of developing an overt structure that is clearly signposted and apparent to and agreed with the client, enabling the veterinarian to plan a path through a complex situation and the client to understand and if necessary influence the proposed course of action. We have seen how focusing on structure and making that structure overt benefit both veterinarian and client. The skills of structuring allow veterinarians to order their consultations, clients to feel more comfortable and clear about what will happen next and both parties to move through the consultations with greater confidence.

CHAPTER 5

Building the relationship

An unmistakable theme runs throughout this book: relationship matters. It makes a difference to communication in veterinary medicine, to the people who are involved, to the care of the animals and the outcome of that care. And it makes a difference in teaching and learning.

As shown in Figure 5.1, five tasks of the interview follow a natural sequence as the consultation evolves. In contrast, both building the relationship and providing structure are continuous threads that occur throughout the interview. Building the relationship runs in parallel to the five sequential tasks. It is the cement that binds the consultation together.

Nearly all of the communication skills we advocate in this book with respect to the sequential tasks also contribute to building a solid relationship with the client. However, we deliberately include this all-pervasive task as a separate category and devote a chapter to it here to emphasize its significance and to highlight important relationship-building skills that apply throughout the consultation rather than fitting under just one task heading.

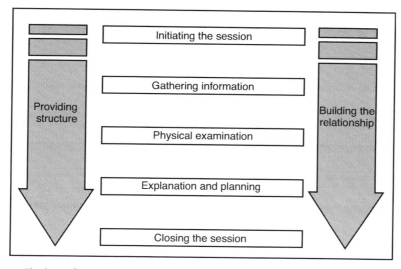

FIGURE 5.1 The basic framework

Building the relationship is a task that is easily taken for granted or forgotten. The sequential components of the interview often dominate as the veterinarian moves through the consultation trying to make sense of the patient's problems or issues and the client's concerns. Yet without paying specific attention to the skills of relationship building, these more "concrete" tasks become much more difficult to achieve. Relationship building in the consultation can be an end in itself – the veterinarian's role is sometimes that of support alone. But in the majority of consultations, relationship building contributes substantively to achieving all the goals of clinical communication that we have outlined in Chapter 1 – namely, accuracy, efficiency and supportiveness, increased satisfaction for both client and veterinarian, promotion of partnership and collaboration. Relationship building enables the client to tell their story and explain their own concerns, it promotes adherence and prevents or reduces misunderstanding and conflict. Ultimately, if indirectly, the relationship between veterinarian and client impacts health outcomes for the animal. Clearly it is important to relate to the animal, too, but the focus of this chapter is on building relationships with people. And, of course, how well you relate to the animal, while important in and of itself, can influence the development of your relationship with the client.

As many veterinary studies demonstrate, forging a relationship with the client is central to the success of every consultation whatever the context.

- Using a survey of 319 small animal clients' expectations, Case (1988) found that client satisfaction was more highly correlated with how the veterinarian interacted with the client than with how the veterinarian treated the animal.
- Stoewen et al. (2014a) found that clients of dogs with life-threatening cancer valued positivity, compassion, empathy, and a non-judgmental stance from veterinarians and staff with whom they have a relationship.
- Shaw et al. (2012a) showed that veterinarians who used communication skills that build relationship with clients, including the use of empathy and greater amounts of conversation, were more satisfied than those who did not. Veterinarians felt more competent and their satisfaction was higher in well-patient visits. Veterinarian satisfaction in these visits was then significantly correlated with the quality of the veterinary/client/patient relationship and with veterinarian positive talk, self-esteem, lower verbal dominance, and more balanced interaction between veterinarian and client. In problem visits veterinarian satisfaction was associated with more rapport building, greater client social discussion, fewer client negative statements and greater client cooperation. In this study the most common factors contributing to veterinary visit satisfaction were long-term relationships with the client and the number of client visits per year.
- Best (2015) used focus groups to explore equine caretakers' (n=46 across 9 focus groups) expectations of the veterinarian–client relationship and equine veterinarians' (n=25 across 4 focus groups) perceptions of caretakers' expectations of that relationship. Both clients and veterinarians identified communication as a way that their relationship was developed and that a good veterinarian–client relationship was important. Clients perceived that their relationship with the veterinarian appeared to influence the care horses received. Several study participants said they had more tolerance for poor treatment outcomes if they had a strong relationship with their veterinarian.
- In a randomized telephone interview study with 2000 dog and cat owners across the USA, Lue et al. (2008) found that the level of pet care received was strongly

linked to the client–veterinarian bond, which the study measured in terms of: the amount of education provided about pet care, the veterinarian's communication skills, the client's perception that the veterinarian was recommending products and services that the pet needed and that the veterinarian interacted with the patient. Eighty percent of dog owners who said they had a strong bond with their veterinarian said that they always follow their veterinarian's recommendations, compared to 48% of dog owners who said they had a weak relationship with their veterinarian.

- Based on an online survey measuring veterinary visit practice trends, Volk et al. (2011b) found that 34% of respondents said their number of patient visits had increased in the preceding 2 years and that there was a significant association between an increase in the number of patient visits and clients seeing the same veterinarian in every visit. The researchers deduced that a strong veterinary–client bond contributed substantially to practice growth.
- Shaw et al. (2012b) found that female veterinarians were more relationship-centered than males and that female veterinarians' rapport-building statements (e.g. expressions of empathy, partnership, concern, reassurance and self-disclosure) strengthened their relationships with clients.
- Kanji et al. (2012) found that clients who adhered to a dentistry recommendation, surgery recommendation or both were more satisfied with the consultations and also the consultations had higher scores for relationship-centered care than those interactions leading to non-adherence.
- Similarly in human medicine, attention to relationship building offers the potential prize of patients who are more satisfied with their physicians and physicians who feel less frustrated and more satisfied in their work (Levinson et al. 1993).
- Commentators on large animal veterinary medicine underscore the importance of relationship in this setting. For example, Kleen (2011) indicates that one type of communication in veterinary advisory practice is the development of personal relationship, including discussion with the client of personal matters like needs and wishes, and that this is the foundation for mutual understanding and respect.

Clients wish their veterinarians to be competent and knowledgeable but they also need to be able to relate to their veterinarian, to feel understood and to be supported. Attention to relationship building offers the potential prize of clients who are more satisfied with their veterinarian and veterinarians who feel less frustrated and more satisfied in their work. In a cross-sectional, descriptive study of 200 video-recorded veterinarian–client–pet interactions, Coe (2008) showed that interactions that scored higher for relationship-centered communication versus veterinarian-centered communication resulted in significantly higher client satisfaction immediately following the visit. This study also found that clients with an established veterinary–client relationship were significantly more satisfied than clients who sometimes saw the same veterinarian or were seeing the veterinarian for the first time.

The relationship between veterinarian and client can be short term in nature, for example in some emergency practice settings. Here developing rapport is still of vital importance – it enables the client to feel comfortable in discussing problems with an unfamiliar person and to benefit fully from the consultation. Yet similar to findings in human medicine (Barnett 2001), the veterinarian faces the added difficulty of having to accomplish the task of relationship building in a short period of time and often in the face of considerable complexity, concern and anxiety.

Building the relationship is also the entry point to a longer term view of medical practice than we have considered so far. In many circumstances, the relationship between veterinarian and client extends beyond a single interview into a continuing association over many meetings. There is a need to maintain a reliable, trusting relationship over time. Many veterinarians see the development of relationships over several years as a rewarding aspect of their work.

Relationship-building skills are increasingly important not only in the context of veterinarian–client consultations but also between veterinary care providers themselves. In her book reporting on a series of studies which show the power of relationships to achieve high performance in the airline industry, Gittell (2003) includes a chapter that discusses a large study (Gittell et al. 2000) she and her colleagues conducted comparing the efficiency and outcomes of nine hospitals (located in Boston, New York and Dallas) with respect to joint replacement surgery. Some of these hospitals invested heavily in hiring and subsequent training for "relational competence," that is, the ability to interact with others to accomplish common goals. Others looked instead for the most highly qualified individuals: the tendency in this group of hospitals to neglect relational competence was most pronounced in physician hiring. This study found significant differences between hospitals in the strength of relational coordination demonstrated by their care providers. Relational coordination is defined as the coordination of work through relationships of shared goals, shared knowledge and mutual respect. Higher relational coordination significantly improved the patient care process. In a later publication summarizing that study, Gittell (2003, p. 48) reported that a 100% increase in relational coordination enabled a 31% reduction in the length of hospital stay, a 22% increase in the quality of service patients perceived, a 7% increase in postoperative freedom from pain and a 5% increase in postoperative mobility. As Gittell et al. (2000) concluded, those in positions that require high levels of functional expertise also tend to need high levels of relational competence to integrate their work with others. A participant in their study put it this way: "We've moved from patients experiencing individuals as caregivers to patients experiencing systems as caregivers. … It's not just individual brilliance that matters anymore. It's a coordinated effort."

Relational competence is necessary to achieve what Gittell and her colleagues call relational coordination (Gittell et al. 2000; Gittell 2009). Applying relational coordination to interpersonal relationships, teamwork and the functioning of organizations, Gittell and others have used this model worldwide to improve outcomes of healthcare, productivity, economic viability, workplace satisfaction, etc. Relational coordination is comprised of the seven elements in Box 5.1 (Gittell 2009). These elements are essential in all veterinary contexts involving relationships between people, whether we apply the elements to our work with individual clients, producers and their employees, our own practice teams and interprofessional interactions, or to our work with students, interns and residents.

Box 5.1 Definition of relational coordination

The coordination of work through relationships of :
- shared goals
- shared knowledge
- mutual respect.

Communication that is:
- frequent
- timely
- accurate
- geared toward problem solving.

Veterinary researchers are beginning to look at the link between communication, relationships and outcomes in veterinary medicine.

- McDermott et al. (2015) used a questionnaire looking at the importance of communication skills to aspects of veterinarians' personal and practice success. The results showed that 88.2% of respondents assigned a score of 5/5 to the importance of communication skills for client relationships and 64.3% assigned 5/5 to the importance of communication skills for colleague relationships (where 1 = not at all important and 5 = extremely important).
- Moore et al. (2014) conducted a study of 48 veterinary clinics (274 team members) regarding the role of veterinary team effectiveness. The four factors of team effectiveness that she measured were coordinated team environment, toxic team environment, team engagement, and individual engagement. They found that coordinated team environment – i.e. team members communicating about their work (conversations, written policies, newsletters), having an opportunity to provide input in challenging situations, and recognizing individual contributions – was associated with decreased cynicism, less burnout, greater job satisfaction and increased professional efficacy.
- In a commentary on interprofessional practice, Kinnison et al. (2014) also highlight the importance of teams in veterinary practice, noting that understanding how to work collaboratively and interprofessionally with others on the veterinary team improves team performance and, ultimately, outcomes for patient, client and veterinarian.
- Jansen and Lam (2012) call our attention to another aspect of relational coordination. Reporting on a series of studies of mastitis control programs in the Netherlands, Jansen and Lam conclude that the prevention of complex disease requires customized communication strategies as well as integrated communication between stakeholders and different scientific disciplines.
- In a study exploring the effect of toxic attitudes and environment on the veterinary healthcare team, Moore et al. (2015) found that a toxic environment contributed

to broken communication and tension between staff members. A theme reflected in all veterinarian and veterinary technician focus groups was that in the absence of good communication everything else fell apart.

- Moore (pers. comm. 2016) assessed the relationship between relational coordination and job satisfaction, intent to stay on the job, and burnout in small animal veterinary practice. Preliminary findings showed that relational coordination was positively correlated with job satisfaction, intent to stay on the job and professional efficacy, and negatively correlated with exhaustion and cynicism for all employment categories. For this study, Moore and her colleagues drew on work done in human medicine (Gittell et al. 2000; Gittell et al. 2008a and b; Bae and Fried 2010; Carmeli and Gittell 2010).

- Best (2015) concludes her study of the communication expectations of equine referral veterinarians and specialists by saying that a focus on relational coordination may improve the outcomes for equine patients, clients and veterinary care providers by focusing on all dimensions of relational coordination, noted in Box 5.1.

So in healthcare relationship-building skills, relational competence and relational coordination are important to patient–physician and veterinarian–client–patient consultations per se and also to relationships between team members in both human and veterinary medicine. Whether it be with clients or co-workers, we agree with Gittell that relational competence is necessary to realize the potential contributions of individual experts.

This chapter focuses on building the relationship between veterinarian and client in the veterinary consultation. The skills we present here are also relevant to building relationships throughout the broader contexts of veterinary heathcare, for example with co-workers or anyone else responsible for the care or health of the animal(s).

The paragraphs above give support to relationship-centered care. Drawn from the biopsychosocial paradigm and akin to patient-centered medicine, relationship-centered care has been concerned with bringing a personalized, partnership-oriented approach to medical care (Suchman et al. 2002). As discussed in Chapter 1, it is an approach to healthcare and healing that places relationship at the core of the therapeutic process. Initially developed in human medicine, this way of conceptualizing the consultation and the broader context of healthcare helps focus attention on the very basic need for relationships between patients, physicians, family members, other caregivers, their health care organizations and their communities (Tresolini and the Pew-Fetzer Task Force 1994; Beach and Inui 2006). It recognizes that clinician–patient communication and relationship take place within organizational contexts and are therefore influenced not only by the needs and skills of the individuals but also by the values expressed in the organization's policies and processes and by the way people within the organization treat each other and are treated (Suchman 2001).

This resonates with the work of Towell et al. (2010). Their cross-sectional study of 1430 US referring and 98 teaching hospital veterinarians regarding discharge communication practices, timely information exchange, and attitudes toward nutritional product recommendations underscores the importance of forming relationships beyond the client. The study shows significant communication gaps between referring and specialist veterinarians. Findings suggest that inadequate information exchange between these veterinarians runs the risk of impairing the diagnostic process, leading to additional patient visits or redundant testing, dissatisfied clients and a loss of confidence in the profession. In an American focus group study of equine referring veterinarians' expectations of equine specialists, Best (2015) found that communication and a relationship between the referring veterinarian and the specialist was essential and likely to support positive outcomes for all involved which includes clients and patients. Suchman and his colleagues' recent book on leading change in healthcare offers excellent, in-depth explanations of relationship-centered care and relationship-centered administration along with several detailed case studies demonstrating how to apply these paradigms to promote change and enhance healthcare in a variety of settings (Suchman et al. 2011). As Aita et al. (2005) showed, individual physicians function within personal and professional value systems as well as within practice systems.

The skills and concepts we discuss throughout this chapter, along with those related to relationship building that are specific to the sequential tasks of the consultation, offer the means for veterinarians to enhance their relational competence and their ability to engage in relationship-centered care. Again referring to Gittel's (2000) work: "The first step is to become a caring person – the second step is to find ways to communicate this caring on an everyday basis as well as in times of extreme crisis."

Sluyter (2004), a past officer of the Fetzer Institute and editor of a book on emotional intelligence, adds further insight to this discussion by adding the notion of personal capacity, which may be innate but can be developed. Sluyter suggests that "… it is really necessary to have both the capacity, which can perhaps be developed through personal development and personal growth processes, and the skills to communicate that capacity to others, which is more of a skills training issue and which would probably be taught differently." He offers the following example: "a person could be very loving and forgiving (capacities) but not very good at loving and forgiving. That is, they may lack the skills to put [the capacity] into practice." We find it appealing to think of compassion or caring as capacities rather than as attributes or qualities – somehow capacity suggests more room for growth and development.

Problems in building the relationship

From the very earliest research into medical communication, relationship problems have featured highly as predictors of poor outcome. In Korsch et al.'s (1968) seminal study of 800 visits to a pediatric walk-in outpatients in Los Angeles, physician lack of warmth and friendliness was one of the most important variables related to poor levels of patient satisfaction and compliance. Another variable that was important was failing to discover and acknowledge the parents' expectations for the visit.

In a UK study of 125 dairy farmers and 132 farm veterinarians using on-farm audio recordings, interviews and a questionnaire, Hall and Wapenaar (2012) found a difference between how the veterinarian defined their role and what the farmer thought the veterinarian's role should be. While 66% of veterinarians preferred a "friend of the farmer" approach for communicating with the farmers, only 33% of farmers preferred this approach.

Morse et al. (2008) found that physicians missed 90% of the opportunities to express empathy in a study in cancer care. Empathy seems to be similarly underutilized in veterinary medicine. In a cross-sectional Canadian study of 300 veterinary–client–patient interactions, veterinarians made empathic statements in 7% of the appointments (Shaw et al. 2004b). In an Australian study of 64 visits, McArthur and Fitzgerald (2013) found that veterinarians expressed empathy less than once per appointment.

In a study of Finnish production animal veterinarians and veterinary students in preclinical and clinical years, Norring et al. (2014) found that respondents' empathy toward animals was greater than their empathy toward humans. Although respondents' empathy scores toward humans and animals and their scoring of patients' pain associated with conditions (e.g. broken bone) or procedures (e.g. disbudding) were all positively correlated, when respondents had higher human empathy scores there was a significant increase in respondents' scoring of patients' pain.

A Malaysian study of 440 veterinary students showed that the majority of students' empathy scores regarding humans were high, but that regardless of their empathy scores the majority of students had poor attitudes toward animal welfare – averaged across all four years, 75% were anti-animal welfare and 25% were pro (Azahar et al. 2014).

In a national randomized mail survey in Canada, Hewson et al. (2007) reported that veterinarians who assumed that owners were unwilling to pay were less likely to perceive dehorning as painful. Their unchecked assumptions led veterinarians in this study to rationalize non-use of analgesics. This despite unequivocal evidence that dehorning calves without pain management causes significant distress.

In a British study, Paul and Podberscek (2000) found that veterinary students in their later years of study rated dogs, cats and cows as having lower levels of sentience than these same students in their early years. Females maintained relatively higher levels of emotional empathy with animals throughout their training, while males' levels declined in their later years of study.

A qualitative Canadian study based on interviews with 44 veterinary clients done 10 days post death of their pets, and 3, 6, and 12 months later revealed that veterinarians' approaches to dealing with the client often resulted in the client feeling confused, inadequate and frustrated (Adams et al. 1999). Limited support was offered. Instead the message conveyed to the clients was that they should be able to cope.

A more recent study shows both progress and ongoing difficulties in this area. In an 18-month ethnographic study of veterinary practices in two US teaching hospitals and an emergency practice, Morris (2012) showed that veterinarians had a growing commitment to recognize clients' emotions. Although veterinarians have often considered dealing with emotion to be outside of their professional responsibility, the research revealed that many veterinarians are rethinking this position. She found that some veterinarians were caring for the emotional needs of clients well while others were not. Some were making empathic statements appropriately, inviting clients to talk about their feelings, and touching a shoulder or offering a hug. However, others "tightly managed" emotion such as grief or guilt by medicalizing or ignoring, disregarding or avoiding the emotion or by reinterpreting, redirecting or rationalizing it.

Commentators have linked the relative lack of development regarding veterinarians' relationship-building skills with what veterinarians in training are often taught about remaining objective. This happens in human medicine, too. As we have seen in Chapter 3, the traditional clinical method is based on scientific reasoning and values emotional detachment. Students are brought up in the world of scientific objectivity and technology. They do need to learn to protect themselves from the negative emotions associated with certain aspects of veterinary practice where feelings are painful for both client and veterinarian. Impassive objectivity is sometimes seen as a strength, a coping mechanism. All of these aspects of veterinary medicine *are* important. On the other hand in this milieu relationship-building skills can easily be compromised.

A. Suchman and P. Williamson. (pers. comm. 2003) offer further insights in their commentary on how human medical schools impact the development of students' relationship skills:

> Students of medicine learn first and foremost from what they see and experience, rather than from what's written in the syllabus. If they witness respectful and collaborative interactions; if they experience listening, empathy, and support; and if they see difference approached with curious inquiry and dialogue rather than conflict and domination, then these interactions will frame their expectations for the nature of relationships in medicine. But if instead they see powerful figures in medicine routinely entering into non-healing or even negative relationships with one another and their patients; if they see their mentors emphasizing the importance of expert technical knowledge above all else, especially above knowledge of self and other; and if they experience hazing or humiliation as standard techniques of medical pedagogy, then they will develop a very different template for their lifelong practice.

Pollard-Williams et al. (2014) conducted a study in Australia surveying 150 veterinary students that focused on the influence of workplace learning (i.e. learning that occurs in veterinary placements outside the classroom). Their findings indicated that empathy for animals declines between the first and fifth years and that specific factors relating to workplace learning negatively influenced the students' beliefs on animal welfare. The researchers recommend taking a closer look at workplace placements to better understand the changes in students' empathy for animals.

Although this is not a book about veterinary medical education, we wonder if this discussion of relationship, empathy and emotion presents an opportunity to open the discussion about the ways that we teach students to deal with some of the more emotionally laden aspects of veterinary practice such as euthanasia, animal handling and mortality in food animal and equine facilities. Are we taking advantage of the opportunities these situations offer to deal with students' emotional reactions, to learn how to channel their own strong emotions effectively, to use their newfound understanding as they learn to respond more effectively in emotional situations with clients or colleagues, even to challenge practices that apparently do not meet high standards of care? As educators and clinicians are we modeling effective emotional support as students encounter these situations and experience emotional reactions to them?

Two studies regarding veterinarians' or veterinary teams' perceptions of "difficult clients" shed light on another potential problem that can impact our effectiveness in building relationships and communicating with clients. In a study of a major veterinary hospital in New England involving semi-structured interviews with 9 veterinarians, 24 technicians, and administrative personnel, Sanders (1994b) found that "problematic veterinary clients" were defined as ignorant (failing to exercise control over their pet or to warn veterinarians of aggression, having ambivalent feelings toward their animal), inattentive and demanding (inattentive or so talkative veterinarians had to interrupt to get a word in), neglectful (not taking care of their pet), over-involved (emotional or "animal nuts" who took extra time and unnecessary attention) or cost focused (more concerned about cost than welfare of animal). In an interview study of 17 small, large, mixed and equine veterinarians done 20 years later, Owens (2015) found that veterinarians identified the following people as "difficult:" those who seek care long after their animals become sick, request euthanasia of healthy animals for a behavioral problem, are "pathologically" attached to their animals, or hear only what they want to hear regardless of the veterinarian doing everything they could to get points across.

These studies remind us of potentially harmful ways in which we categorize people. How we think about and "label" the client (perceptual) can interfere with our ability to relate to and communicate effectively (process and possibly content) with that client. We may think in terms of a particular individual being a "difficult client" that in turn colours our relationship and interaction with that client. As part of their "In the Eye of the Beholder" module, the Institute for Healthcare Communication, Veterinary Communication Project (2004) underscored this problem and offered a solution for it. They showed 12 vignettes of supposedly "difficult clients" to groups of veterinarians and asked them to rank order the vignettes in terms of how difficult each vignette was for them. There was a great deal of variability between veterinarians in terms of what they found to be "difficult" or "not so difficult." It is not the client that is "difficult" but the situation or the relationship and the way that we react to it. Changing our perspective from "difficult clients" to "situations (or relationships) that I find difficult" enhances our ability to work together and communicate more effectively in such situations.

Objectives

The objectives that we seek to accomplish in building the relationship with the client can be summarized as:

- developing rapport to enable the client to feel understood, valued and supported
- establishing trust between veterinarian and client, laying down the foundation for a professional relationship

- encouraging an environment that maximizes accurate and efficient initiation, information gathering, and explanation and planning
- enabling the provision of support as an end in itself
- developing and maintaining a continuing relationship over time
- involving clients so that they understand and are comfortable with participating fully in the process of the consultation
- reducing potential conflict between veterinarian and client
- increasing both the veterinarian's and the client's satisfaction with the consultation.

These objectives encompass many of the tasks and checkpoints mentioned in other well-known guides to the consultation – *see* Appendix C.

Skills

> ### Box 5.2 Building the relationship
>
> **Using appropriate nonverbal communication**
> - **Demonstrates appropriate nonverbal behavior**
>   — eye contact, facial expression
>   — posture, position and movement
>   — vocal cues, e.g. rate, volume, intonation
> - **Use of notes:** if reads, writes notes or uses computer, does so in a manner that does not interfere with dialogue or rapport
> - **Picks up client's nonverbal cues** (body language, speech, facial expression, affect); checks them out and acknowledges as appropriate.
>
> **Developing rapport**
> - **Acceptance:** accepts legitimacy of client's views and feelings; **is not judgmental**
> - **Empathy:** uses empathy to communicate understanding and appreciation of the client's feelings or predicament; overtly acknowledges client's views and feelings
> - **Support:** expresses concern, understanding, willingness to help; acknowledges coping efforts; offers partnership
> - **Sensitivity:** deals sensitively with embarrassing and disturbing topics, animal pain, and animal behavior, including when associated with physical examination.
>
> **Involving the client**
> - **Sharing of thoughts:** shares thinking with client to encourage client's involvement (e.g. *"What I'm thinking now is … "*)
> - **Provides rationale:** explains rationale for questions or parts of physical examination that could appear to be non-sequiturs
> - **Examination:** explains physical examination while performing it, including why; asks permission.

Many of the skills related to building the relationship pertain to animals. For example, as Radford et al. (2006) point out, it is important to acknowledge and alert the animal to your presence, to approach and handle the animal sensitively, and to relate to the animal, taking into account the relationship between client and animal.

What to teach and learn about building the relationship: the evidence for the skills

Next we examine in detail the individual skills for building the relationship that are listed in Box 5.2 and explore the evidence from theory and research that validates their use in the consultation.

Using appropriate nonverbal communication

Nonverbal communication is of major importance throughout the veterinary consultation. Clinicians need to pay as much attention to the effect of their non-verbal interaction with clients and patients as they do to the impact of their words (Friedman 1979; Hall et al. 1995; Roter et al. 2006; Shaw et al. 2008; Kanji et al. 2012).

In veterinary medicine we need to recognize clients' and animals' vocal cues, facial expression or eye behavior, affect and body posture. But we also need to be aware of our own nonverbal behavior, since how we use eye contact, body position and posture, movement, facial expression and vocal cues can all influence the success of the consultation (MacDonald 2009; McArthur and Fitzgerald 2013). Box 5.3 describes the variety of behaviors and cues that contribute to human nonverbal communication (Mehrabian 1972; Gazda et al. 1995). Many of these items also relate to the nonverbal behavior of animals.

Box 5.3 What do we mean by nonverbal communication?

- **Posture:** sitting, standing, erect, relaxed
- **Proximity:** use of space, physical distance between and positioning of communicators
- **Touch:** handshake, pat, touch on the shoulder
- **Body movements:** hand and arm gestures, fidgeting, nodding, foot and leg movements
- **Facial expression:** raised eyebrows, frown, smiles, crying
- **Eye behavior:** eye contact, gaze, stares
- **Vocal cues:** pitch, rate, volume, rhythm, silence, pause, intonation, speech errors
- **Use of time:** early, late, on time, overtime, rushed, slow to respond
- **Physical presence:** race, gender, body shape, clothing, grooming
- **Environmental cues:** location, furniture placement, lighting, temperature, color.

The difference between verbal and nonverbal communication

What are the differences between verbal and nonverbal communication? (Verderber and Verderber 1980):

- Verbal communication is discrete with clear endpoints – we know when the message has come to an end. In contrast, nonverbal communication is continuous – it goes on for as long as the communicators are in each other's presence. We cannot stop communicating nonverbally (Watzlawick et al. 1967): even when people are together in silence, the atmosphere is filled with messages. The difference between comfortable and uncomfortable silence is mediated by our nonverbal communication.
- Verbal communication generally occurs in a single mode, either auditory (spoken) or visual (written), whereas nonverbal communication can occur in several modes at once. We can send and receive all the nonverbal cues listed in Box 5.3 simultaneously; all of our senses can be receiving signals at once even if we are not consciously aware of all of them.
- Verbal communication is mostly under voluntary control whereas nonverbal communication operates at the edge of or beyond our conscious awareness. Nonverbal communication can be amenable to deliberate control: for instance we use nonverbal cues from voice, body, head and eye movement deliberately to help coordinate the taking of turns in conversation. However, nonverbal communication also operates at a less conscious level. Our nonverbal communication may be "leaking" spontaneous cues to the receiver that we are not even aware of and may be providing a better representation of our true feelings than our more considered verbal comments. DiMatteo et al. (1980) have shown that this is particularly true for body posture and movement.
- Verbal messages are more effective in communicating discrete pieces of information and in conveying our intellectual ideas and thoughts. In contrast, nonverbal communication is the channel most responsible for communicating our attitudes, emotions and affect, for conveying the way we present ourselves and how we relate. Considerably more information about liking, responsiveness and dominance is provided by nonverbal than verbal means. Nonverbal communication plays an increasingly important role when someone is unable or unwilling to explicitly express feelings verbally, for example when cultural taboos dictate against disagreeing with a superior or where words are inadequate to describe love or grief or pain (Ekman et al. 1972; Mehrabian 1972; Argyle 1975).

Why understanding nonverbal communication can make a difference in the consultation

Nonverbal communication can work to accent, qualify, regulate, take the place of or contradict verbal communication. In most circumstances, verbal and nonverbal communication work together to reinforce one another. Nonverbal cues enable verbal messages to be delivered more accurately and efficiently by strengthening the verbal message. For example, after the veterinarian has summarized and asked *"Have I got that right?"* the client says *"Yes, that's exactly right"* and smiles, leans forward and uses an animated voice; or as the client talks of her fears about her dog's surgery, she looks down, talks more slowly and plays with her fingers.

When we are deprived of accompanying nonverbal confirmation, our verbal conversation is more liable to misunderstanding. We have all encountered problems communicating over the telephone where we are denied so many nonverbal cues.

We can intentionally use nonverbal communication to reduce uncertainty and misunderstanding in our verbal communication. *"Are you happy with that plan?"* accompanied by eye contact, hands opened out and an inquiring facial expression will indicate your genuine interest. Alternatively, the same phrase accompanied by a closure of the notes, hands banged on the table and a quick look at the client and then away all suggests that you don't want to know if the answer is no.

As we can see from the last example, the two channels can also work to contradict each other. Communication research has shown that when the two are inconsistent or contradictory, nonverbal messages tend to override verbal messages (Koch 1971; McCroskey et al. 1971). If the verbal statement is *"Tell me about what's going on with Rex"* while your nonverbal cues are speaking quickly and looking agitated, the client will make the correct interpretation that time is at a premium today. If the veterinarian says there is nothing to worry about but hesitates in their speech as they deliver this verbal message, the client will assume that perhaps there is some concern and that information is being withheld. However, this generalization about contradictory messages may apply only to normal adults. Young children and emotionally disturbed adults or adolescents tend to believe the verbal message when faced with contradictions or inconsistencies (Reilly and Muzarkara 1978).

A further use of nonverbal behavior relates to the reinforcement theory of social interaction (Mehrabian and Ksionsky 1974) and to nonverbal synchrony (DeVito 1988). People tend to act in ways which reinforce their general expectations. People also tend to mirror or imitate each other's nonverbal behavior – to move or talk in synchronization – as a gesture of affiliation. Veterinarians can use these concepts to advantage, first by anticipating a positive experience and second by modeling relaxed attentive listening skills. Unconscious mirroring and reinforcement of this behavior by clients will enable them also to relax and become more attentive. We can affect others positively through our behavior. On the other hand, if we act disinterested, our nonverbal behavior will be picked up by the client and communication can deteriorate.

What is the research evidence that nonverbal communication makes a difference to the consultation?

As described throughout this book, a number of studies in veterinary medicine highlight nonverbal cues and behaviors as major factors influencing what veterinarians and clients hear and the sense they make of things as well as client and veterinarian satisfaction and even client adherence. Aspects of interaction where nonverbal behavior or cues are an important part of the communication include attentiveness, interest, respect, friendliness, warmth, responsiveness, engagement, non-anxious presence, anxiety and nervousness, distress, irritation and anger, assertiveness or dominance, emotional tone, empathy, confidence. Here we add additional literature demonstrating how nonverbal cues and behaviors make a difference.

Building on the work of Sullivan (1953), Winnicott (1986), Bowen (1985) and Friedman (1985), Strand (2006) describes three factors of non-anxious presence that veterinarians need to develop in order to enhance veterinary communication skills and practice effective veterinary medicine. Nonverbal cues and behaviors play a role in each of the factors:

- the *diagnostic mind* – that part of the veterinarian that pays attention to diagnosing what the other person (client, colleague or team member) is experiencing, i.e. understanding the internal experience of another person through exploration of the other's verbal and nonverbal cues
- the *interpersonal mind* – that part of the veterinarian that pays attention to what he or she is saying both verbally and nonverbally
- the *self-aware/self-monitoring mind* – that part of the veterinarian that pays attention to what he or she is experiencing internally, in the moment while interacting with another person, so as to be able to respond to both self and the other.

Shaw et al. (2008) found that veterinarians were significantly more hurried and rushed during problem appointments than during wellness appointments. Nonverbal behaviors that indicated being rushed included rapid pace of speech, less pause, and less space between taking turns.

In a study on client adherence to dentistry and surgery recommendations, Kanji et al. (2012) showed that veterinarians' use of laughter as well as positive rapport-building statements, such as approval, compliments and agreement, played a role in client adherence.

McArthur and Fitzgerald (2013) found that the veterinarian's tone of voice made a difference regarding clients' ratings of their own satisfaction and perceptions of their veterinarian's relational communication. These ratings were higher when the veterinarian's tone of voice demonstrated warmth. Based on this and other results of their study, the researchers concluded that a focus on nonverbal communication in veterinary medical education may enhance the veterinary–client relationship and outcomes.

MacMartin et al. (2014) found that when animals signaled distress or discomfort using vocalizations, veterinarians responded. Animals' nonverbal signals included the vocal channel (e.g. growling, hissing, crying), physical movement (e.g. leaping off the table, flinching, ear flicking, jerking of head or body, twitching, trembling, non-voiced snarling, freezing), changes in posture (e.g. crouching), and gaze changes (e.g. shifting gaze away from the veterinarian). Veterinarians responded to these non-verbal cues with verbal empathy, for example, by saying "*I know*" and adding "*relax*," "*hang on*," or "*shshshsh*." This happened frequently. The researchers suggested that the veterinarian's pet-directed talk also potentially played a role in ameliorating the negative effect of the animal's distress on the veterinary–client relationship.

In a qualitative study of the communication expectations of veterinary clients accessing oncology care for their dogs, Stoewen et al. (2014a) showed that clients screen their service providers (specialists, technicians, etc.) in an effort to look for subtle cues that indicate the seriousness of the situation. They report that service providers must focus on their nonverbal behavior and consider its effect on clients.

Several studies on nonverbal communication in human medicine have potentially useful implications for veterinarians. Harrigan et al. (1985) have demonstrated that physicians who face their patents directly, have more eye contact and maintain open arm postures are regarded as more empathic, interested and warm.

Larsen and Smith (1981) have demonstrated in family medicine that nonverbal immediacy, defined in terms of touch,[11] closer distance, leaning forward, body orientation and gaze, is related to patient satisfaction as well as patient understanding.

Hall et al. (1981) used the technique of filtered speech to separate verbal messages from vocal cues. In electronically manipulated recordings, vocal expression could be heard but not the content of words. The researchers showed that patients and physicians in a family and community health clinic reciprocated their emotions in their voice quality. If one party appeared satisfied or angry or anxious, so did the other. This reciprocation was far more apparent in filtered speech than in non-filtered speech or written transcripts. The researchers inferred that much of the affective communication actively responded to in the interaction takes place via nonverbal cues.

Haskard et al. (2008) also used filtered speech and found that affect in physicians' voices was correlated with patients' satisfaction, perceptions of choice/control, medication adherence, mental and physical health, and with physicians' satisfaction.

Hall et al. (1987) demonstrated that physicians in primary care who were high information givers were also rated highly on their voice tone by independent observers: they were more interested, more anxious and less bored. In contrast, physicians who gave less information spent more time in pleasantries and had voices that were perceived as bored or calm. Again, the researchers conclude that anxiety in the physician's voice is perceived as anxious regard. DiMatteo et al. (1980, 1986) have shown that internal medicine residents and family practice residents who tested highly on objective laboratory tests of their ability to communicate emotion through their faces and voices ("encoding") had patients who were more satisfied with their medical care and, interestingly, more patients on their lists! Physicians who tested highly on their ability to recognize the meanings of patients' nonverbal cues ("decoding") had more satisfied patients who were better at keeping their appointments!

Ambady et al. (2002) have shown a relationship between judgments of surgeons' voice tone and their malpractice claims history. Surgeons were audiotaped while speaking to their patients during office visits, and very brief samples of the conversations were rated by coders blind to surgeons' claims status. Two 10-second clips were extracted for each surgeon from the first and last minute of their interactions with two different patients. Controlling for content, ratings of higher dominance and lower concern/anxiety in their voice tones significantly identified surgeons with previous claims compared with those who had no claims. This study underscores the potency of vocal cues in medical interactions.

Unfortunately, there is still evidence that physicians respond to increased patient participation with nonverbal blocking behaviors, like breaking eye contact as patients begin to talk (Zandbelt et al. 2007).

In a simulation study in a US teaching hospital where patients observed a pre-recorded simulated consultation involving disclosure of error, Hannawa (2012)

---

11   As in human medicine, the way we touch clients in veterinary medicine or whether to touch at all is an important judgment call.

demonstrated that physicians' nonverbal behaviors had a significant impact above and beyond what physicians *said*. Physicians' nonverbal behavior impacted patients' ratings of trust, closeness, empathy, forgiveness, avoidance, distress, and satisfaction.

Swayden et al. (2012) showed that something as simple as sitting rather than standing has a positive impact. In a prospective, randomized, controlled study of inpatients admitted for spinal surgery, Swayden and colleagues found that patients whose providers sat during brief postoperative consultations perceived that the provider was present at the bedside longer than when the provider stood. This was the case even though the actual time the physician spent at the bedside did not change significantly. Patients with whom the physician sat reported a more positive interaction and a better understanding of their condition. In some veterinary contexts it would seem impractical to sit, but we wonder if it might be useful to move some parts of the consultation to places where veterinarians and clients can sit down. Alternatively, might there be a way to mimic sitting? For example, kneeling down to be at the animal's level, leaning on a fence or the back of a truck, etc. In places where veterinarians can influence the layout, consider planning the exam room with enough benches, chairs and rolling stools to accommodate everyone.

What then are the lessons for veterinarians?
Reading the nonverbal cues of clients

Being able to "decode" nonverbal cues is essential if we wish to understand our clients' feelings and perspectives. The cultural norms of the veterinary setting militate against clients' expressing their feelings verbally – clients may be reluctant to express their thoughts or feelings openly, but instead use indirect or tacit messages. Nonverbal cues may therefore be one of the few indicators to the veterinarian of a client's desire to contribute their own thoughts or concerns about a problem.

Picking up on nonverbal cues helps the veterinarian begin to understand the client's perspective and the impact of the patient's problems on the client. However, just because spontaneous cues representing true feelings are being sent does not mean that you can interpret those cues accurately simply by noticing them – there are many sources of possible distortion and misunderstanding inherent in receiving nonverbal messages. To ensure accurate interpretation of *nonverbal* behavior, it is important not only to observe carefully but also to verify our perceptions *verbally*. Your interpretations and assumptions about what the client's nonverbal cues mean may or may not be right – they need to be checked out with the client. Checking your assumptions encourages clients to talk further about what they are thinking or feeling and has a double payoff – both veterinarian and client avoid possible misinterpretation and discover more information.

The skills of picking up nonverbal cues and checking them out verbally (*"You seem unsure – would you like to tell me what you're thinking?"*) are described in Chapter 3.

Transmitting your own nonverbal cues

Similarly, without attention to your own nonverbal communication skills and the messages that you are transmitting through the nonverbal channel ("encoding"), many of your other efforts to communicate may be undone. If your verbal and nonverbal signals are contradictory, at the very least you risk confusion or misinterpretation, and at worst your nonverbal message will win out. Nonverbal skills signaled through eye contact, posture, position, movement, facial expression, timing and voice can assist in demonstrating attentiveness to the client and facilitate the formation of a helping relationship; ineffective attending behavior in contrast closes off the interaction and prohibits relationship building (Gazda et al. 1995). Again, the disparity in power and control between client and veterinarian leads clients to be particularly attentive to nonverbal cues regarding veterinarians' attitudes and meanings. Clients rarely ask for verbal confirmation of cues that they pick up and commonly base their impressions primarily on nonverbal messages.

Use of notes and computers

One of the most important of all nonverbal skills is eye contact. Yet so often, veterinarians lose eye contact when they refer to the patient's written or computer record during the consultation while the client is speaking. In a qualitative study in British general practice, Heath (1984) examined the consequences of physicians attempting to read the patient's records and listen to the patient at the same time. She demonstrated how instead of increasing efficiency, quite the opposite occurs:

- patients withhold their initial reply to the physician's solicitation until eye contact is given
- patients pause in mid-utterance when the physician looks at the notes and resume when eye contact is regained
- patients use body movement to catch the physician's gaze if the physician is reading the notes while the patient is talking
- patients' fluency deteriorates as the physician looks away and recovers on reestablishment of gaze
- physicians frequently miss or forget information given to them while they are reading their notes.

Similarly in veterinary contexts, eye contact allows the client to infer that the veterinarian is prepared to participate and listen. In the absence of eye contact, the client makes nonverbal efforts to encourage the veterinarian to realign their gaze and there is a reduction in quality and quantity of information provided. Heath's study concludes that using records while the patient is speaking is not an efficient way to conduct the consultation for either patient or physician. The patient will give their information more slowly and less completely and the physician may well not "hear" the information provided. Heath suggests various strategies to overcome the common problem of needing to both hear the patient's story and examine their records:

- deliberately postpone using the records until the patient has completed their opening statement
- wait for opportune moments before looking at the notes
- separate listening from note reading by signposting both your intention to look at the records and when you have finished, so that the patient understands the process.

These findings have been replicated more recently by Robinson (1998) and Ruusuvuori (2001). Ruusuvuori also showed that gaze withdrawal is more disruptive at critical moments when human patients are describing points of particular importance to them. Eye contact is not necessary throughout the interview (and, indeed, veterinarians do need to look at their notes at times) but at certain points in the client's storytelling, eye contact is critical.

Perhaps the most important lesson for veterinarians to grasp is the skill of structuring the consultation into separate elements, with a deliberate attempt to start the interview by giving full attention to the client and patient and then explaining to the client when attention has to be given to records. In this way, a happy medium can be reached where the veterinarian has both the skills to communicate well with the client and is also able to manage the consultation in such a way as to refer to the records when appropriate and record the necessary data. The same counsel could apply to trying to get a history and perform physical examination at the same time. If you are looking at, or otherwise focusing attention on, the animal rather than the client, that is likely to negatively impact the effectiveness of communication between you and the client.

Veterinarians are using computers as an adjunct to handwritten records and in many situations computers have replaced written notes entirely. Although veterinarians often wait until the end of the appointment to update their records, increasingly they are using computers during the consultation. Even more care with regard to eye contact and body positioning needs to be taken to consult effectively while using a computer (Greatbatch et al. 1993; Als 1997; Makoul et al. 2001; Frankel et al. 2005; McGrath et al. 2007; Pearce et al. 2008; Shachak and Reis 2009; Shachak et al. 2009; Silverman and Kinnersley 2010; Noordman et al. 2010), although many advantages can also ensue (Mitchell and Sullivan 2001; Booth et al. 2002). Communication benefits of using the computer collaboratively in the consultation include:

- sharing information, e.g. digital radiographs, a body condition score chart
- discussing prompts, e.g. *"I see it is time I rechecked your herd's vaccine protocol – shall we also do that today?"*
- recording agreed plans and follow-up.

However, Bensing et al. (2006) observed that communication between Dutch general practitioners during the period 1986 to 2002 had become more task oriented with the physicians less likely to engage in building partnerships with their patients, less likely to express concern for their patients and less likely to provide a structure to the consultation. Bensing and colleagues considered that a likely cause of the deterioration in communication they observed was GPs' increasing use of computers. This is a useful heads-up as the veterinary profession makes more frequent use of computers during consultations.

Duke et al. (2013) have very helpfully reviewed the literature on use of computers within the consulting room. The major strategy that they identified to improve physicians' communication skills while consulting with the electronic health record (EHR) was dividing the encounter into patient- and computer-focused stages that are clearly demarcated from one another and signaled both verbally and by changes in body language and focus of gaze. Another key strategy was engaging patients by sharing the screen with them or reading out loud while typing. The authors of this article modified "ten tips" for physicians on how to incorporate the computer into consultations as originally suggested by Ventres et al. (2006) and have also formulated a model to help clinicians, residents, and students improve physician–patient communication while using the electronic health record (EHR). This model integrates patient-centered interview skills and aims to empower physicians to remain patient centered while effectively using EHRs.

Developing rapport
Acceptance
In Chapter 3, we looked at the importance of understanding the client's perspective. We examined the need to elicit clients' *thoughts* (their ideas, concerns and expectations) and take note of their *feelings*. But having discovered these thoughts and feelings, what should be our first response? The concept of acceptance as proposed by Briggs and Banahan (1979) is helpful here. It suggests that instead of immediate reassurance, rebuttal or even agreement, our initial response to clients' contributions should be to give an "accepting response."

The accepting response
Also called the "supportive response" or the "acknowledging response" elsewhere in the literature, the accepting response provides a practical and specific way of:

- accepting nonjudgmentally what the client says
- acknowledging the legitimacy of the client to hold their own views and feelings
- valuing the client's contributions.

The accepting response acknowledges and accepts both the client and the client's emotions or thoughts wherever and whatever they are. Note that acceptance here does not mean that you necessarily agree with the client but rather that you hear and acknowledge the patient's emotion or point of view. This approach is effective in relationship building because it establishes common ground between veterinarian and client through a shared understanding of the client's perspective. Acceptance is at the root of trust and trust is the bedrock of successful relationships (Briggs and Banahan 1979; Gibb 1961).

Accepting clients' ideas and emotions without initial judgment may not be easy – especially if they do not accord with your own perceptions. However, by acknowledging and valuing the client's point of view rather than countering immediately with your own ideas, you set the stage for understanding and enhance your relationship. The key concept here is acknowledging the client's rights to hold their own views and feelings. It helps for clients to understand that not only is it reasonable for them to have thoughts and emotions about their animal's problems but also it is important to you as a veterinarian for these to be expressed so that you can be aware of and appreciate the client's perspective and needs.

In their qualitative study done in Finland, Steihaug et al. (2012) showed that recognizing a human patient's perspectives through skills similar to those of the accepting response may also help to reduce potential conflict and make it easier to tolerate disagreement when, for example, patients have values and perspectives that conflict with the physician's or with sound medical practice. Based on the work of Schibbye (1993), Stiehaug et al. (2012) usefully called these skills and behaviors "recognizing interactions" or a "recognizing attitude."

Functions of the accepting response

The accepting response has three valuable functions:

1. to respond supportively to the client's expression of feelings or thoughts
2. to act as a facilitative response to obtain a better understanding of these thoughts and feelings
3. to value the client and their ideas even when their feelings or concerns seem unjustified or perhaps even wrong.

Skills of the accepting response

The following set of skills can be used in the sequence shown to signal acceptance to the client. In this example, the client has expressed his thoughts by saying, *"I think my horse has gastric ulcers and that is causing his weight loss."*

- **Acknowledge the client's thought or feeling by naming, restating or summarizing:** *"You are worried about your horse's weight loss and want to have him evaluated for gastric ulcers."*
- **Acknowledge the client's right to feel or think as they do by using legitimizing comments:** *"The weight loss is concerning. It will be important for us to figure out what is causing it and gastric ulcers are a reasonable concern."*
- **Come to a "full stop":** the use of attentive silence and appropriate nonverbal behavior here makes space for the client to tell you more. *"My farrier and trainer both told me I should have you treat him for gastric ulcers. We had a horse in the barn colic really badly two weeks ago and he had an ulcer."*
- **Avoid the tendency to counter with "yes but …".**

Although not a necessary part of every accepting response, it can also be helpful to:

- **Acknowledge the value of the client expressing their views:** *"Thank you for telling me that – it's very helpful to know your concerns."*

Responding to overt feelings and emotions

In the example just given, we use the accepting response to respond to a client's belief. Acceptance is equally valuable as our initial response to feelings and emotions. For instance consider this accepting response to a bereaved client dealing with the death of her husband saying: *"I am not even sure what I am going to do with all these horses."*

We never got around to talking about the plan of what to do when he was gone. Now I just feel stuck."

Veterinarian: *"You have twelve horses and two new babies on the way and no idea what your husband's wishes were, now you feel stuck. That has to be a difficult set of emotions."*

(Pause – a "full stop" gives the client time/space to go on)

Client: *"I want to honor his love of the horses and keep going with his breeding plan, but it is so hard to keep up with by myself. Sometimes I wish it had been me ..."*
Veterinarian: *"Those are strong emotions to deal with – I'm glad you mentioned them."*

(Pause)

or

Veterinarian: *"You are dealing with a lot right now. I am glad you told me what is going on."*

(Pause)

Responding to indirectly expressed feelings and emotions

The next two examples demonstrate that the accepting response can be useful when the feeling or thought is indirectly expressed, for instance through nonverbal behavior alone. Here we can combine picking up a cue to the client's feelings (as we discussed in Chapter 3) with the accepting response:

Veterinarian: *"I sense that you feel anxious about having to come to see me [the veterinarian is an oncologist], am I right? That's OK, many people feel that way when they first come here ..."*

(Pause/full stop)

or

Veterinarian: *"I can see you're delighted with these test results; I'm glad they're so good too ..."*

(Pause/full stop)

An important part of the accepting response is to come to a *full stop* after giving the initial acknowledgment, to wait briefly and attentively in silence and to avoid saying "yes, but ..." which automatically negates the acceptance. This is almost a knee jerk reaction for most of us. We are so eager to help that instead of waiting we say "yes, but ..." and then quickly go on to give our point of view or correction to erroneous thinking or reassurance before we give the client a chance to feel the acceptance or to say anything further. All of this can come later, perhaps considerably later in the interview, *after* the client has had an opportunity to respond to our statement of acceptance. It is of course imperative that we correct, advise and reassure – the question is when.

What happens if we make a full stop rather than adding the "but ..." clause? Usually clients will respond with a brief outpouring of whatever thought or feeling has been acknowledged, share the burden or exhilaration briefly, and get "back" to being less overwhelmed with the emotion or thought so that they can either talk about it further or go on to focus on other matters.

Acceptance is not agreement

It is important to differentiate acceptance from agreement. Acknowledging that a client would like their horse to have additional hock injections or prefers not to vaccinate their pet is not the same as agreeing to inject or agreeing not to vaccinate. It is a two-stage process. First, identify and acknowledge a client's beliefs without immediately countering. This enables you to understand the client without provoking initial defensiveness. If the clients' thoughts do not fit with your own, later on in the consultation and after due consideration go to the second stage: offer your own perspective and correct misapprehensions.

Contrast the following possible replies to this statement "I think my cat is mad at me – she keeps peeing on my bed when I'm not in the house."

Veterinarian: *"Oh, this happens sometimes with cats. She's not mad at you. What exactly have you noticed?"*

Client: *"Well, three times in the past two weeks, I've come home from work to find she has peed on my bed. I swear she is doing it because she is mad at me for leaving."*

Veterinarian: *"Not to worry, she is not mad at you."*

This approach devalues the importance of the client's views and although most probably correct, the reassurance comes too early in the consultation to be accepted by the client. The client will not be encouraged to propose their own theories in the future.

If instead, we follow the plan we proposed earlier:

Veterinarian: *"So, you're worried her peeing on the bed might be because she is mad at you."*

(Pause/full stop)

Client: *"Yes, she only seems to do it when I'm not home."*

Veterinarian: *"I can appreciate your concern – we'll check her out carefully. Tell me about any changes in routine that have occurred for you or Lily in the past month."*

Here instead of countering the client's view or giving premature or ineffective reassurance, the importance to you of hearing and explicitly acknowledging the client's concerns is emphasized. You can explain and correct misconceptions later. In fact, Donovan et al. (2000) found that the key to reassurance was the physician's ability to acknowledge the patient's perspectives of their difficulties or concerns: patients who felt their problems were acknowledged felt more reassured.

Acceptance is the second stage in the three-stage process of discovering clients' beliefs that we introduced in Chapter 3:

1. **identification** – discover and listen to the client's ideas, concerns and expectations
2. **acceptance** – acknowledge the client's views and their right to hold them, without necessarily agreeing with them; then pause so the client can say more
3. **explanation** – explain your understanding of the problem in relation to the client's understanding and reach mutually understood common ground; this might occur immediately or, if strong emotion is present, later after a cool down period.

Acceptance makes it possible to remain open to the client. It precludes judgmental remarks. It reinforces a tentative frame of mind, prevents premature closure or defensive reactions and instead establishes mutually understood common ground. It is this that ultimately allows for change even if the mutually understood common ground is that we disagree.

The problem of premature reassurance

Acceptance also enables us to avoid the trap of premature or ineffective reassurance. Simple reassurance by itself may not be an effective supportive response (Wasserman et al. 1984). Often reassurance is given before adequate information has been obtained, before clients' concerns have been discovered and before rapport has been developed. Unless we obtain sufficient information first, reassurance may sound false or in fact be inappropriately optimistic. Unless we understand our clients' fears, we may be addressing the wrong concern. Unless we have developed rapport with the client, reassurance may well be interpreted as indifference or as being dismissive. And, lastly, unless appropriate and relevant information is provided to back up our reassurance, people will not understand the basis for our assertions (Kessel 1979). Acceptance prevents premature reassurance – by discovering and accepting the client's concerns, trust is developed and more information can be obtained about the patient's problems and the client's concerns before an opinion is offered. Reassurance when it comes can then be appropriately timed, properly explained and matched to the client's concerns. Schein's (2011) book, entitled *Helping: How to Offer, Give, and Receive Help*, is a useful resource that reinforces the ideas in this paragraph.

Before we have collected further information or ordered tests we may not be in a position to provide reassurance that there is nothing to worry about. But we still have much to offer. We can accept the client's concern and then use reassurance in other more appropriate ways. Instead of offering reassuring about the animal's problem, we can for instance reassure the client about our intent: we can offer our support by demonstrating that we wish to work with the client and that we will give careful attention to their concerns.

Emotional and cognitive empathy

One of the key skills in building relationships with others is the use of empathy (Spiro 1992; Garden 2009). Empathy is a capacity that you continue to develop. Skilled communication is what allows you to demonstrate that empathy to others. In a recent review of the literature, Neumann et al. (2009) go much further by suggesting that clinical empathy is a fundamental determinant of quality in medical care that enables the clinician to fulfill key medical tasks more accurately and thereby leads to enhanced health outcomes. As we have already seen veterinarians may (or may not) direct empathy toward clients and animals (Shaw et al. 2008; McArthur and Fitzgerald 2013; MacMartin et al. 2014).

Goleman (2011), whose work focuses on emotional and social intelligence, calls empathy the essential building block for compassion. His work helps us conceptualize empathy more accurately. Goleman describes three interdependent varieties of empathy, three ways of sensing another person's thoughts and feelings. The first variety is *cognitive empathy*, which is the capacity to understand others' perspectives, to see how others think about things and to know at a cognitive or mental level how they are feeling. Clearly this is an important capacity for veterinarians to develop. However, Goleman also points out a downside: if I do not care about you and have only this kind of empathy, I can use it to manipulate or take advantage of you. So cognitive empathy alone is insufficient. The second variety is *emotional empathy*, which is the capacity to sense how the other person is reacting, to feel with the other, to have an emotional connection. As essential as this kind of empathy is, it too has a downside: I can internalize another's emotion to the point that it overwhelms or leads me to emotional exhaustion and burnout. The antidote here is not to stop feeling emotional empathy but to learn what Goleman calls "emotional self-management skills" which allow you to keep emotional empathy in balance. The third variety is *empathic concern*. This is the capacity not only to understand the other's predicament and to feel with them, but also to spontaneously want to take action to help them.

Of all the skills in the consultation, empathy is the one most often thought by learners to be a matter of personality rather than skill. Certainly, a first step in empathy is the internal motivation and commitment to understand the client's perspective, and this must be present along with appropriate communication skills (Norfolk et al. 2007). Although some of us may naturally be better at demonstrating empathy than others, the skills of empathy can be learned. The challenge is to identify the building blocks of the empathic response and enable learners to integrate the elements of empathy into their natural style so that it appears genuine to both veterinarian and client (Bellet and Maloney 1991; Platt and Keller 1994; Gazda et al. 1995; Coulehan et al. 2001; Buckman 2002; Frankel 2009).

Empathy is a three-stage process:

1. gaining the understanding and sensitive appreciation of another person's predicament or feelings

2. communicating that understanding back to the other person in a supportive way
3. pausing – coming to full stop for a few seconds to let the empathy sink in, to give the other person a chance to say more or just feel your concern, caring and presence.

Again, the key to empathy is not only being sensitive but also overtly demonstrating that sensitivity to the client so that they appreciate your understanding and support. It's not good enough to think empathically – you must show it too. *Demonstrating* empathy in this way overcomes the isolation of the individual in their thoughts and feelings and can be therapeutic for the client in its own right. It also acts as a strong facilitative opening, enabling the client to divulge more of their thoughts and concerns. What then are the building blocks of the empathic response?

Understanding the client's predicament and feelings

Many of the skills that we discuss throughout this book demonstrate to clients that we are genuinely interested in hearing about their thoughts. Together these skills provide an atmosphere that facilitates disclosure and enables the first step of empathy – understanding the client's predicament – to take place:

- welcoming the client warmly
- clarifying the client's agenda and expectations
- attentive listening
- facilitation especially via repetition and paraphrasing of content and feelings
- encouraging the expression of feelings and thoughts
- picking up cues, checking out our interpretations or assumptions
- internal summary
- acceptance
- nonjudgmental response
- use of silence
- encouraging the client to contribute as an equal
- offering choices.

Having set up a climate conducive to client disclosure, the veterinarian has to pick up clients' verbal and nonverbal cues, become aware of their predicament and consider their feelings and emotions. In a descriptive qualitative study of medical interviews in a variety of settings, Suchman et al. (1997) demonstrated that patients seldom verbalized their emotions directly. Instead they offered clues in statements about situations or concerns that might plausibly be associated with an emotion. Physicians needed to pick up these "potential empathic opportunities" by inviting elaboration (a "potential empathic opportunity continuer") in order for the patient to directly express their emotional concern. Only then could the physicians respond by communicating empathy. In many instances that they observed, physicians used "potential empathic opportunity terminators," redirecting the interview with an unrelated biomedical question or comment and thereby preventing the patient's emotion from being voiced. Levinson et al. (2000) similarly found that physicians only responded positively to patient cues in 38% of cases in surgery and 21% in primary care and in the remainder missed the opportunity to respond to the patients' cues and acknowledge their feelings. Morse et al. (2008) in a study of patients with lung cancer and their thoracic surgeons or oncologists found that physicians responded empathically to 10% of empathic opportunities and provided little emotional support, often shifting to biomedical questions and statements. When empathy was provided, 50% of these statements occurred in the last one-third of the encounter, whereas patients' concerns were evenly raised throughout the encounter. Anecdotally in the hundreds of veterinary interviews that we have observed, the expression of empathy seems similarly to come later in the interview. Considering the value of acknowledgment from the standpoint of relationship building, both the infrequency and delay seem particularly unfortunate.

Communicating empathy to the client

The skills outlined above do not complete the second step of empathy, which is communicating your understanding back to the client so that they know that you appreciate and are sensitive to their difficulty. Both nonverbal and verbal skills can help us here.

Empathic nonverbal communication is valuable. Facial expression, proximity, touch, tone of voice or use of silence in response to a client's expression of feelings can clearly signal to the client that you are sensitive to their predicament. But what are the verbal skills that we can use to demonstrate empathy?

Empathic statements are supportive comments that specifically link the "I" of the veterinarian and the "you" of the client. They both name and appreciate the client's affect or predicament (Platt and Keller 1994).

- *"I can tell **you** are very attached to your flock and proud of the progress **you** have made in improving their genetics."*
- *"I can appreciate **you** were not anticipating the costs that have resulted from Rory's accident today."*
- *"I can see that **you** are angry at how things have turned out following Riley's treatment."*
- *"I sense that this is a frustrating situation for **you**."*
- *"It sounds to me like **you** feel that you are completely on your own to make this difficult decision."*
- *"I hear that **you** were planning to get on the fields early today with this nice weather and two DA [displaced abomasum] surgeries was not part of the plan."*

It is not necessary to have shared an experience to empathize, nor to feel yourself that you would find that experience hard. It is necessary, however, to see the problem *from the client's position* and communicate your understanding back to the client. Empathy should not be confused with sympathy which is a feeling of pity or concern from *outside of the client's position*.

Using a nine-item evaluation scale developed by Truax and Carkhuff (1967), Poole and Sanson-Fisher (1979) have clearly shown that empathy is a construct that can be learned. Poole and Sanson-Fisher showed that without specific training medical students' ability to empathize did not improve over their medical school training. Both first and final year students scored poorly on the evaluation scale (av. 2.1). However, after participating in eight 2-hour workshops using audiotapes, students' scale ratings significantly improved to an average level of 4.5. After training, students also:

- used less jargon
- made clear attempts to understand the unique meaning of events, words and symptoms to patients
- blocked off emotional-laden areas less frequently
- obtained descriptions of more of their patients' problem areas
- matched their voice tone to their patients more often
- did less talking
- responded more in an understanding mode
- offered less advice
- were reported by patients to be understanding and caring.

More recently, Hojat et al. (2009) and Newton et al. (2008) found that empathy levels are continuing to decline as students progress through medical school.

Nunes et al. 2011 showed that out of 355 students at a Carribean university who were enrolled in dentistry, pharmacy, nursing, medicine, and veterinary medicine, the pharmacy and veterinary students were found to have the lowest empathy scores on entering their training. All students had lower empathy scores at the end of their first year than at the beginning. In an American study of veterinary students, Schoenfeld-Tacher et al. (2015) found a sharp decline in perspective taking scores between first and second year veterinary students. Empathy scores declined even further during third year.

Bonvicini et al. (2009) have demonstrated that communication training with practicing physicians made a significant difference in physician empathic expression during patient interactions 6 months after the training as demonstrated by outside observer measurements.

Bylund and Makoul (2002) developed a measure of empathic communication in the physician–patient encounter and confirmed that female physicians tend to communicate higher degrees of empathy in response to empathic opportunities created by patients. Shaw et al. (2012b) examined gender differences in veterinary medicine and found that the number of expressions of empathy were greatest between female veterinarians and female clients.

Interestingly, Bylund and Makoul (2005) demonstrated that patients provide empathic opportunities irrespective of familiarity with the clinician and length of relationship.

There has been debate about whether skills-based training and assessment of empathy trivializes the very qualities we are trying to instill by reducing them to surface behaviors, potentially preventing learners from acquiring the habits of mind and sensitivity needed for genuine attempts to understand and relate to patients' or clients' stories. Others believe that surface manifestations of behavioral empathy should be assessed and taught because these are essential skills for the compassionate and effective care of patients and clients. A student who is unable to display these basic communication skills is likely to be deficient in the other, deeper components of empathy as well. Clearly skills-based training should be complemented by other approaches which enhance students' capacities for compassion and authentic presence and enable students to more readily identify with the feelings of others (Stepien and Baernstein 2006; Steele and Hulsman 2008; Wear and Varley 2008; Teherani et al. 2008).

In addition to how we educate medical and veterinary students, what other reasons might account for the repeated finding that providers in human medicine miss 70–90% of opportunities to express empathy (Morse et al. 2008; Bylund and Makoul 2005; Levinson et al. 2000) and in veterinary medicine 59–93% (McArthur and Fitzgerald 2013, Shaw et al. 2004b). Hsu et al. (2012) found that when opportunities arose to respond empathically, clinicians did attempt to respond. However, they did not offer acknowledgment (i.e. explicit empathic support). Instead they tried to solve the underlying problem (i.e. instrumental support). The study found that in human medicine providers "… rarely ignore the patient's cue altogether; rather, they recognize and acknowledge the patient's cue but may fail to respond adequately." Hsu et al. suggest that a better alternative for clinicians would be to recognize the importance of both kinds of support. By offering both problem solving and empathic responses "… providers may build stronger relationships and achieve better health outcomes …."

Others suggest additional reasons for missing opportunities to express empathy in veterinary contexts. Carson (2007) suggests that veterinarians may avoid empathy because once they open the conversation to emotion, they get stuck there right along with their client (what Carson refers to as "synchrony") and then don't know how to move out of that emotion; the consequence can be that by the end of the day they feel emotionally drained and don't want to go there again.

Another frequently heard rationale for avoiding empathy is: "I don't go there because I am not a psychologist; it's not my job." The response to this is that we are not talking about psychological counseling or about having to fix emotions if they come up. We are talking about emotional intelligence, about the ability to pick up on and acknowledge emotions – our own and those that our clients may be feeling. As Adams et al. (1999) found in their study, clients identified veterinarians as the best people to provide support regarding matters pertaining to an animal's end of life but did not expect veterinarians to be counselors. Rather they wanted the opportunity to spend time with their veterinarian; discuss next steps; have their veterinarians answer questions, show sensitivity, reduce embarrassment, and "normalize" their feelings of guilt, grief, or being fine.

A third reason for missing empathic opportunities with clients is that veterinarians may be inclined to direct their empathy toward the animal and in so doing miss seeing the need to direct additional empathy toward the client. In a UK study of 10 videotaped veterinary clinic visits, Roberts (2004) set out to determine the function of utterances directed at or said on behalf of animals in a veterinary setting. She concluded that addressing the animal and speaking for it appeared to be in the service of managing professional relations. She notes that much of the pet-directed talk went to managing professionally delicate interactional moments like critiquing the client's care of the pet, deflating client complaints, or palliating client concerns. She also showed that pet-directed talk was used to begin interacting with the client and manage apologies such as those needed for keeping a client waiting past the originally scheduled appointment time. This study does not comment on whether talking to the animal is more useful than talking directly to the client. However, an Australian study of 64 small animal visits shows that 5% of the talk was directed toward the patient (McArthur and Fitzgerald 2013) and that client satisfaction was not affected regardless of whether the veterinarian did or did not direct an empathy statement toward the animal. Interestingly, veterinarians directed 73% of the empathy statements they made to the animal.

Shaw et al. (2004a) indicate that 8% of the talk across 300 visits was directed toward the patient, including empathic statements.

MacMartin et al. (2014) found that within 284 visits, veterinarians responded to animal distress using pet-directed "I know" statements in 110 of the visits. Patients included dogs, cats, iguanas, a bearded dragon lizard and a snake. The researchers suggest that animal distress or reluctance can elicit anxiety for clients on many levels. The veterinarian's pet-directed "I know" response is a resource for addressing the various reasons for not just the patient's distress but also the client's, for calming the animal as well as alleviating the client's (and, we would add, the veterinarian's) anxiety regarding procedures or the animal's pain. It may indirectly build rapport with the client. Based on this research, veterinarians seem to use "I know" (an empathic response) and reassurance statements directed to the animal so much more frequently than empathic responses to the client that it may behoove us to ask ourselves if we are inadvertently substituting reassurance and pet-directed empathy for client-directed empathy.

Of course, emotional and/or cognitive empathy may not always be necessary. The context and nature of the problem may require more or less empathy regarding the client's thinking and more or less emotional engagement. Again, one size does not fit all (Lussier and Richard 2008).

All of these reasons for not responding to empathic opportunities are justifiable. Yet given the literature related throughout this chapter, avoiding empathy is not the answer. Rather we need to:

- understand that talking about emotion or otherwise making space for a client to express emotion does not mean we need to "fix" that emotion, only that we need to acknowledge it
- keep in mind that two kinds of opportunities for empathy arise in most interviews – cognitive (related to what the client is thinking) and emotional (related to what the client is feeling)
- master the skills of attentive listening, nonverbal facilitation and response, and, perhaps above all, the accepting response, including the highly important pause that is necessary afterwards

- master the skills of verbally structuring the consultation and using appropriate nonverbal skills, so that we can assist the client in moving forward, returning to what else needs to be discussed and done during the interview
- be knowledgeable about and plugged in to the network of community resources in order to be able to refer clients to these services or support groups when the client's needs or difficulties (e.g. severe depression or grief, suicide, abuse etc.) go beyond the help that veterinarians can provide.

Support

Several other supportive approaches contribute to relationship building and the development of rapport (Rogers 1980; Egan 1990). They are often used to complete the empathic response:

concern

"I'm concerned Duke might lick open his stitches and so I would like to send him home wearing an E-collar if possible, to prevent this from happening."

or

"Getting ointments into Trigger's eye three times a day might be challenging when he is not sedated. I am worried that this might not go well for either of you."

understanding

"I can understand this is not the outcome you were hoping for following her surgery."

or

"I understand your time is valuable and we have kept you waiting 30 minutes."

willingness to help

"Please do not hesitate to give me a call if you have questions or if there is anything else I can do."

or

"Although we can't cure the cancer at this point, we can make Luke comfortable during this time. So please call me right away if he appears worse or if you have concerns."

or

"I have some ideas of how we might improve production and cow comfort at the same time if that would be helpful."

partnership

> *"It is going to take both of us working with our teams to get a handle on this outbreak."*
>
> or
>
> *"Let's work together to try different approaches to manage Thunder's back pain."*
>
> or
>
> *"Let's explore some other options to see if we can find something that will work within your budget."*

acknowledging coping efforts

> *"You have done the right thing calling us out and it is clear that you have been doing everything in your power to address the situation."*
>
> or
>
> *"With the amount of experience you have in the industry, I can appreciate how frustrating it must be not to have anything you have tried work."*
>
> or
>
> *"You've really done the right thing by bringing in Lady this morning."*
>
> or
>
> *"I think you have done everything you could have for Marcel despite some very challenging moments."*

sensitivity

> *"I recognize not everyone is comfortable being present when their pet is euthanized. You are welcome to stay and be with Toby or I can come and get you once she is gone."*
>
> or
>
> *"I know the prepurchase examination of the horse did not turn out the way you hoped."*
>
> or
>
> *"I suspect you might feel like your reputation is on the line if we don't get this handled quickly."*

The key point here is that our thoughts and acknowledgments need to be verbalized to be supportive. Communication must be overt to be truly effective and not liable to misinterpretation. Without explicit comment, the client may well not be fully aware of your support.

Pilgrim (2010) conducted a qualitative study in the USA examining veterinarians' perceptions of giving social support to grieving clients. The study showed that veterinarians communicate social support in three ways: 1) emotional support (e.g. acknowledging emotion, telling clients that it was OK to euthanize their pet); 2) informational support (e.g. being clear about the pet's prognosis and outlining recommendations for treatment [or not]); 3) instrumental support (e. g. scheduling euthanasia appointments at quiet times in the practice, encouraging clients to depart the clinic following their pet's euthanasia using a private exit, and conducting home euthanasia when appropriate).

Stoewen (2012) discusses managing uncertainty as an important aspect of support. In a qualitative study of veterinary oncology settings based on 30 audio-recorded and transcribed interviews with 43 dog owners, she unexpectedly found that uncertainty was an overarching psychological feature that dominated clients' experience throughout the course of cancer care for their dog. The diagnosis of the dog's life-threatening cancer shifted clients from stability, orderliness and predictability to ambiguity, unpredictability and ominous probabilities.

Stoewen identified two kinds of uncertainty: relational and informational. Both can be managed through skilled communication. The ongoing relationships that clients develop with service providers is the foremost means to prevent relational uncertainty, not only minimizing relational uncertainty, but also building trust and confidence, which reduces the overall burden of uncertainty. Veterinarians can manage informational uncertainty by determining clients' needs for information, their information preferences, and their perceptions of uncertainty, followed by attending to the quality and structure of the information provided. Stoewen suggests that many animals could benefit from treatment but do not get that treatment or are euthanized as a result of owners receiving inadequate or no information about the possibilities for the care of the animal.

On the other hand, uncertainty per se is not inherently good or bad, depending on the individual's dispositions, beliefs and experiences (Lazarus and Folkman 1984 in Stoewen 2012). Stoewen suggests that uncertainty can sometimes be a coping strategy, a source of hope (*"I know I'm hoping for a miracle but my dog may be the exception"*).

As Stoewen says, this discussion of uncertainty is sure to be relevant not only to cancer care but to many other animal illnesses and conditions. She argues effectively that if veterinarians could better understand the psychology of the illness experience – including how something as supposedly innocuous and pervasive as uncertainty influences clients – and support clients through the design and delivery of services, clients and their animals most certainly would benefit.

Kedrowicz (2015) used a questionnaire to assess clients' satisfaction with veterinary interactions and support during cancer management of their animals. Ninety-four clients completed the survey. Findings revealed that clients needed three kinds of support: problem-focused informational support (e.g. providing information about disease and prognosis that was understandable, answering questions, providing options), problem-focused tangible support (e.g. being accessible and available, referrals to grief counselors, being genuinely interested in the animal, knowing the animal's history), emotion-focused support (e.g. showing compassion, empathy, listening). Clients favored support that empowered them and enhanced their sense of control. The need for emotional support was less prevalent in clients' responses than their need for problem-focused informational or tangible support. Kendrowicz suggested that this could have been because clients do not expect to receive emotional support from veterinarians.

Williamson (in Suchman et al. 2011) has provided the PEARLS acronym to help with remembering the variety of relationship-building statements available to us. Although empathy is listed as an individual statement in this acronym, the discussion of empathy on the preceding pages demonstrates that all of these statements contribute to empathy as well as to relationship building.

- Partnership
- Empathy
- Acknowledgment
- Respect
- Legitimization
- Support.

What is the research evidence that rapport-building skills make a difference to the consultation?

Throughout this chapter we have summarized numerous studies demonstrating how relationship matters. Here we sample additional research regarding the impact of rapport-building skills on the consultation and outcomes of care in human medicine, because this research underscores a number of important lessons. Some of the more provocative findings below stimulate our thinking about relationship building and possibly our veterinary research going forward.

Buller and Buller (1987) described two general styles displayed by physicians in medical interviews. The first, affiliation, was composed of behaviors designed to establish and maintain a positive physician–patient relationship. Many of these behaviors were those discussed in the sections above including friendliness, interest, attentiveness, empathy, nonjudgmental attitude and social orientation. The second style included behaviors that established the physician's power, status, authority and professional distance. Patient satisfaction was found to be significantly higher when physicians in both specialist and family practice adopted the affiliative style.

Hall et al. (1988), in a meta-analysis of 41 independent studies, reported that patient satisfaction was related to the amount of information given by physicians, technical and interpersonal competence, more partnership building, more positive talk, more positive nonverbal behavior and more social conversation. The definitions used to group behaviors together under "partnership building" and "positive talk" include many of the rapport-building skills discussed this chapter.

Wasserman et al. (1984) analyzed the effect of supportive statements made to mothers during pediatric visits. They found that empathic statements led to increased satisfaction and reduction in maternal concerns. Encouragement (such as acknowledging coping efforts and appropriate self-care) led to increased satisfaction and higher opinions of physicians. In contrast, simple reassurance which was the commonest intervention led to no improvements in outcome. This confirms the suggestion that reassurance without understanding the patient's concerns or providing adequate information may be of little value.

In an audiotape study of 461 discussions of weight, Cox et al. (2011) showed that when physicians expressed empathy along with other patient-centered techniques, patients' weight-related attitudes and behaviors improved.

Research evidence points increasingly to the impact of relationship and relationship-building skills on multiple outcomes. This influence may, as Street et al. (2009) suggest, follow an indirect pathway. The skills that contribute to building relationship may for instance enhance trust and accuracy of understanding, which in turn influence client satisfaction and involvement, clinical reasoning, quality decision making and client adherence which then influence patient health and other outcomes. Whether direct or indirect, the influence is unmistakably there. These findings concerning the impact of relationship on health outcomes represent another confirmation of the interdependence of communication content, process and perceptual skills that we discussed in Chapter 1.

Involving the client

One of the principles of effective communication that we presented in Chapter 1 and examined more carefully in this chapter was ***reducing unnecessary uncertainty***. This is not a simple concept. Uncertainty may take the form of ambiguity concerning the state of the illness; unpredictability concerning the course of the illness and prognosis; lack of information about the illness, its treatment and the system of care; complexity or lack of clarity regarding what information exists (Mishel 1981, 1983, 1997 in Stoewen 2012). To this we would add that clients may be uncertain about what to expect during a given interview, about the significance of a line of questioning, about the role of a particular member of the veterinary team, or about the attitudes, intentions or trustworthiness of the other individual. Unresolved uncertainties can lead to lack of concentration, distraction or anxiety that in turn can block effective communication. Therefore one important aspect of building the relationship during the consultation is to employ skills that limit the uncertainty that can so easily block communication and client involvement.

Distractions associated with uncertainty can be particularly evident in emergency situations or settings. Slade et al. (2015) conducted a series of studies on interactions in human medical emergency departments in Australia that offer valuable insights applicable to veterinary emergencies. As Slade et al. point out, in emergency settings urgency is a factor, medical problems can be dire, multiple people are involved, and emotion is at heightened levels. Furthermore, interactions can be rushed with little opportunity given for asking questions, interruptions are common, the consultation may become fragmented, multiple clinicians may be interacting with the patient and others during the same visit, people may have limited understanding and be given little explanation of what is happening. All of these distractions amplify uncertainty and have substantial potential for interfering with communication.

Sharing of thoughts

Throughout this book, we have espoused a system of clinical communication that encourages a collaborative understanding between client and veterinarian. We have seen how important it is for client and veterinarian to understand each other and the steps that we can take to ensure that communication in the consultation is an interaction rather than a one-way transmission. Techniques such as *the use of internal summary* in information gathering and *checking understanding* in information giving not only ensure accuracy but also act as facilitative openings by encouraging a truly interactive process.

Sharing your thinking with the client is another example of encouraging the client's involvement, including their ability to think with you:

> Veterinarian: *"Sometimes it's difficult to work out what causes these ear infections. What I'm thinking is that it may be due to Dooley swimming in the river, as you suggested, or it could be due to a food allergy or some other cause."*

Sharing your thought processes in this way allows the client to understand the reasons for some questions but also acts as a facilitative probe. If you leave a space after the example in the previous box, the client may well add:

> Client: *"Well, we are feeding him a no-name dog food from the grocery store and freeze-dried liver treats we get there as well. Do you think that could be it?"*

This overt approach allows the client insight into the process of the interview, enabling them to understand the drift of your questioning and providing a very open-ended method of eliciting further information.

Let's start the same case over again. The client has brought Dooley in to have you check out what looks to the client like an ear infection. You think through the dilemma internally without saying anything about your thinking to the client and then ask a closed-ended question:

> Veterinarian: *"What kind of food are you feeding him?"*

This closed question would likely give you similar information but would seem like a non-sequitur to the client. As a result the client is less able to be involved in the interaction and unable to think with you since this line of questioning about an ear infection would make little sense because of uncertainty about what lies behind the veterinarian's choice of direction. In this case, the client might even then be thinking with some defensiveness:

> *"We are feeding him no-name dog kibble, but we just can't afford anything more at this time."*

Apart from a few previously presented studies that describe the amount of time spent on orientation and transition statements, we are not aware of research on veterinary–client communication regarding shared thinking. Research from human medicine offers insights. Peräkylä (2002) used conversation analysis to explore the effect of physicians explaining overtly their reasoning for a diagnosis. Patients talked about the diagnosis more often and became more involved than after diagnostic statements in which such explication was not done. Robins et al. (2011) explore the concept of transparency, of clear signaling to the patient about the process as well as the content of the interview, so that not only the physician but also the patient understands where the interview is going and why. They clarify how this promotes relationship building, reduces uncertainty for the patient and enables a more collaborative consultation. They particularly comment about the importance of sharing thinking and providing a meta-commentary to the patient about why the physician is exploring a particular pathway. Robins et al. demonstrate in their study that physicians spent little time using such process-related transparency.

Providing rationale

Explaining the rationale for questions or parts of the physical examination is another specific example of transparency and the principle of reducing uncertainty. Many of our questions and examinations remain a mystery to the client unless explained – why pass a nasogastric tube in a horse that is colicky, why ask about deworming or nutrition in cases where that is not the primary problem, why ask about exposure to plants or toxins?

Providing a rationale resolves the confusion. For example, when taking a history from a client whose dog is coughing, you might ask:

> *"How is he during the night?"*

This appears to the client to make no sense as a line of inquiry. Why is Dr. Jones asking about how is he doing at night? Alternatively, you could so easily have asked:

> *"Do you notice him coughing more at night or when sleeping?"*
>
> followed if necessary by
>
> *"Do you notice his coughing is worse when he is lying down?"*

Similarly, without explaining why we are requesting various tests, especially if they are perceived to be expensive, we may leave the client in confusion and may even lay ourselves open to the suspicion that we are attempting to make extra money.

Summary

In this chapter, we have examined the skills of building the relationship, a task that is central to the success of the consultation. Without attention to both our own and our clients' nonverbal communication, without efforts to develop rapport, without taking pains to involve the client in the process of the consultation, many problems will arise. Not only will our long-term relationships with the clients suffer, but even in the short term our clients will feel less understood and supported, the other tasks of the interview will become much more difficult to achieve and client satisfaction, adherence and follow-through will diminish.

Throughout the interview, it is important to pay specific attention to the skills of relationship building while completing the more sequential tasks of the consultation. By keeping in mind the skills outlined in this section of the Calgary–Cambridge guides, you will be rewarded with higher personal satisfaction as well as a more accurate, efficient and supportive consultation that paves the way for a the development of a trusting and productive long-term relationship.

CHAPTER 6

Explanation and planning

Explanation and planning is the Cinderella subject of communication skills teaching. Many teaching programs concentrate on the first half of the interview and tend to neglect or underplay this vital next stage in the consultation. To some extent, this emphasis is understandable as so many problems in communication arise from the beginning or information-gathering phases of the interview. Also, as we show in this chapter, the successful implementation of explanation and planning skills depends on how effectively you have gathered information and developed relationship before you get to this point in the consultation. Effective explanation and planning needs to be based on information gathered about the patient's problems and also to be framed in terms that take into account the client's perspective, including ideas, concerns and expectations.

Undoubtedly explanation and planning is of utmost importance to successful consultations. There is little point in being able to discover what the client wishes to discuss, in taking a good history and in being highly knowledgeable if you cannot make a joint management plan that the client feels comfortable with, understands and is prepared to adhere to. Making recommendations that the client does not follow through with wastes all our clinical reasoning and diagnostic efforts. And of course, here again you need to decide who the "client" is. For example, as Abood (2008) points out in her commentary on nutritional assessment it is important to find out who actually feeds the animal(s) not only so you can gather the most accurate information but also so that you know who needs to be involved with treatment planning and follow-through. If the first half of the consultation represents the foundations of veterinary medical communication, explanation and planning is the roof.

Problems in clinical communication

Research identifies substantial difficulties in the explanation and planning phase of the interview. In fact, the studies concerning these problems pose worrying questions about the value of much of our everyday activity!

Are there problems with the timing of explanation and planning?

Stivers' (1998) study showed that even in the initiation or early history-taking phases of the consultation, veterinarians started explanation and/or planning whenever clients asked a question. Too easily this amounted to giving information, reassurance or advice prematurely, before we have enough information to do so. Everitt et al. (2013) found that veterinarians responded to the clients' concerns whether those concerns had anything to do with the medical problem at hand or not. This disrupted the flow of the consultation.

Are we building strong enough foundations to support the roof?

- Have we gathered the necessary information to be able to interpret physical examination findings and diagnostic test results before we move into explaining and planning?
- Are we getting enough information about client perspective in the very short amount of time that we spend gathering information, considering how important this information turns out to be for relationship building and effective explanation and planning?

Recall the findings of Shaw et al. (2004a) and McArthur and Fitzgerald (2013) showing that small animal veterinarians spend between 6% and 9% of the consultation gathering information and close to half giving information.

Are there problems with the amount of information that we give?

Takeuchi et al. (2000) evaluated owner compliance and treatment outcomes for 52 dogs with separation anxiety. The study also examined clients' perceptions of the effectiveness of discharge instructions. Dogs with owners who were given more than five discharge instructions were significantly less likely to improve or be cured compared with dogs whose owners were given fewer instructions. The researchers concluded that owners who received many instructions may have been confused or reluctant to comply. Owners who complied were given easy instructions such as "no punishment," increase activity, or special toy for the animal.

In a Canadian study of 218 dairy producers and their veterinarians, Giger et al. (1994) found that veterinarians overestimated the degree to which they were involved in nutrition consulting and heifer rearing. Veterinarians said their involvement in these areas was "fairly comprehensive," but farmers indicated veterinarian involvement regarding nutrition was "at best occasional" and 50.7% of farmers said they rarely or never received advice on heifer rearing.

In a telephone survey of 238 Canadian dairy producers Sorge et al. (2010) found producers thought their veterinarians made too many recommendations at once and failed to highlight the most important feature of their recommendations. As Atkinson (2010a, p 115) put it: "[Veterinarians'] knowledge is their stock and trade, and it is no surprise that they tend to spout it!"

Waitzkin (1984) demonstrated in human medicine that American internists devoted little more than 1 minute on average to the task of patient education in interviews lasting 20 minutes and overestimated the amount of time that they spent on this task by a factor of nine.

Makoul et al. (1995) found that physicians in British general practice overestimated the extent to which they accomplished the following key tasks in explanation and planning: discussing the risks of medication, discussing the patient's ability to follow the treatment plan and eliciting the patient's opinion about medication prescribed.

Richard and Lussier (2003) studied the discussion of medications in Canadian general practice. They assessed audiotapes of 40 experienced physicians engaging in 462 patient encounters. Several of their findings echo and extend those from earlier research. In instances of the prescription of new medications, instructions were discussed in 75.9% of cases, warnings and side effects were rarely discussed and reasons to re-consult were discussed in only 35.4% of cases. Discussion of compliance issues regarding these new prescriptions occurred in only 5% of cases.

Using a coding system for communication research called MEDICODE, Richard and Lussier (2006) determined that physician initiation and monologues dominated during interactions with patients. In a subsequent study of 442 encounters involving 1492 discussions of medications, these researchers found that when discussing medications physician and patient often talked past each other rather than engaging in real dialogue (Richard and Lusseier 2007). Patients had little opportunity to discuss their concerns and perspectives.

Are there problems with the type of information that we give?

- In a UK study of 125 dairy farmers and 132 veterinarians, Hall and Wapenaar (2012) found that 81% of the farmers valued discussions with their veterinarian about persistent herd problems, herd welfare issues, cost–benefit interventions and finances, but only 26% of veterinarians instigated such discussions.
- In a British study Kindelan and Kent (1987) showed that human patients placed the highest value on information about diagnosis, prognosis and causation of their condition. However, physicians greatly underestimated their patients' desire for information about prognosis and causation and overestimated their desire for information concerning treatment and drug therapy. Patients' individual information needs were not elicited.
- Jenkins et al. (2011) discovered that 50% of human oncologists reported discussing prognosis in the consultation, but only12% of patients and 20% of researchers looking at these interactions agreed that it had been mentioned.
- A qualitative Canadian study by Coe et al. (2008) found that the two most common reasons for a breakdown in veterinarian–client communication were: a) the client not feeling adequately informed about the medical procedure, the cost, or the possible outcomes including the long-term implications for the owner and pet, and b) that their concerns had not been heard. This study also found that pet owners and veterinarians differed in the kind of information they perceived to be meaningful and useful and that these differences in perception could impede effective communication.
- In a study of six pet owner and four veterinarian focus groups, Coe et al. (2007) showed that clients expect to have conversations with veterinarians about the costs of veterinary care but that such conversations are uncommon. Clients expected veterinarians to initiate these discussions but veterinarians rarely did so.
- In a cross-sectional videotape study of 350 Canadian veterinarian–client–patient interactions, Coe et al. (2009) randomly selected 200 for analysis. Discussions of cost were again found to be relatively uncommon. When they did occur,

veterinarians focused on the cost to clients in terms of the veterinarian's time and services rather than on the information that could be obtained through diagnostic tests or as a result of the procedure or benefits to the animal. The researchers suggest that this lack of common ground can compromise client decision making, as cost discussions are often a factor to assist clients with decision making and understanding about the clinical benefit of money spent. Coe et al. suggest that the problem is exacerbated when support staff rather than the veterinarian discuss cost with clients. They also indicate that delegating this discussion to support staff inhibits the discussion of options and prognosis within the context of the cost and clients then have greater difficulty understanding how money spent contributes to the health and welfare of the animal.

- In a Dutch study Derks et al. (2013) report that dairy farm veterinarians seldom suggest a cooperative strategy, summarize important points given or follow up.
- Roche et al. (2016, in review) conducted a Canadian study on Johne's disease and its control involving six focus groups consisting of dairy producers and two of bovine veterinarians. Their findings show that the producers thought that recommendations veterinarians made (i.e. keeping a closed herd or buying from low-risk herds) were unrealistic, too difficult to do, and often disrupted their routines. In contrast, veterinarians thought nearly all of their recommendations were practical and they routinely recommended them.

Are there problems with the language we use?

Many studies have shown that clinicians not only use language that clients/patients do not understand but also appear to use it to control the other person's involvement in the interview:

- Volk et al. (2011a) found that 43% of clients surveyed did not completely agree with the statement: "My veterinarian communicates with me using language I understand."
- Coe et al. (2008) found that clients expect veterinarians to use lay terms, perceived that jargon was a potential barrier to transfer of information, and indicated that when the veterinarian used words that were outside their understanding it could be condescending.
- Stoewen et al. (2014a) found that clients were frustrated and had difficulty understanding when the veterinarian used complicated medical terminology in situations that were emotionally charged.
- Taking a different tack, Paul (2012) points out that some of the language we use in veterinary medicine, such as "compliance" or "noncompliance," sets us up to see clients in a negative light or make negative judgments about their commitment to their animal's health, and in turn increases the chance of a defensive or adversarial conversation. Paul suggests that alternative terms such as "concordance" and "adherence," noted by Silverman et al. (2005) in human medicine, might be better choices. Recognizing that choice of words can make a difference, health professionals are moving away from the use of the word "compliance" with its overtones of passive clients who are unquestioning recipients of advice. The connotation

is that noncompliers are somehow "negligent" or "bad" animal owners and the blame for noncompliance is primarily the client's. The word "compliance" does not fit well with modern approaches to planning and shared decision making.

- Svarstad (1974) suggested that physicians and patients engage in a "communication conspiracy." In only 15% of visits where unfamiliar terms were used did the patient admit that they did not understand. Physicians in turn seemed to speak as if their patients understood all that they said. Physicians deliberately used highly technical language to control communication and to limit patient questions – such behavior occurred twice as often when doctors were under pressure of time.
- McKinlay (1975), in a study of British obstetricians and gynecologists, showed that physicians were well aware of the difficulties patients had in understanding physicians in general. Despite this, physicians continued to use terms that they had previously identified were the very ones they would not expect their patients to understand.
- Korsch et al. (1968) found that pediatricians' use of technical language (e.g. "edema") and medical shorthand (e.g. "history") was a barrier to communication in more than half of the 800 visits studied. Mothers were confused by the terms used by doctors yet rarely asked for clarification of unfamiliar terms.

Do people recall and understand the information that we give?

In both human and veterinary medicine it is clear that people do not recall everything that clinicians tell them nor do they make sense of difficult messages. Earlier studies in human medicine showed that only 50 to 60% of information given was recalled. Later studies in both fields have suggested that in fact much more is remembered and that the real difficulty is that people do not always understand the meaning of key messages nor are they necessarily committed to the clinician's view.

- Braddock et al. (1997) showed in a study of audiotaped patient encounters with primary care physicians in the US that physicians assessed patient understanding only 2% of the time.
- Dunn et al. (1993) found that human cancer patients in their first interview with an oncologist remembered only 45% of "key points" as determined by the oncologist.
- Jansen et al. (2008) looked at the recall of information presented to newly referred human patients with cancer and showed that younger and older patients correctly recalled 49.5% and 48.4% of information, respectively. Although age decreased recall of information, this effect was only present when total amount of information presented was taken into account. Older patients had more trouble remembering information if more information was presented.
- In a qualitative study of 30 interviews with clients whose dogs had life-threatening cancer, Stoewen et al. (2014a) showed that the manner in which information was communicated to clients facilitated understanding while providing a safe and supportive environment. Clients preferred forthright provision of information, understandable language, use of multiple formats, and an unrushed environment where time was afforded by the veterinary team to listen, answer all questions, respond to concerns, and repeat important parts of the message.

- Rohrbach et al. (2011) surveyed 708 members of a national hunting dog club and found that approximately 87% of study participants had given their dogs heartworm medication within the year, 78% had tested their dogs for heartworm one or more times during that year, and 10% had not tested their dogs at all. Only 64% tested newly acquired dogs; only 21% of these dogs had a second test. The study concluded that in their discussions with clients veterinarians need to place more emphasis on frequency and timing of heartworm tests and to underscore that year round treatment does not eliminate the need for annual testing.
- Latham and Morris (2007) assessed accuracy of clients' recall of information given to them by British veterinary students following the students' participation in different levels of communication skills training. Higher levels of student training resulted in higher levels of client recall.

Are there problems knowing whom to involve in explanation and planning?

When multiple people are involved in the care of the animal(s), the question of who needs to be involved is just as important for explanation and planning as it is for gathering information and relationship building. For example, in small animal medicine this might involve family members; in equine medicine it might involve owners, riders, trainers and groomers; in production animal settings, particularly in large operations, it might include owners, managers, herdsmen, nutritionists, calf feeders, calf treaters and others.

- Atkinson (2010a) indicated that a common problem encountered on farms is identifying whom to give advice to – the herdsmen, owner, milkers, foreign-speaking workers, or all four? In order to achieve a good outcome, the veterinarian needs to communicate relevant advice to the entire farm team.
- Based on his review of the literature regarding reproduction in dairy cattle, Logue (2004) says it well: "The most important constraint on reproduction on any dairy farm is the level of communication between the practicing veterinarian, the farm staff, other 'advisors', and the farm accountant." (p. 51)
- In their study looking at antibiotic use in dairy calves, Sischo et al. (2016, research in progress) also concluded that veterinarians need to understand the dynamics of information exchange and the organizational structure on any given dairy in order to know who needs to be involved in explanation and planning.
- In a Dutch study of 40 dog or cat owners and 17 horse owners who were prescribed oral antibiotics (n=14 companion animal veterinarians, n=6 equine veterinarians), Verker et al. (2008) found that none of the veterinarians asked whether the person they were talking to would be the person who would administer the medication. In 5 out of 57 consultations the person given the explanation of how the medication worked was not the person who administered the drug and compliance was poor for four of these five owners.
- In a focus group study of veterinary–client communication, Coe et al. (2008) showed that small animal veterinarians felt challenged when more than one client was directly or indirectly involved in the animal's care. Some found

that children in the examination room impeded effective communication with clients.

Are people involved in decision making to the level that they want?

The preceding section suggests that in veterinary medicine some of the people who might usefully be involved in decision making are not. We have found no studies in the veterinary literature regarding the level of involvement people desire, but two studies in human medicine offer useful insights.

- Degner et al. (1997) studied women with a confirmed diagnosis of breast cancer attending hospital oncology clinics, and found that physicians can't assume the level of participation patients want in decision making; 22% wanted to select their own cancer treatment, 44% wanted to select their treatment collaboratively with their doctors, and 34% wanted to delegate this decision making to their doctors. Only 42% of women believed they had achieved their preferred level of control in decision making.
- Audrey et al. (2008) looked at how much oncologists in the UK tell patients about the survival benefit of palliative chemotherapy during consultations in which decisions about treatment are made: most patients were not given clear information about the survival gain of palliative chemotherapy, preventing them from being fully involved in decision making.

Do people follow through with the plans that we make?[12]

Here the research is clear-cut and demonstrates that adherence is clearly connected to good communication:

- In an early study of 26 dogs and their owners, Bomzon (1978) found that 73% of the owners did not adhere to the instructions given regarding the administration of antibiotics. The major reason given by the owners for their non-adherence to the instructions was that they were at work during the day and were unable to treat the dog in the middle of the day.
- A Canadian dairy study (Giger et al. 1994) reported that the major reason farmers gave for non-adoption of herd health services was non-availability of the veterinarian. The study found that frequency of veterinary visits (at least monthly) increased dairy producers' sense of being in a herd health program and that those farmers who thought they were in a program thought they received more advice and service.
- Cummings et al. (1995) reviewed records to evaluate the success of implementing heartworm programs during a 12-month period at 50 veterinary clinics located in heartworm-endemic areas of the USA. The study found sufficient medication

---

12   For further information about non-adherence, the following texts provide reviews of the field in human medicine: Haynes et al. (1979), Meichenbaum and Turk (1987), Ley (1988), Coambs et al. (1995), Haynes et al. (1996), Butler et al. (1996), and DiMatteo (2004).

was dispensed to fully protect only 41% of the 116 087 dogs in the database, so the majority of the dogs brought to these veterinary clinics were not placed on the clinic's recommended heartworm preventive program. The authors concluded that there was a sizeable gap between the medicine recommended and medicine practiced.

- In a systematic review of compliance Haynes et al. (1996) indicated that between 10 and 90% of patients prescribed drugs by their physicians (with an average of 50%) did not take their medicine at all or took it incorrectly. Many studies have shown that patients do not follow their physicians' recommendations, with 20–30% non-adherence in medications for acute illness, 30–40% in medications for illness prevention, 50% for long-term medications and 72% for diet. Yet, surprisingly, physicians have had a tendency to ignore non-adherence as a possible cause of poor outcome.

- Stull et al. (2007) surveyed 545 small and mixed animal veterinarians in Western Canada to determine the veterinarians' perception of zoonotic parasites and how they used small animal deworming protocols in client education. Forty-four percent (238/539) of respondents reported that they actively discussed with all clients the zoonotic risk of small animal-derived endoparasites. Close to 10% discussed zoonotic risk with only those at greatest risk (households with children, young animals, immunocompromised individuals), while 40% discussed zoonotic risk with clients only when prompted by the clients or when worms were diagnosed. Six percent of the veterinarians never discussed the zoonotic risk of cat/dog helminthes. Because many of the preventive measures important in the control of zoonotic helminth disease occur outside the veterinary clinic, client education remains vital to the control of these diseases. The researchers conclude that although client education is a crucial service, in busy veterinary practices it is easy to overlook the degree of client education and adequate patient follow-up required to improve owner compliance with recommended protocols. In light of the fact that this book intentionally integrates concepts and research from human and veterinary medicine, it is interesting to note that Stull et al. (2007) make reference to research done by Gauthier and Richardson (2002) and Grant and Olsen (1999) indicating that although physicians could play a role in educating their pediatric patients (and parents) and their immunocompromised patients on zoonotic problems such as helminthes, physicians are even less involved and comfortable with the task than veterinarians.

- Barter et al. (1996a) compared different methods for assessing the compliance of 31 owners from three Sydney veterinary hospitals whose dogs were prescribed amoxicillin-clavulanate two or three times daily, for five to seven days. One method the study examined was veterinarians' estimates of owner compliance. The study showed that veterinarians have poor ability to predict their clients' compliance and should therefore avoid reliance on their ability to predict compliance or noncompliance in their clients.

- In a large compliance study the American Animal Hospital Association (AAHA) (2003) surveyed over 1000 pet owners, carried out in-depth interviews with veterinarians and practice teams in 52 small animal practices, and reviewed records of 1340 patients in 240 practices. Results showed that in almost every case practice teams seriously overestimated their clients' adherence. Veterinarians and staff confused telling the clients what to do with the client accepting and following through with their recommendations. Clients said that their lack of compliance was due to ineffective communication about the need for or benefit of the recommendation. AAHA's 2009 follow-up study showed that compliance had improved overall from 64% to 73%. AAHA also reported a major shift in perception regarding compliance, noting that in their 2003 study, 60% of veterinary professionals interviewed thought that compliance was the client's responsibility, but in their 2009 study, 60% of those interviewed thought that compliance was the responsibility of the practice team.

- In a Norwegian study consisting of 113 dogs and their owners, Grave and Tanem (1999) assessed the compliance of clients via a telephone interview conducted 10 days after the client had been given a prescription for oral antibacterial drugs. The researchers found 16% of owners did not fill the prescription at all and said that they did not think the treatment was necessary or were skeptical of using antibiotics. Only 37% of owners had used as much medication as the veterinarian had recommended at the time of the interview. Of those who filled the prescription, 85% thought the veterinarian had spent enough time with them and their pet during the consultation. This group also reported a significantly higher compliance than the remaining group. The researchers conclude that time spent with owners influences the owners' willingness and ability to comply with the recommended regime. Owners were more compliant with treatment having to do with gastrointestinal issues in their dogs. The researchers suggest that when issues impact the owner more, which would be the case with gastrointestinal issues, these owners may be more invested in maintaining treatment.

- In an Australian study comprised of 11 dogs with conditions assigned to two doses of medication a day and 12 assigned to three doses a day, Barter et al. (1996b) used an electronic monitoring device to assess client compliance regarding medication doses given, timing of the dose, and number of doses per day. The study found that owners gave 84% of the prescribed number of doses per day, but only 32% of the doses were given within the designated optimum time periods. Clients gave medication the correct number of times a day 56–59% of the time. Clients whose pets were prescribed a two-dose-a-day regime gave the medication within the optimum interval 43% of the time whereas clients in the three-dose-a-day group did so 22% of the time. Clients gave an incorrect number of tablets per day on 43% of the treatment days and they gave 66% of doses outside of optimum time periods.

- Kanji et al. (2012) showed that only 30% of Canadian small animal clients followed through with dental or surgery recommendations or both (25 out of the 83 visits in the study where such recommendations were made). The odds for adherence were seven times greater when clients received a clear rather than an ambiguous recommendation. Adherence was also significantly greater when veterinarians provided a rationale for the recommendation, were more sympathetic and empathetic, were less hurried and gave clients ample opportunity to speak, used positive rapport building statements/actions (i.e. laughter, approval, compliments, agreement), and had higher scores for relationship-centered care (i.e. worked collaboratively with clients). Interestingly, the researchers also found that when veterinarians used more than 45 positive rapport-building statements, client adherence began to decrease.

- In a study of 238 Canadian dairy producers, Sorge et al. (2010) found that although the majority of dairy producers found the recommendations made by the veterinarian to be reasonable and feasible, on average they implemented two recommendations out of six.
- In a study of 2000 dog and cat owners across the USA, Lue et al. (2008) found that 71% of clients who believed that their veterinarian was a good communicator said that they followed their veterinarian's advice. That number decreased significantly to 51% when clients thought their veterinarian was not good at communicating. In addition this study showed that 30% of owners did not follow their veterinarian's recommendation because they did not believe the recommended treatment was necessary.
- In a review of selected veterinary literature, Loftus (2012) identified several reasons for poor compliance, including inadequate demonstration, information or length of appointment; lack of written information, follow-up telephone calls or reminders for chronic medication; inadequate continuity of care.
- In an equine management survey study, Loftus (2011) found that owners often had difficulty in applying or maintaining dressings as requested by the veterinarian. Fearful of applying the dressing incorrectly, many owners left the areas undressed. On the other hand 60% of veterinarians in the study reported that clients removed dressings prematurely resulting in problems with wound healing.
- Based on findings in veterinary studies and what can be extrapolated from human studies, Maddison (2011) offers a useful compilation of practical information and suggestions for improving communication related to medication compliance in small animal practice, what it is, how it can be measured, how compliant small animal owners are, barriers to compliance, and factors in veterinary practice that can improve compliance.
- In an analysis of published research in human medicine, Zolnierek and DiMatteo (2009) showed that effective communication is highly correlated with better patient adherence, and that training physicians to communicate better enhances their patients' adherence.

How does all of this relate to Internet use and health literacy?

There is increasing and considerable interest and research regarding health literacy (Kripalani and Weiss 2006; Sudore and Schillinger 2009; Coleman 2011). The Institute of Medicine defines health literacy as "the degree to which individuals have the capacity to obtain, process and understand basic health information and services needed to make appropriate health decisions" (Nielsen-Bohlman et al. 2004). Low health literacy contributes to possible communication gaps between clinicians and patients or clients. People with low health literacy may have less familiarity with medical concepts and vocabulary and ask fewer questions. They may also hide their limited understanding from shame or embarrassment. Clinicians commonly overestimate people's literacy levels. Clearly, in all consultations, there is a need to tailor information giving to each individual patient or client and actively discover what will be helpful.

Are there problems in teaching and learning explanation and planning?

In her study of Dutch veterinarians' perceptions regarding udder health management, Jansen (2010) collected 91 surveys and conducted 10 in-depth interviews. Veterinarians in this study perceived a lack of confidence, competence and knowledge in their advisory capability. Some veterinarians doubted the usefulness of veterinary advice – they did not see giving advice to farmers as part of their job or thought it was too difficult to convince farmers to change what they were doing. This study has potentially important implications for veterinary education regarding explanation and planning, including postgraduate education.

Maguire et al. (1986) looked at the information-giving skills of young physicians who 5 years previously had completed training in interviewing skills at medical school. This training had, however, not included any specific training in information giving per se. The results were disturbing. Physicians were weakest in many of the very techniques that have been found to increase patients' satisfaction and adherence with advice and treatment, namely:

- discovering the patient's views and expectations (70% no attempt)
- negotiation (90% no attempt)
- encouraging questions (70% no attempt)
- repetition of advice (63% no attempt)
- checking understanding (89% no attempt)
- categorizing information (90% no attempt).

No difference at all was detected in information-giving skills between those who had completed the course on interviewing skills at medical school and controls. Yet the same students had maintained their superiority over controls in key information-gathering skills. This demonstrates the need for teaching not only information-gathering skills but also the specific skills of explanation and planning if we wish clinicians to become effective in information transfer in the consultation.

Campion et al. (2002) looked at 2094 human medicine candidates' scores on the consulting skills module of the examination for membership of the Royal College of General Practitioners in the UK. For this national high stakes examination, residents nearing completion of their 3-year residency program submitted a videotape of seven actual consultations with their own patients – the first five of these were assessed for each candidate. Even in this highly select set of consultations where candidates were fully aware of the performance criterion, Campion et al. found significant deficits in four patient-centered competencies related to explanation and planning:

- exploring patients' beliefs about the illness was not seen in 14% of the candidates – only 39% met this performance criterion in three or more of their five consultations

- using patients' beliefs in explanation was not seen in 31% of the candidates – only 17% met this criterion in three or more of the five
- checking patients' understanding of explanations was not seen in 45% of the candidates – only 9% met this criterion in three or more of the five
- involving patients in decisions was not seen in 14% of the candidates – only 36% met this criterion in three or more of the five.

In a UK study of fifth-year veterinary students Latham and Morris (2007) compared the effectiveness of small group teaching of communication to minimal training or no training. Small group training consisted of a 6-hour seminar comprised of discussion, analysis of videotaped consultations and interactions with simulated clients for the purpose of practicing communication skills. This group was also taught the structure of a consultation by way of the Calgary–Cambridge model for the medical consultation. The students in the small group teaching cohort showed significant improvement in building a relationship with a client, aiding recall and incorporating clients' views compared with the groups that received minimal or no training. There was no significant difference between the three groups with regard to providing information, one of the skills inherent to the explanation and planning phase of the Calgary–Cambridge model. These findings raise important questions:

- Was there enough time devoted to teaching the students how to give clients information?
- Were the people involved in teaching the small groups adequately prepared to coach these students on how to give information?
- Did the students at this point in their training have enough information to give?

As evidenced above and throughout, even with residency training or years of practice, clinicians continue to have problems with explanation and planning. Learners receive little focused training regarding how to give explanations and plan with clients and patients. In both human and veterinary medicine, we seem to assume that clinicians will learn this on their own once they are in practice. It is not surprising then that we have problems in this area. While we are making progress in our teaching and learning regarding explanation and planning, consider the following.

- Too often, veterinary schools do not teach explanation and planning in any depth – we run out of time in the curriculum to do this. Faculty often have limited training in this area and understandably focus attention on teaching medical content.
- Students are early in development of their experience, knowledge base and skills even during their final years of training; consequently careful consideration needs to be given to the contexts in which they practice these skills and the level of supervision they need. Depending on their level of training and experience they may not really be "ready" to do what is needed with explanation and planning during even their final years in veterinary school.
- Interns, residents and new graduates who go directly into practice seem to have few opportunities to develop these skills with feedback from supervisors or colleagues.

- Both teaching hospital faculty and community practitioners who precept rotations have had limited if any formal training regarding communication process skills related to explanation and planning.
- Few substantive continuing education opportunities are available regarding evidence-based explanation and planning process skills training.

Objectives

Our objectives for explanation and planning can be summarized as:

- gauging the correct amount and type of information to give to each individual
- providing explanations the client can remember and understand
- providing explanations that relate to the client's perspective
- using an interactive approach to ensure a shared understanding of the problem with the client
- involving the client and planning collaboratively to the level the client wishes, so as to increase the client's commitment and adherence to plans made
- continuing to build a relationship and provide a supportive environment.

These objectives encompass many of the tasks and checkpoints mentioned in other well-known guides to the consultation – *see* Appendix C.

The content of explanation and planning

In Chapter 3 we described how the process skills for gathering information that are on the Calgary–Cambridge Guides relate to the content guide. The process skills for explanation and planning also correspond to specific areas of the content guide. Box 6.1 shows these content guide components:

Box 6.1 The content of explanation and planning

Differential Diagnosis – Hypotheses
Including both veterinarian's and client's ideas regarding problems and issues

Veterinarian's Plan of Management
Investigations
Treatment alternatives

Explanation and Planning with Client
What the client has been told
Plan of action negotiated

These content components include aspects of the veterinarian's internal thinking and planning as well as the explanation and planning that occurs jointly with the client. Throughout the rest of this chapter on explanation and planning, it will be useful to keep in mind how process and content skills work together during this important part of the consultation.

The process skills of explanation and planning

Box 6.2 The process skills for explanation and planning

Providing the correct amount and type of information
Aims: to give appropriate information, neither restricting nor overloading
        to assess each individual client's information needs
- **Chunks and checks**: gives information in manageable chunks, checks for understanding, uses client's response as a guide to how to proceed
- **Assesses client's starting point**: asks for client's prior knowledge early on when giving information, ascertains extent of client's wish for information
- **Asks clients what other information would be helpful**, e.g. etiology, prognosis
- **Gives explanation at appropriate times**: avoids giving advice, information or reassurance prematurely.

Aiding accurate recall and understanding
Aims: to make information easier for clients to remember and understand
- **Organizes explanation**: divides into discrete sections, develops a logical sequence
- **Uses explicit categorization and other signposting** (e.g. *"There are three important things that I would like to discuss. First ..."* *"Now, shall we move on to ..."*)
- **Uses repetition and summarizing** to reinforce information
- **Uses** concise, **easily understood language**; avoids or explains jargon
- **Uses visual methods of conveying information**: diagrams, models, written information and instructions
- **Checks client's understanding of information given** or plans made (e.g. by asking client to restate in own words; clarifies as necessary)

Achieving a shared understanding: incorporating the client's perspective
Aims: to provide explanations and plans that relate to the client's perspective
        to discover the client's thoughts and feelings about the information given
        to encourage an interaction rather than one-way transmission
- **Relates explanations to client's perspective**: to previously elicited ideas, concerns and expectations
- **Provides opportunities and encourages client to contribute**: to ask questions, seek clarification or express doubts; responds appropriately
- **Picks up and responds to verbal and nonverbal cues**, e.g. client's need to contribute information or ask questions, information overload, distress

- **Elicits client's beliefs, reactions and feelings** re information given, terms used; acknowledges and addresses where necessary.

Planning: shared decision making
Aims: to allow clients to understand the decision-making process
to involve clients in decision making to the level they wish
to increase clients' commitment to plans made
- **Shares own thinking as appropriate**: ideas, thought processes and dilemmas
- **Involves the client**:
  — offers suggestions and choices rather than directives
  — encourages client to contribute their ideas, suggestions
- **Explores management options**
- **Ascertains** level of **involvement client wishes** re decision making
- **Negotiates a mutually acceptable plan**:
  — signposts own position of equipoise or preference regarding available options
  — determines client's preferences
- **Checks with client**:
  — if accepts plans
  — if concerns have been addressed.

Options for explanation and planning

(includes content and process skills)

If offering opinion and discussing significance of problems
- Offers opinion of what is going on and names if possible
- Reveals rationale for opinion
- Explains causation, seriousness, expected outcome, short- and long-term consequences
- Elicits client's beliefs, reactions and concerns (e.g. if opinion matches client's thoughts, acceptability, feelings)

If negotiating mutual plan of action
- Discusses options (e.g. no action, investigation, medication, non-drug treatments, fluids, surgery, behavioral consult, preventive measures, euthanasia/cull)
- Provides information on action or treatment offered
  a) name
  b) steps involved, how it works
  c) benefits and advantages
  d) possible side effects
- Obtains client's view of need for action, perceived benefits, barriers, motivation
- Accepts client's views, advocates alternative viewpoint as necessary
- Elicits client's reactions and concerns about plans and treatments including acceptability

- Takes client's lifestyle, beliefs, cultural background and abilities into consideration
- Encourages client to be involved in implementing plans and to follow through
- Asks about client support networks, discusses other options.

If discussing investigations and procedures
- Provides clear information on procedures including what client and animal might experience and how client will be informed of results
- Relates procedures to treatment plan: value and purpose
- Encourages questions about and discussion of potential anxieties or negative outcomes.

What to teach and learn about explanation and planning: the underlying concepts and evidence for the skills

We now explore the individual skills for explanation and planning listed in Box 6.2 and examine the evidence from theory and research that validates their use in the consultation. In other sections of the consultation the skills we present are used more or less in any interaction. However, the numerous skills for explanation and planning are more case specific – you will select the appropriate skills to use on a case-to-case basis. For example, you would rarely use all of the possible alternatives for improving recall and understanding, in some cases shared decision making is not appropriate and so those skills would not be used, and a given consultation may not take up all of the topics in the "Options" section.

We have divided the skills of explanation and planning into five sections and will look at each in turn:

1. Providing the correct amount and type of information
2. Aiding accurate recall and understanding
3. Achieving a shared understanding: incorporating the client's perspective
4. Planning: shared decision making
5. Options in explanation and planning.

As we progress through these sections, we will illuminate the explanation skills veterinarians use with clients by considering the skills involved in delivering a lecture. Thinking about the poorly delivered lecture provides us with many insights into the skills required in information giving in the veterinary consultation. Most of us have attended many lectures in our lifetime, not all of them of the highest quality, in which some or all of the following apply:

- the lecture has no apparent structure and as a listener you cannot tell where it is going
- the lecturer uses language or jargon you cannot understand
- the lecturer loses you early on and you struggle to keep up from then on
- the information given is either way below or above your current understanding

- you are given too much or too little new information
- the lecturer has made assumptions about your personal needs which are incorrect and the questions you wish to be answered are not addressed
- you are not sure what the key points are at the end.

At its worst, the following scenario ensues. The lecturer speaks for 45 minutes without interruption in a darkened room with poor-quality slides. You concentrate for a while and a question enters your head that needs clarifying in order for you to make sense of what has been said so far. While you are thinking about this, you miss the next few minutes of the speech. You start to drift into a day-dream and return to concentrate on the lecture after an unclear amount of time. When you wake up, the rest of the lecture does not quite make sense. At the end, the lecturer asks for any questions but you are too embarrassed to ask the question you thought of earlier as you do not know if it was answered when you were asleep. You say nothing.

We can apply lessons learned from this scenario not only to giving a lecture but also to conducting the explanation and planning component of the veterinarian–client consultation. To optimize information giving in both of these settings, it is useful to revisit two approaches to communication outlined in Chapter 2 of the companion book, *Teaching and Learning Communication Skills in Medicine*. Barbour (2000) metaphorically labeled these approaches:

- the shot-put approach
- the Frisbee approach.

The shot-put approach defines communication simply as *the well-conceived, well-delivered message*. From the classical Greek times of its origins right through to the mid-twentieth century, formal communication training in the professions has focused almost entirely on the shot-put approach. Effective communication meant content, delivery and persuasion. An early communication model developed by a telephone company reflects the shot-put approach: the sender puts together a clear, well argued message and transmits it, the receiver picks it up and that is perceived to be the end of the communication.

The traditional lecture in its most basic form exemplifies the shot-put approach. The skills that make for effective lecturing are part of what makes for effective communication in the veterinarian–client relationship – we need to know how to deliver a message effectively and how to package and articulate the message we want to get across to the client so that it can be both remembered and understood. However, the shot-put approach is only part of what is needed.

In the 1940s, our understanding of effective communication began to shift toward a more interactive, give-and-take approach. This new perspective – appropriately dubbed the Frisbee approach – finally caught on in the 1960s. In this approach *mutually understood common ground* is perceived as a necessary foundation for both trust and accuracy, so achieving this common ground is one of the central concepts of the approach. If mutually understood common ground is important to effective communication then our time-honored, one-dimensional focus on the well-conceived, well-delivered message falls short. In the interpersonal or Frisbee perspective the message is still important, of course, but the emphasis shifts to interaction, feedback and collaboration.

This brings us back to one of the principles of communication that we have outlined earlier: *effective communication ensures an interaction rather than a direct transmission process*. If communication is viewed as direct transmission, the senders of messages assume that their responsibilities as communicators are fulfilled once they have formulated and sent a message. However, if communication is viewed as an interactive process, the interaction is complete only if the sender receives feedback about how the message is interpreted, whether it is understood and what impact it has on the receiver. Just imparting information is not enough – responding to feedback about the impact of the message becomes crucial and the emphasis moves to the interdependence of sender and receiver in establishing mutually understood common ground (Dance and Larson 1972).

In the veterinarian–client consultation, we need to take an even more interactive approach. As we shall see, we need to take into account each client's individual requirements, their different capacity to take in information and their different needs and concerns. What does this client know already, how much information would the client like, what do they need to know to care for their animals, what is the client most concerned about and how much would the client like to be involved in decision making? And we have to do all of this without sacrificing the important organizational and linguistic skills learned from the shot-put approach.

Providing the correct amount and type of information

If the research shows that clients and patients tend to want more information, why do their clinicians persist in giving them less? Why is there such a wide gulf between what clinicians think clients and patients want and what they tell us they need? And how can clinicians determine just how much information each individual would like in each situation? Much of the disparity between the amount of information that clinicians give and the amount clients and patients would prefer to receive has its roots in the traditional view of the doctor–client/patient relationship.

And what about the type of information? For example, Harvey et al. (1991) surveyed 450 small and mixed animal veterinarians about their perceptions and practices with respect to control of roundworms and hookworms in dogs. Thirty-three percent said they routinely discussed zoonotic concerns with all clients. Twenty-nine percent of the veterinarians said they never discussed potential zoonotic hazards of roundworms or discussed them only when asked. Thirty-eight percent discussed them when roundworms were diagnosed.

In a US study of 2188 dog and cat owners aimed at understanding the reasons for the decline in the number of veterinary visits, Volk et al. (2011a) found that owners did not understand the need for or value of routine wellness visits, thought veterinary costs were too high or were unwilling to put up with the stress to the animal and themselves involved with taking their pet to the veterinary hospital. In a follow-up study of 400 practice owners, Volk et al. (2014) reported that many veterinarians recognized that transporting cats to the veterinary practice was challenging for clients but only twenty-four percent of respondents said they provided specific instructions to clients on making the visit less stressful. These findings raise important questions: are we providing clients with enough information about why regular visits are important or how to prepare their animals for such visits?

In Chapter 3, we contrasted the traditional method of history taking with the integrated clinical method. We now take a similar approach to explanation and planning by comparing the traditional view of information giving with more recent concepts that mirror changes in society as a whole. We would like to start with a look at theoretical underpinnings and research that have impacted this aspect of explanation and planning.

Underlying concepts

While the ideas we discuss in this section have particular relevance to explanation and planning, keep in mind that these concepts affect all aspects of communication in veterinary medicine.

The "traditional" view of the veterinarian–client relationship

A PERCEIVED KNOWLEDGE AND COMPETENCE GAP

Veterinarians may tend to take a more doctor-centered approach in some contexts than in others. For example, Shaw et al. (2006) showed that in small animal practices the veterinarians adopted a variety of approaches to their interaction with clients. Doctor-centered was the predominant pattern, i.e. veterinarians were verbally dominant throughout all the appointments, which may have left clients little time to comment or ask questions (the study did not assess clients' preferences).

Stoewen et al. (2014b) studied expectations of clients accessing oncology care at a tertiary referral center for dogs with life-limiting cancer. They found that a central expectation was for information to be the truth. In their discussion the researchers pointed out that truth telling in the oncological setting is actually a fairly recent phenomenon. Prior to the 1990s, it was commonplace to supposedly protect human patients (and most probably veterinary clients) from the psychological impact of the cancer diagnosis by withholding information (Faden et al. 1981; Nekolaichuk and Bruera 1998; Baile and Beale 2001). The finding that clients in the study repeatedly raised truth telling suggested the possibility of an ongoing current of public distrust. The researchers concluded that veterinarians could provide clients with verbal assurance by underscoring the principle of truth telling early in the service encounter.

The more "traditional," paternalistic view of the veterinarian–client relationship suggests that there is a knowledge and competence gap that makes it difficult to explain complex issues to clients appropriately and achieve true client understanding. Furthermore such knowledge and understanding is thought to be somewhat unnecessary – all clients have to do is follow the recommended advice. Lam et al. (2011) offer additional insight from large animal settings when they suggest that it is a misconception to think that simply communicating expert technical knowledge leads to a change in [farmers'] behavior – it does not. This more "traditional" view likely emanated from the eighteenth century with the onset of the scientific method. So what else justifies this "traditional" approach?

EMOTION IN THE CONSULTATION

In veterinary medicine we have tended to view clients' outward displays of emotion in a negative light. One reason given for this being an appropriate stance is that as veterinarians became more involved in small animal care the presence of client emotion accompanying animal illness or injury interferes with objective communication and understanding. Following on from this argument, veterinarians have withheld information from clients so as to avoid upsetting them. Veterinarians have also viewed client expression of emotion negatively because of its potential effect on the animal.

PROFESSIONAL AUTHORITY

An alternative, if possibly dated, view in human medicine (Freidson 1970) is that the difference between the medical interview and other information-giving circumstances is not due to any emotional difficulty within the consultation but more an inevitable result of physicians' desire to retain their high status within society. This analysis suggests a much less altruistic reason for withholding information. If the difference in social standing between physician and patient is something that the profession wishes to preserve, in part this can be achieved by limiting the provision of information to the lay population. Mystification of the physician's and devaluation of the patient's knowledge might be said to be more powerful driving forces than the higher motive of creating informed and autonomous patients. Maintaining clear water between professional and client necessitates a degree of ownership of information by the clinician. The use of Latin terms can be seen as one part of this complicated process of obfuscation – the patient presents a sore throat, the doctor advises that it is acute pharyngitis. Of course, this impressive title is simply a translation of the patient's words into an unshared medical language (Bouhris et al. 1989).

Reflecting on Shaw et al.'s (2006) work showing that veterinarians were verbally dominant and tended toward paternalism, it seems appropriate to think about how professional authority plays out in the veterinary profession.

The perceived knowledge/competence gap, the possible presence of emotion and the need to preserve professional authority may have predisposed healthcare professionals in both fields to withhold information and clients/patients to remain passive bystanders in the explanation and planning phase of the interview.

What recent trends in society have influenced veterinary medical practice?

CHANGES IN SOCIETY AT LARGE

Recent decades have brought many changes in society and the breaking down of a multitude of class and social barriers. Moves toward freedom of speech, gender and racial equality and freedom of information have changed society irrevocably. As educational standards and personal wealth have increased, expectations have followed suit and demands have escalated on many services including human and animal health. Changes away from a focus on curative medicine toward prevention of illness and maintenance of health have led to an increased awareness of both human and animal health issues in the population. The mushrooming of articles and programs in the written and broadcast media and the explosion of information on the Internet has led to much greater availability of information about health and disease, and the emergence of consumer and advocacy groups has changed people's awareness and their influence on the consultation. Our attitudes toward animal rights and welfare are also changing. Jaak Panksepp's extensive research regarding emotion in animals (e.g. 2011, 2013), Temple Grandin's success in changing attitudes toward animal welfare and food animal handling (e.g. 2005, 2010, 2013), and Franklin McMillan's (2002) work promoting the development of mental wellness programs for animals are only three examples of these societal changes regarding how we perceive animals. Legislation focusing on human patient rights and on animal and veterinary client rights have followed these changes and cemented their influence.

Society has not stood still nor has the clinician–client/patient relationship: the public routinely questions both the knowledge and motivation of physicians and veterinarians and no longer demonstrates a blind faith in either profession. These changes are clearly impacting interactions in both human and veterinary medicine. A brief look at some of the literature in both fields offers additional useful insights.

Hay et al. (2008) showed that 87.5% of human patients attending their first appointment in rheumatology outpatients looked up their symptoms or suspected condition prior to their first appointment, with 62.5% of all patients seeking that information on the Internet. Only 20% of online information seekers discussed that information with their physicians during the consultation. Bylund et al. (2007) looked at patients' experiences of talking to their providers about Internet health information. The provider taking the information seriously was associated with higher patient satisfaction. Bowes et al. (2012) showed patients used the Internet to become better informed about their health and hence make best use of the limited time available with their GP and to enable the GP to take their problem more seriously. Patients expected their GP to acknowledge the information; discuss, explain, or contextualize it; and offer a professional opinion. Patients tended to prioritize GP opinion over Internet information. However, if the GP appeared disinterested, dismissive or patronizing patients reported damage to the doctor–patient relationship, occasionally to the extent of seeking a second opinion or changing their doctor.

A study by Kogan et al. (2008) of 412 veterinary clients across 17 small animal veterinary clinics shows that the most frequently used sources of pet health information reported by participants using a 5-point scale were as follows: veterinarian visited in person (X=3.28), veterinarian contacted by telephone (X=2.86), friends or family (X=2.77) and the World Wide Web (X=2.53). Also in 2008, Hofmeister et al. found that veterinary clients rated the Internet as the third most likely source of information after veterinary general practitioners and specialists. In 2011, Volk et al. found that increased use of the Internet by pet owners was one of three factors related to the decline in veterinary primary patient visits and less reliance on their veterinarians. As a result of checking the Internet, many pet owners delayed taking their sick or injured animal to the veterinarian or did not go at all – in some cases the animal's problem resolved but in others the condition worsened. Showing a continuation of this trend, Kogan et al. (2012) found that 94.4% of the 1687 clients surveyed in their study reported using the Internet. The two most common reasons cited for using the Internet were the desire for a second opinion and disagreement with the veterinarian.

In a subsequent study, Kogan et al. (2014) assessed the impact of providing clients with a URL to a general veterinary medicine website. A third of the 367 clients who returned a follow-up survey said they had accessed the URL and 86% of that group said they found it very or somewhat helpful in: making better decisions (88%), talking with their veterinarian (90%), or improving their understanding of an illness or condition (41%). Since Internet use is likely to continue to increase, veterinarians may want to take a more active role in helping their clients access pet health information from reliable sites, thereby overtly acknowledging clients' use of sources other than the veterinarian and opening up discussion about Internet information and use.

Other societal changes, for example regarding how people view animals and veterinary medicine itself, also influence veterinary–client–patient interactions. Decades ago Blau and Duncan (1967) pointed out that the veterinary profession is situated in societies that have very contradictory attitudes and practices toward animals. This becomes even more obvious when we look at the current global picture. Bryant (1979) and Arluke (1997) have argued that as animals' moral value increases, clients' expectations from veterinarians also increase. As Owens (2015) points out, veterinary medicine has undergone major transformations over the past century and the perceptions that humans construct regarding the animals to whom they are attached impacts interactions between veterinarians and clients. This research underscores the need for veterinarians to ascertain clients' perspectives about their animals. It also raises awareness of the need for veterinarians to stay in touch with their own perceptions about the animals and clients they serve.

CHANGES IN VETERINARY MEDICINE ITSELF

As is the case in human healthcare, both veterinary medicine and surgery have become increasingly advanced and complex. For example, advances in veterinary medicine include back injury treatment, limb sparing surgery, cancer treatment, vision surgery, heart repair, kidney and cartilage transplants, stem cell therapies – the list is long. And then there are the wellness options and the preventive treatments and services. With so much more information to wade through, so many more diagnostic aids available, and so many more treatment options possible, communication with clients and decision making have also become increasingly complicated. All of this has changed the nature of and need for skilled communication in veterinary medicine. The magnitude and complexity of the information that can be disseminated and that clients need to understand as well as the involvement of clients in decision making have changed considerably.

Do all clients want more information?

But do all individuals want more information and if not, how can we adapt our information giving to match their needs and preferences? A number of studies reported on in previous chapters of this book indicate that clients and human patients often do want more information so that they can make more informed decisions. The following studies offer additional insights.

AAHA's (2003) study found that in small animal practice 90% of clients wanted to be informed about all of their options for patient care regardless of whether they could afford it.

Coe et al. (2008) found that rather than giving clients multiple options, veterinarians generally present clients with what the veterinarian thinks is the best option and then modify this option based on the client's response. The researchers also found that animal owners expect information up front from their veterinarian so that they can make decisions regarding the care of their pet, information provided in various forms including reading material and discharge instructions, information regarding the options that are available regarding the animal's treatment.

Stoewen et al. (2014b) found that some clients with dogs in oncology care wanted a lot of information and others wanted substantially less. Individual clients' expectations regarding the amount of information they wanted varied over time. So veterinarians cannot just ask about this once.

Jansen et al. (2009) show that farmers' motivation to improve udder health is linked to the provision of the latest udder health information and educational products described by their veterinarian.

In Pinder's (1990) study of information giving to patients with Parkinson's disease, physicians adopted a set style with all patients despite individual patients varying greatly in the amount of information that they wished to know. Most patients wanted to hear more information about their illness and medication, but not all. Jenkins et al. (2001) in a large study of 2331 patients with cancer showed that 87% of patients wanted as much information as possible while 13% preferred to leave disclosure of details up to the physician. Many other studies have shown that patients can be divided into seekers (around 80%) and avoiders (around 20%) concerning information, with seekers coping better with more information and avoiders with less (Miller and Mangan 1983; Deber 1994). Steptoe et al. (1991) showed that information avoiders report a better understanding and satisfaction with doctor–patient communication than seekers but paradoxically have a worse understanding: seekers on the other hand are less satisfied with communication and would like even more information despite having already gained a better understanding.

While most people do want more information, a minority would like less. But it is not at all easy to predict which individual is in which group. For instance, as Waitzkin (1985) has said, "research has clearly shown that the commonly expressed assumption that working-class patients do not want a full explanation of their illness seems to derive from the hesitancy of human patients to ask questions rather than from any actual disinterest in information." Repeated studies have also shown that the assumption that elderly people do not wish to receive information about their illness is unfounded. Although slightly more elderly than younger people prefer to receive less information, by far the majority of older people want to be kept very well informed (Davis et al.1999).

Skills to help gauge the correct amount and type of information

One of the key issues of explanation and planning is how to gauge just what information to share with the client. How do we negotiate the delicate path between not giving enough information and overloading the client with too much? How do we ascertain the individual information needs of each client and tailor our information giving accordingly? How do we discover what information each client requires to make sense of the situation rather than give a predetermined lecture based on our assumptions of what the client needs? How do we take into account clients' pre-existing knowledge and discover what information they would like along with information that we think they need to have?

Returning to the comparison with lecturing, how could you personalize a lecture to the needs of the audience rather than give a predetermined speech based on your assumptions of the audience's requirements? First, you could start on the path that you had planned, but break the lecture up into discrete sections and ask the audience for questions about what you have said within each section – this would allow you to answer questions as you go and equally importantly gauge the learners' level of understanding and their further requirements. Second, you could deliberately ask the audience early on what they already know about the topic, what problems they have in this area and what specific questions they would like answered. And you could repeat the process as the lecture proceeds, constantly asking what further information would be helpful. In other words, you could increase the interactivity and thereby move from the shot-put to the Frisbee approach. This is exactly what is helpful in the context of the veterinary consultation.

Chunking and checking

Chunking and checking is a vital skill throughout the explanation and planning phase of the consultation, not only for gauging the correct amount of information to give but also as an aid to *accurate recall* and to *achieving a shared understanding*.

In chunking and checking, the veterinarian gives information in small pieces, pausing and checking for understanding before proceeding and being guided by the client's reactions to see what information is required next. This technique is a vital if indirect component of assessing the client's overall information needs. If you give information in small chunks and give clients ample opportunity to contribute they are more likely to respond with clear signals about what they require.

> Veterinarian: *"So, given the ping I pick up on #301's right side, her rapid heart rate and just how tough she looks right now, I feel confident she has a right displacement that has twisted on itself, putting her in pretty rough shape. We'll need to make a decision whether to do surgery or cull her right away. What are your thoughts on that?"*
> Client: *"Hmm – what do you think her chances are if we do surgery?"*

Assessing the client's starting point

One key interactive approach to giving information to clients involves *assessing the client's prior knowledge*. How can you determine at what level to pitch information unless you take active steps to find out the client's starting point? How can you assess the degree to which your view of the problem differs from that of the client and the approach that you will need to take to achieve mutual understanding unless you discover early on the client's understanding of the issues and problems?

Explaining a new diagnosis of diabetes in a cat to either a university professor or a manual laborer is apparently not the same task, with potentially very different levels of understanding and different capabilities of processing information. However, making this assumption without directly asking for the client's prior knowledge is dangerous. The professor may have almost no understanding of diabetes in cats. The laborer may have looked after a cat with diabetes for several years and have a high level of understanding of the condition. It would therefore be helpful before proceeding too far into a detailed explanation to say:

Veterinarian: *"I don't know how much you know about diabetes in cats."*

Client: *"Well, I know a little about it in people – my best friend at college had it."*

Veterinarian: *"It would be helpful for me to understand a little of what you already know about diabetes from that experience, then I can try to fill in any gaps from there."*

Similarly, it is important to *ascertain each individual client's overall preference for information*. As we have already seen, while many clients wish their veterinarians to provide more information, some would prefer less. How can we discover if a particular client is a seeker or avoider of information? Chunking and checking and asking for clients' questions are indirect approaches to assessing a client's overall information needs. A more direct approach is to ask the client early on in the process:

Veterinarian: *"There's a lot more information that I'd be happy to share with you about hypothyroidism in dogs and our approach to testing for and managing it. Some clients like to know a lot about these things and some prefer to keep it to a minimum – how much information would you prefer?"*

Client: *"Well, I'm not sure I need to hear a lot more right now. Perhaps we can just test him then if you have a pamphlet I can give it to my wife to read."*

or

Veterinarian: *"We have a number of vaccine recommendations that will help keep Trooper safe from diseases he may encounter in his day-to-day life. Some people like to know the ins and outs of how and why we make those recommendations and others just want to get the vaccines and get going. Which fits with your point of view?"*

Client: *"I have heard so much on the news about the problems with vaccines and I don't really know what to think. Could you explain more about what they do and why, and also if they are dangerous to my dog?"*

Lue et al. (2008) found that one in eight pet owners had little or no previous experience caring for a pet. These people will have information needs that are different from those who have substantial previous experience. Also remember that a client's preference and need for information may change over time and from situation to situation. Stoewen et al. (2014b) reinforced this point and showed that when ascertaining a client's preferences/needs regarding cancer, it was important for veterinarians to ask about clients' previous experience with cancer. In large animal practice, Brennan and Christley (2013) showed that cattle producers' understanding of biosecurity may not be constant and could vary over time depending on the messaging that ensues after an outbreak, proximity of the outbreak, and kind of outbreak that occurs. Consequently, the information they need at one time will differ from what they need at another. We need to be aware of these possibilities and not assume that the answer to questions regarding preference and need for information will be the same for all individuals or that it will remain constant for any one individual.

Finding out about the client's prior knowledge and experience are important aspects of assessing their starting point. It is also essential to ascertain clients' attitudes. Taking obesity as an example, Bland and Hill (2011) assert that an owner's attitudes toward obesity, particular feeding or exercise regimes, etc. contribute to the cause of an animal's obesity and a greater understanding of those attitudes on the part of the veterinarian will help the veterinarian work more effectively with the client to treat or prevent the animal's obesity. We continue examining the importance of client attitudes later in this chapter when we take up client motivation.

Asking clients what other information would be helpful

As we have seen clinicians often misconstrue the types of information the client/patient requires. They often do not address the "what has happened, why has it happened, why to me/to my animal(s), why now, what would happen if nothing were done about it?" questions that clients/patients would like to have answered in preference to information about treatment (Helman 1978; Coe et al. 2008).

It is difficult to guess each client's individual needs and asking directly is an obvious way to prevent the omission of important information.

Veterinarian: *"Are there other questions you'd like me to answer or points I haven't covered?"*

Client: *"Do you think she could give it to the other cat – I mean is it infectious?"*

or

Veterinarian: *"We have covered a lot of ground this afternoon in figuring out what is going on with your herd and what we might need to do about it. I want to stop here and ask you what questions have come up for you or what you would like me to explain differently."*

Client: *"Well doc, I think you lost me back where we were talking about why this is happening. I am not sure I understand well enough to share that with my business partners."*

Giving explanations at appropriate times

As we saw in Chapter 3, a common difficulty in veterinary consultations arises from giving advice, information or reassurance prematurely (Stivers 1998) not only during the explanation and planning phase of the consultation but even during history taking. For example, a client who has discovered new lumps on their dog says:

Client: *"Sophie has a couple of new lumps on her side – I was hoping you could check them out. Do you think they'll be okay?"*

Veterinarian: *"I'm sure they're just a couple more lipomas. For a dog at her age, it is not uncommon for them to develop lumps which are just growths of fat. They rarely cause any problems unless they are in a place, and grow large enough, to impede movement."*

You deliver your standard lecture. You then assess the lump and take a fine needle aspirate to discover one of the new lumps contains mast cells. You start back-tracking and feel you have lost the client's confidence.

Veterinarian: *"Ah, despite what I said about them being just growths of fat, one of them is actually what is called a mast cell tumor. We should discuss having it removed as well as sending it off to a specialist to assess how serious it is."*

or

Client: *"I think the calves need antibiotics. We have been losing quite a few to the diarrhea."*

Veterinarian: *"Antibiotics are not going to fix this problem. We need to look at the colostrum protocol …"*

You deliver your standard lecture. You then take more history, find that the protocol is being followed and that, based on the physical examination findings there seems to be a problem with infected umbilicus, which probably does warrant antibiotics. Examination reveals unilateral signs. You start back-tracking and feel you have lost the owner's confidence.

Veterinarian: *"Well, on second thought you might be right with the calves needing antibiotics."*

Instead, you could simply acknowledge the client's question and deal with it later after you have all the facts at your disposal:

Veterinarian: *"I appreciate you letting me know about the new lumps. I hear your concern and I'll make sure to pay particular attention to them during my examination of Sophie. I'll likely take a fine needle aspirate of each lump as well, and then we can discuss what I think they are and what it means for Sophie. Is that okay?"*

Then after you have gathered the relevant information and completed your assessment of the animal:

Veterinarian: *"Coming back to the lumps you were concerned and had questions about – I do have a concern with one of the lumps on her. The fine needle aspirate we took of the lump just behind her left elbow contained what we call mast cells. This is indicative of a mast cell tumor which are very unpredictable growths for dogs. We should discuss having it removed as well as having it sent off to a specialist to assess how serious it is."*

or

Veterinarian: *"I heard your comment and I would like to hold off responding until I take a look at the calves and get a little more information."*

Then after you have looked at the calves:

Veterinarian: *"About treating the calves with antibiotics. I think we have two problems going on. The diarrhea will not be effectively addressed with antibiotics. On the other hand, I think that antibiotics would be helpful to address the belly button infections."*

These examples underscore the importance of giving explanations and engaging in planning at appropriate times. One issue with timing is the temptation to respond to clients' questions fully as soon as they ask them and regardless of where we are in information gathering. Conceptualizing how we time explanation and planning in terms of the tri-level model in Figure 6.1 is helpful here (Riccardi and Kurtz 1983).

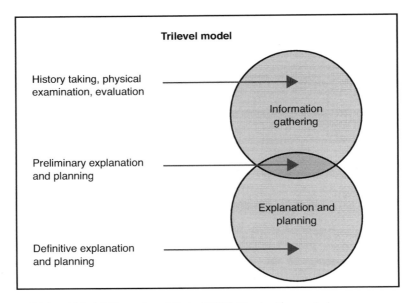

FIGURE 6.1 Tri-Level Model. Riccardi and Kurtz (1983). Used with permission

In this model, preliminary explanation and planning takes into account what is going on in the broader context of what veterinarians are doing. The goals of preliminary explanation and planning are to enhance gathering additional information and to set the stage for later, more complete explanation and planning. These goals are different from those of the full-blown explanation and planning that occurs after completion of history taking and return of results regarding diagnostic procedures and investigations. Preliminary explanation and planning allows the veterinarian to give more limited preliminary information and then to return later to provide more detailed information or to set up a transition for the next steps in the diagnostic process and the planning that will follow. It can be as simple as telling clients what you are doing during physical examination or thanking them for a question and indicating that you would like to answer it later after you have more information. Or preliminary explanation might be given during physical examination to help the client understand abnormalities that you find that might need further investigative tests or more complete explanation later: *"I can feel a small lump on the side of his leg and a few more on his side."* Another kind of example might be if you are called out to see a horse at a boarding facility where the client has concerns about their horse's feet. As you approach the facility you notice that the paddocks are extremely wet. While you are doing the physical examination you might comment out loud to the client that it has been a very rainy month and the fields are very wet. This can lead to gathering further information about length of time the horse is turned out and into which paddock, which then allows you to plan for the horse's care going forward.

Aiding accurate recall and understanding
Underlying concepts

Another important area in explanation and planning is how to give information that can be more easily remembered and understood. In the previous section on providing the correct amount and type of information, we explored the need to move toward a highly interactive, "Frisbee" approach to information giving in order to tailor our message to the needs of the client. But that does not mean that we abandon the lessons learned from the shot-put approach. The way in which we give information can lead to excellent recall and understanding or to an extremely unsatisfactory learning experience.

So how do you achieve the *well-conceived, well-delivered message*? How do you give information so that clients can understand and remember what you say? The old adage from lecturing, "Say what you are going to say, say it and then say what you have said," identifies some of the organizational and structuring tools that can make information giving effective. To these we need to add the appropriate use of language and of visual aids as well as the skills involved in checking for understanding.

Skills that improve recall and understanding

Ley (1988) undertook comprehensive research in human medicine to establish which communication skills could improve patients' recall of information. Many of the skills in this section are based on his seminal work.

Organizing explanation

A key skill to improve recall and understanding is organizing what you want to say so as to avoid giving a large amount of information all at once. A long monologue will produce a strong primacy effect – the client is still thinking about the first point as the next three are being presented and is distracted from listening to later pieces of information. If the aim is to increase recall, understanding and commitment to plans, reducing the likelihood of a primacy effect occurring in the first place is a better way to go.

This can be achieved by chunking and checking, i.e. giving information in small pieces, pausing and checking for understanding before proceeding and being guided by the client's reactions to see what information is required next. Only then is it likely that clients will both recall and understand. As they assimilate each section of information, clients will become ready for the next. This technique is also a vital component of assessing the client's overall information needs. If you give information in small chunks and give the client ample opportunity to contribute, you will generally get clear verbal or nonverbal signals about the amount and type of information the client still requires.

Using explicit categorization: an example of signposting

Categorization is an example of signposting. In this technique, the veterinarian forewarns the client about which categories of information are to be provided and then presents the information category by category:

Veterinarian: *"There are three important things I want to explain. First I want to tell you what I think is wrong, second, what tests we should do and, third, what the treatment might be. First, I think your pet has …"*

or

Veterinarian: *"There are three important things we need to discuss relating to the possible source of your high somatic cell count. First I want to tell you what I think may be wrong, second, what we need to do to investigate it further and, third, what the possible solutions might be. First I think …"*

Ley (1988) demonstrated that recall was higher using this method in both laboratory and clinical experiments, with typical increases in recall rates from 50% to 64%.

There are two processes at work here. The first is the organization of information giving. Categorization allows the information to be divided into discrete sections or "chunks" and enables a logical sequence to be followed. The second is making that categorization explicit to the client. In this case, signposting is the process of explaining to the client where the interview might go next and perhaps why. Providing an overt structure to the consultation reduces uncertainty and anxiety which can otherwise block effective communication and reduce recall and understanding. This is similar to effective lecturers having an outline that they make explicit to their audience at the beginning of the lecture.

Labeling important information: another example of signposting

A more subtle aspect of signposting that Ley emphasized is the primacy effect – that people remember best or perceive to be most important what they are told first. While this primacy effect can make a difference to recall and therefore to adherence, other factors may be more influential in the context of veterinary and human medicine. What if the client remembers exactly what the veterinarian said but has no intention of complying or following through because he has little understanding of the problems involved or commitment to the veterinarian's recommendations:

> *"The veterinarian told me to keep her on antibiotics twice a day for the next ten days; however, she seems fine now, so I stopped them."*
>
> or
>
> *"The veterinarian said to give the insulin twice a day for the foreseeable future. Now that Milo is not using the litter box as much, I think I can maybe give the insulin every few days instead of twice a day."*

Clearly, recall is not everything. And who is to say what is the most "important" information? What the client and veterinarian think is important might be completely different. As Tuckett et al. (1985) found a few years after Ley's research, discovering and addressing each person's very individual needs is one way to overcome this dilemma.

One further message of value here is Ley's finding that it may help if the clinician labels certain pieces of information as important to raise the individual's awareness of the clinician's point of view. This verbal highlighting is an example of another kind of signposting:

> *"This part of the treatment is crucial and failing to follow it could be life-threatening."*
>
> or
>
> *"It is very important to remember this, that you must give the antibiotics two times a day even if she feels better."*

Using repetition and summarizing

Two elements of repetition can make a considerable difference to client recall:

- repetition of important points by the veterinarian
- restatement of information by the client.

In human medicine, repetition by the physician of important points has been shown to be of value in assisting recall (Ley 1988; Kupst et al. 1975). Kupst showed immediate recall to be 76% for single presentation and 90% after physician repetition.

In their study of companion animal and equine veterinarians, Verker et al. (2008) observed client–veterinarian consultations and afterwards asked the veterinarians if they thought the client would comply. Owners completed a questionnaire regarding their opinion about the consultation. Assessing compliance via a telephone survey, the researchers found that 30 clients (52.6%) were compliant. Veterinarians' overestimated their client's compliance significantly. Two variables significantly improved owners' compliance: the veterinarian repeating the most important instructions and explaining the effect of the medication. Of the 13 owners who were given the most important instructions more than once, 76.9% were compliant compared with 45.5% of owners that were given the instructions just once.

Consider this example:

> Veterinarian: *"So just to recap: there does not appear to be any abrasion to the surface of the eye, although it is very irritated. At this point we have agreed to try a topical ointment including an antibiotic and steroid for the next seven days. We plan to have you treat the eye twice a day, around your work schedule. We've also planned for you to bring her back for a recheck seven days from now to see how the eye has come along before you stop treatment."*

Client restatement is also a highly effective technique. Here the veterinarian checks the client's understanding of information given by asking them to restate in their own words what they have understood. The veterinarian then clarifies as necessary. In Kupst's work in human medicine patient restatement achieved 91% immediate recall, which matched physician repetition. However, for recall at 1 month, patient restatement with feedback was shown to be the most effective method. Client restatement has the added benefit of giving you and the client early insight into what the client understands or what you may not have explained well enough.

Restatement also impacts satisfaction. Bertakis (1977) found that when family practice residents were trained in this technique, patients were more satisfied and showed an increase from 61% to 83% in retention of information.

Bravo et al. (2010) also demonstrated that patients leaving the consultation remembered more of the recommendations if they had been asked by the physician to restate them during the consultation.

Fink et al. (2010) looked at enhancing surgical informed consent by adding patient repeat back. This large multi-center, randomized clinical trial showed that patient restatement significantly improved patient understanding following informed consent discussions.

The difficulty of requesting client restatement is all in the phrasing and tone of voice. It is so easy to sound patronizing by implying that the client has limited capacity to understand what the clever veterinarian has said! Practicing phrases that work for you is all important:

Veterinarian: *"I know I've given you a lot of information today and I'm concerned that I might not have made it very clear – it would help me if you repeated back to me what we have agreed on so far so I can make sure we are on the same track."*

or

Veterinarian: *"I know this is a lot of information to take in and that you will need to pass it on to the trainer after we finish here. It would be helpful to me for you to give me a sense of what you think are the important points we have covered so I know we are on the same page."*

Kemp et al. (2008) looked at which approaches to assessing human patients' understanding were preferred and perceived to be most effective by a panel of patients observing pre-prepared videos of physician behaviors. Three options (that we've also seen veterinarians using) were presented:

1. Yes–no: *"I've given you a lot of information. Do you understand?"*
2. Tell back–collaborative: *"I imagine you're really worried about this lump. I've given you a lot of information. It would be helpful to me to hear your understanding about this lump and its treatment."*
3. Tell back–directive: *"It's really important that you do this exactly the way I explained. What do you understand?"*

The "tell back–collaborative" option, involving both patient restatement and a patient-centered approach, was significantly preferred over the other two approaches.

Keller and Kemp-White's (2001) "Ask-Tell-Ask" tool combines asking for client restatement with assessing the client's starting point. First, *ask* the client for their current knowledge. Then *tell* the client information in clear, concise language. Finally, *ask* the client to restate in order to ensure that the client understands and (we would add) that the veterinarian has explained adequately. The Ask-Tell-Ask model has been useful in both human and veterinary medicine.

Using concise, easily understood language

We have seen that the use of jargon is a problem in communication and that clients might be reluctant to ask for clarification for fear of appearing ignorant. It is not just technical language that is the problem as even simple everyday words in a medical context can be ambiguous. An example from human medicine showed that 52% of people thought that a drug prescribed *for* fluid retention would *cause* fluid retention (Mazzullo et al. 1974). Similarly in veterinary medicine, telling a client their animal has been "put to sleep" can be misconstrued, particularly by young children, to mean the animal still has the ability to return to consciousness (i.e. "wake up"). Ley's

(1988) advice for simplifying information to aid recall and understanding continues to be useful:

- reduce the use of jargon
- explain jargon when used
- use shorter words
- use shorter sentences.

Another aspect of language use is to make explanations or advice specific enough for the client to understand or act upon. Ley quotes Bradshaw et al. (1975) to demonstrate that specific statements are more easily recalled than general statements – obese women given dietary advice remembered 16% of general and 51% of specific statements. Making advice more specific clearly works in veterinary situations too. As Kanji et al. (2012) found, adherence to dental and surgical recommendations was seven times greater when the recommendation was clear (i.e. specific versus ambiguous).

As we shall see, additional evidence from human medicine favors a collaborative model of explanation and planning where patients are involved in choices and physicians offer options and suggestions rather than directives. Also relevant to veterinary medicine, this collaborative approach includes making suggestions, eliciting reactions and negotiating. The final step in this process is clarifying *explicitly* what the agreed upon plan involves. How to "be specific" therefore depends upon the complexity of the task. In simple instructions, being specific is relatively easy. Being specific is also relatively easy when there are few instructions. But as complexity increases it becomes more difficult to be specific. For example, when you are conveying the long-term value of regular veterinary healthcare visits for dogs and cats (or on dairy operations the long-term value of participating in a Johne's disease prevention program), it is pointless to ensure excellent recall without attending to client motivation and understanding. Being specific needs to be balanced by the skills associated with accurate understanding, negotiation and motivational interviewing, which we discuss at the end of this chapter.

Using visual methods of conveying information

Many studies in human medicine have shown that the use of diagrams, models, written information and instructions, and audio or video recordings, can improve recall, understanding and adherence (Ley 1988; Tattersall et al. 1997; McConnell et al. 1999; Sowden et al. 2001; Scott et al. 2001; Hack et al. 2007; Minhas 2007; Van der Meulen et al. 2008; De Morgan et al. 2011). Both veterinary and human medicine have promoted the use of written and other visual materials as a way to convey information to clients and patients. This material can be very helpful, but a few cautionary notes are in order with respect to their use:

- Written or audio material does not work well as a stand alone or substitute for interaction with the veterinarian. To optimize its use, veterinarians need to:
  — introduce, follow up and personalize the materials for the individual client

- — set up opportunities for clients to ask questions after they have looked at or listened to it.
- While provision of audio or video recordings of the actual interview, where appropriate, has been shown to improve human patient understanding, recall and follow-through, providing a general audiotape about a condition did not increase recall of information from the interview and in some cases actually decreased recall.
- Audio, video and print materials may be inappropriate when the client is not fluent in the language in which the materials are presented (Brown et al. 2007; Kurtz and Adams 2009).
- Written materials (including written instructions on medications) are inappropriate when the client is functionally illiterate (for illiterate people, this generally includes diagrams as well as the written word). Even in countries where education is widespread, the percentages of functionally illiterate people are much higher than many healthcare professionals realize.

Achieving a shared understanding: incorporating the client's perspective

Underlying concepts

In the above analysis, we have looked in detail at the skills that can be employed to improve clients' recall of information. This approach is concerned primarily with the client's recall and understanding of information and explanations that veterinarians consider to be important. Veterinarians are clearly perceived to be credible and reliable sources of information (Brennan and Cristley 2013; Garforth et al. 2013; Ellis-Iversen 2009; Gunn et al. 2008; Kogan et al. 2008; Kuiper et al. 2005; Ritter et al. 2015). However, as we have already suggested, what the client and veterinarian think is important is not always the same. So looking at what veterinarians think their clients should be told and discovering the best ways to give that information is only half the story. What about the information needs from the client's perspective?

Asking this question does not negate the findings of Kanji et al. (2012), Ley (1988) and others who present important skills that clinicians can use to make information giving clearer and that can lead to better client and patient recall. However, a further analysis is needed of how to match information giving to clients' perspectives and life circumstances. How do you provide information and explanations that relate to the client's perceived needs and their perspectives of the problems or issues? How do you ascertain the client's thoughts about the information that you have given? How do you achieve a shared understanding with your clients?

In previous chapters we presented theoretical and research evidence in support of identifying and acknowledging the client's perspectives as part of initiating the consultation, gathering information and building relationship. Here we look at underlying concepts and research in support of incorporating those perspectives during explanation and planning, and continuing to work at achieving shared understanding between veterinarian and client. Based on this evidence we examine the communication skills that contribute to achieving these important tasks.

What is the evidence to support achieving shared understanding and incorporating the client's perspective?

Described in their book *Meetings Between Experts: An Approach to Sharing Ideas in Medical Consultations* (1985),[13] Tuckett et al.'s research remains central to our understanding of a shared approach to information giving. They studied 1302 consultations conducted by 16 physicians in the UK in considerable depth. Because their findings and methodological approach greatly extended our understanding and challenged previous perceptions about explanation and planning during the consultation, we draw on their findings frequently in this chapter. Tuckett et al. set out with the following three principles in mind:

1. **Not all information is of equal importance.** We need to consider what information has been imparted and whether people can remember and understand the key points rather than simply how much has been imparted and remembered.
2. **Recall does not necessarily imply understanding or commitment** – three outcome measures are important:
   - recall – did the person remember information accurately?
   - understanding – did the person make correct sense of what they were told?
   - commitment – did the person agree with the clinician's key ideas and were these ideas in conflict with the person's own explanatory models?
3. **Information giving needs to be looked at from the patient's (client's) perspective as well as the clinician's.** This idea corresponds to the integrated clinical method model that we explored in Chapter 3 and moves toward the all-important concept of mutually understood common ground.

What does research show about the information given by clinicians?

Looking at human medicine, Tuckett et al. (1985) found that:

- in only a small percentage of occasions were physicians' views presented clearly
- physicians almost never related their explanations to patients' views or beliefs – in only 12 out of 405 consultations were physicians' explanations related to their patients' beliefs at all. In only 6% of consultations were patients' ideas and explanatory beliefs elicited in the first place.
- even when patients volunteered their ideas either as hinted cues or as spontaneous outright statements, physicians still only asked patients to elaborate on their ideas in 7% of consultations; not only were patients not asked to elaborate on their ideas, physicians often evaded them, interrupted them or deliberately inhibited their expression.
- in only 7% of consultations did physicians in any way check their patients' understanding of what had been said.

In summary, Tuckett et al.'s extensive research showed that physicians rarely exhibited

---

13 Researchers may find it particularly useful to look at the methodology that Tuckett et al. used in their extensive study since it represents a useful approach for veterinary medicine that we have seldom applied.

the organizational and other communication skills to make their efforts clear to patients. They also showed little interest in their patients' theories, hypotheses or understanding.

In veterinary medicine a series of three studies (Coe et al. 2007, 2008, 2009) showed that:

- a number of breakdowns in veterinarian communication impacted the clients, including owners feeling that they had not been given all the options, that their concerns had not been heard, and that they were misinformed
- clients wanted their veterinarians to focus on how costs related to future health or function of the pet, but this occurred in only 10 of 58 appointments
- in 38 of 58 appointments with discussions of cost, veterinarians focused on how costs related to their time and service.

Do patients and clients attempt to influence clinicians' information giving and if so, how?

To assess how often patients tried to play an active role in this part of the consultation, Tuckett et al. examined strategies that patients could use to influence the information obtained from their physicians. They found a remarkably high level of participation, although this participation was mostly indirect, using hints and vague questions rather than direct questions or clear statements. In any case, 85% of patients engaged in at least one of the following:

- seeking clarification of a physician's views and instructions
- asking for a physician's reasons and rationales
- expressing doubts
- indicating their own explanatory models.

Rock and Babinec (2010) offer insight into how explanatory models work. Their research shows that people's experience of human illness such as diabetes influences how they regard (can they treat it?) and respond (will they treat it?) to health problems in their companion animals and vice versa. One participant, for example, said that she attributed improvement in managing her own diabetes to properly caring for and treating her dog's diabetes.

When human patients did ask questions or contribute overtly, they were more likely to receive answers and more detailed information (Svarstad 1974; Boreham and Gibson 1978; Roter 1977). Where physicians did not respond positively to patients asking them for their rationale or expressing doubts, patients were more likely to perceive an increase in tension and to characterize the physician's attitudes and behavior as evasive.

Patients and clients can exert considerable control over how their physicians and veterinarians interact and think and are wise to ask questions openly rather than covertly if they wish to receive more information. In his popular book, *How Doctors Think*, Jerome Groopman (2007) offers another interesting take on question asking.

He identifies three important questions that patients could ask their physicians, to augment physicians' clinical reasoning process and reduce potential cognitive errors:

- What else could it be?
- Is it possible that more than one thing could be going on?
- Is there anything that is at odds with what you are thinking this is?

What would happen if veterinarians asked these questions of themselves consistently during the clinical reasoning process or if we taught veterinary clients to ask these questions of their veterinarians?

Roter (1977) and Kaplan et al. (1989) found that more patient question asking led to increased physician anxiety and anger, although this was interpreted as an indication of being engaged rather than a negative finding. Nevertheless we wonder if this is one reason clinicians do not make more space for their clients and patients to participate.

Do patients and clients feel they would like to ask their physicians and veterinarians questions, and if so why don't they do so more overtly?

In Tuckett et al.'s research, 76% of the patients said afterwards that they had specific doubts or questions during the interview that they did not mention to the physician. Only 19% of patients who exhibited gaps in their knowledge said that they did not ask questions because they were not interested in the answer. Patients in the study gave the following reasons for their behavior:

- not up to them to ask questions, express doubts or behave as if their view was important (36%)
- afraid of being thought less well of by the physician (22%)
- frightened of a negative reaction from the physician (14%)
- too flustered or hurried to ask coherently (27%)
- doubted that the physician could tell them any more at the moment (22%)
- forgot or waiting until next time to ask when they were more certain if what they thought was reasonable to ask (36%)
- fear of the truth (9%).

Anecdotally, we have observed many instances in veterinary medicine where clients ask or tell the receptionist or veterinary technician something important that they did not take up with the veterinarian. The reasons appear to be very similar to those identified with human patients. Consider also the finding in the study of small animal and equine veterinarians done by Verker et al. (2008) that in none of the 57 consultations in the study were owners explicitly asked whether they had questions.

In an Australian study of communication in a human medical emergency department that combined observation with analysis of audiotapes and transcripts, Slade et al. (2008) showed that overwhelmingly physicians asked questions and patients answered. This pattern of physicians' questions dominating occurred not only during history taking but throughout the encounter. With little opportunity to deviate from the question/answer structure, patients and their families rarely asked any questions, suggesting that they did not think it appropriate for them to ask questions or felt too intimidated by the context to do so.

Tying together the findings throughout this section, it appears that the more traditional clinician-centered approach too easily compromises communication. When clinicians ask questions and clients answer, when clients' passive role is confirmed, and when little space is made for clients to respond in other ways, shared understanding is unlikely to occur.

Can clinicians positively influence clients' and patients' participation to ensure a shared understanding?

We have already seen that the more active patients are in the consultation, the more likely they are to obtain the information that they would like. There is also no doubt that clinicians can enable clients and patients to take a more active role. Svarstad (1974) showed that physicians who avoided certain inhibiting behaviors enabled their patients to ask more questions. Inhibiting behaviors included: clock-watching, use of jargon, mumbling incomprehensibly, interrupting, ignoring patients' comments, unfriendliness, ending consultations precipitately. More recently, Dysart et al. (2011) showed that the mean length of time clients spoke before veterinarians interrupted was 15.3 seconds (range 1 to 130 seconds) and that when veterinarians did not interrupt, clients raised more concerns and talked more about what was on their minds.

Do clients and patients make correct sense of explanations?

Surprisingly, Tuckett et al. (1985) found no relationship at all between the clarity of explanation given by the physician and whether patients made correct sense of the physicians' comments! However, attempts to correlate the value of mutual sharing of perspectives to patient understanding did produce evidence of a relationship. Consultations in which the physician inhibited or evaded their patients' ideas were more likely to result in a failure of recall and understanding than those in which physicians did not inhibit or evade. This suggested that paying attention to the patient's explanatory framework increased understanding. In this study it was not possible to assess other aspects of mutual sharing because physicians so rarely demonstrated the appropriate skills required. Patients' understanding was so rarely checked and clarified by the physician, patients' ideas and beliefs were so infrequently actively discovered, and the rationales given were so rarely related to patients' explanatory beliefs that their effect on understanding could not be ascertained.

The key to the problem of understanding appeared to be the detailed ideas that the patient brought to bear on the explanation of the physician – if there was a match with the physician's explanation, good understanding ensued, even if the explanation by the physician had been unclear or sparse. However, if there was a mismatch in the physician's and the patient's explanatory frameworks, understanding was likely to suffer. Not surprisingly it is more difficult to assimilate information that is unfamiliar, unexpected or threatening. In those instances ambiguous or disorganized information giving on the part of clinicians is likely to be particularly unhelpful. If views are divergent and that is overtly discovered, acknowledged and taken into account in subsequent explanation and planning, that, too, is likely to result in better understanding and follow-through.

Are people committed to the clinician's view?

Research from human medicine is helpful here. Tuckett et al. (1985) found that the overwhelming majority (75%) of patients who remembered and made sense of information that they were given were also committed to the physician's views. Consultations in which the physician inhibited or evaded their patients' ideas were more likely to result in lack of commitment to the physician's views than consultations in which physicians did not evade or inhibit patients' ideas. The qualitative analysis showed a major difference between those patients who were committed to a physician's view and those who were not. Those committed usually expected what they heard and already agreed with it. However, if the patient started out with views divergent from the physician, the consultations appeared to do little to change them. Patients rejected their physician's views in favor of their own. As physicians rarely paid attention to patients' ideas, the physicians remained uninformed about their patient's thinking and could not direct explanations precisely to it. Tuckett et al. firmly believe that without establishing what ideas the patient has, there is no possibility of a mutual exchange of views and without this there is little likelihood of increasing commitment.

Tuckett et al. concluded that there is a need for two concerted approaches to encourage success in our goals of patient recall, understanding and commitment:

- clarity, so that the patient can understand what is said and comprehend if there is a difference between the physician's and their own beliefs
- exploration of the patient's beliefs and ideas together with checking the patient's interpretation and reaction to information given. The physician needs to be willing to explore the differences in viewpoint and negotiate a shared explanatory model.

Tuckett et al. suggest that we need to change our approach to explanation and planning to enable a "meeting of experts," an explicit sharing of our explanatory models between two parties with different expertise, one of the medical world and one of the unique experience of the individual. It is clear from the work summarized here that differences in explanatory framework lead to poorer understanding and commitment. Nogueria Borden et al. (2010) found this to be true in veterinary medicine as well. In their study, veterinarians in clinical practice did little exploration of unannounced simulated clients' feeling, ideas and expectations. Consequently it was difficult for the veterinarians to make informed recommendations and formulate a treatment plan that was in the best interests of the client and patient.

Does incorporating the client's perspectives improve understanding and follow-through?

We are still left with the partially unanswered question: if we do elicit our clients' conflicting ideas, take them into account and explain our findings in relation to them, will we improve our clients' understanding, commitment and decisions that are in the best interest of their animal(s)? We have reported some literature responding to this question positively earlier in this chapter and in Chapter 5. A number of additional studies confirm these findings and are helpful.

A Canadian study of 90 consultations showed that dog owners were nine times more likely to be 100% compliant when medications were required once or twice a day versus three times a day (Adams et al. 2005). Based on their findings the researchers made two recommendations to improve compliance: a) ask about the client's lifestyle and home situation to help in choosing a dosing regime that the client is able to follow, and b) check in with the client after the consultation to ask in a non-judgmental way if the client had any trouble with administration of the prescribed medications or had missed any doses.

In their study assessing how veterinarians and clients discuss cost, Coe et al. (2007) suggested that while cost discussions may be challenging, veterinarians can minimize these challenges by exploring the client's belief systems and other perspectives and by improving veterinarian communication. Such exploration puts veterinarians in a better position to recognize and address differences between the client's and the veterinarian's views.

A study by Stoewen et al. (2014b) showed that in small animal oncology information presented forthrightly and without "sugar coating" along with veterinarians taking a client's individual expectations and preferences into account helped to build trust. In turn, this approach enhanced client's confidence necessary to engage in treatment and influenced client's ability to make decisions, face uncertainties and follow through with treatment plans.

In a study by Jansen et al. (2010) 24 farmers that were identified as "hard to reach" with udder health information and uptake of this information took part in a qualitative interview study. The interviews revealed four kinds of "hard to reach" farmers – do-it-yourselfers, proactivists, reclusive traditionalists, and wait-and-seers. The findings suggest that hard-to-reach farmers may not be as difficult to reach as veterinarians often assume.

In a study of 336 Dutch dairy farms, Jansen et al. (2009) report a relationship between farmers' attitudes and mastitis incidence – only when the farmer regards mastitis incidence on their farm as problematic will they take action. A second finding of the study is that farmers' perception of what is "normal" and what constitutes a problem varies. If you are looking for compliance and improved farm management, you have to ask about the farmer's perceptions and tailor your explanation and planning to respond to that farmer's point of view.

In conjunction with a 5-year mastitis program of the Dutch Udder Health Centre, Lam et al. (2011) suggest that "… farmers are fundamentally willing to participate in all kinds of activities but have not been approached in an optimal way, and thus do not participate in study groups or advisory programs on udder health." They add that it would behoove veterinarians to invest in a client-oriented approach and hone their communication skills.

Based on what they discovered in their study regarding Johne's disease and its control, Roche et al. (2016, in review) concluded that veterinarians need to focus on the producer's perspectives and tailor the information they give and their recommendations accordingly. Taking the producers' perspectives into account in this way will in turn make recommended changes more meaningful, doable and sustainable.

In a UK study Garforth et al. (2013) used semi-structured interviews to collect data from nine sheep and six pig enterprises. They found that tailoring risk communication to the different types of livestock farmers and improving communication about risk in the farming press and from veterinarians could increase uptake of disease risk measures.

Heffernan et al. (2008) conducted a qualitative study with 121 cattle and sheep farmers in the UK regarding biosecurity behavior among farmers. They found that even though veterinarians were the primary source of information about biosecurity measures the study participants report that veterinarians were an "occasional" rather than a regular source of information and assistance. Within an outbreak situation, the communication pathways between the veterinarian and the farmer were unlikely to be sufficiently strong to forge high levels of cooperation and behavioral change on the part of the farmer. Heffernan et al. suggest that greater attention needs to be paid to the frequency of contact between farmer and veterinarian not only during but before an outbreak situation occurs.

Eisenthal and Lazare 1976 (see Chapter 3) demonstrated that if physicians in a psychiatric walk-in clinic discovered patients' expectations, those patients were more likely to feel satisfied and to adhere to plans whether their requests were granted or not. In other words, we do not discover expectations just so that we can give people what they want but so that we can base our negotiation on an open understanding of our respective positions. Applied to veterinary medicine, it is not finding out whether the client wants an MRI for her dog and going along with her wishes that is important but finding out the client's ideas and expectations, explaining your position in relation to the client's views and reaching a negotiated plan acceptable to both you and the client.

Inui et al. (1976) showed that discovering human patients' perspectives and using them to achieve shared understanding improved adherence and outcomes of care.

In another outcome study that we describe in more detail in the next section of this chapter, Kaplan et al. (1989) coached patients to voice their questions and concerns in the medical interview. They found that the subsequent change in patient behavior not only produced a dramatic difference to what happened during the interview but also led to improved physiological outcomes, likely because recall, understanding, explicit common ground and adherence were better.

Tuckett et al.'s concept from human medicine regarding "sharing of explanatory models" and Rock and Babinec's finding from veterinary medicine that human sicknesses may serve as prototypical analogies for companion animal sicknesses and that pet sicknesses may become linked through prototypes to human health issues fit very well with the integrated clinical method model and the concept of mutually understood common ground as discussed in Chapter 3.

Keeping conclusions about clarity and shared explanatory models in mind, how do we make the lessons that we have learned from the research above come alive? How do we put them into practice in the consultation? Again the analogy of the lecture helps. The most interactive approach to lecturing is the "learner-centered lecture." Here, in addition to:

- tailoring the presentation to the learners' needs by chunking and checking and assessing the learners' starting point (Frisbee approach)
- paying attention to structure and organization, language and visual aids (shot-put approach)

the lecturer also deliberately encourages the audience to brainstorm their doubts, concerns and expectations early on in the proceedings. Then as the lecture continues, the lecturer repeatedly:

- refers to the learners' doubts and expectations
- checks the response to what they are saying by reading the verbal and nonverbal cues of the audience
- deliberately asks for the audience's reactions to what they are saying.

Note that the lecturer has to be much more flexible here to accommodate the audience's needs and has to be very careful to use structuring and organizational tools at appropriate times to prevent the lecture from becoming too random and disorganized – in other words, as you implement more interactive approaches take care not to lose the useful aspects of the shotput approach.

So far so good. However, the Frisbee approach at its most powerful occurs not in the large group context of a lecturer talking with an entire audience but in the interpersonal context of two or three individuals communicating with each other as partners and collaborators. The Frisbee approach, then, connotes even greater possibilities for interaction and relationship. In the context of the veterinary consultation, it is not just about what the veterinarian says but equally about what the client says. All of the lessons learned from the learner-centered lecture analogy continue to apply but we have even greater opportunity for flexibility and interaction; for veterinarian and client to hear each other, respond to each other and achieve a more shared understanding; and for clearly establishing mutually understood common ground.

Skills for achieving shared understanding with clients
Relating explanations to the client's perspective

In Chapter 3, we discussed gathering information and saw how discovering the client's perspective was an essential component of the effective veterinary consultation. Discovering the client's ideas, concerns, expectations and feelings contributed to the client feeling more supported and understood while at the same time it helped in making an accurate diagnosis and a more effective and efficient interview.

However, perhaps the most important benefit of discovering the client's perspective is the effect this has on explanation and planning. Recall, understanding, satisfaction and adherence are all likely to suffer when an explanation does not address the client's individual ideas, expectations and concerns.

So early on in this phase of the interview, we need to start to relate our explanations to the client's perspectives that we elicited when gathering information:

> Veterinarian: *"When we started this consultation, you brought up a concern about parasite resistance in your flock. That is a completely reasonable concern and something we always need to keep in mind. Fortunately, I don't think that is the case right now and here is why …"*
>
> or
>
> Veterinarian: *"You mentioned earlier that you were concerned that he might have fleas. … Based on your previous experience I can see why you might have thought that. Given what you have told me and my assessment, I think he is more likely to have mange which I'd like to follow up on moving forward. … Let me explain why and what this means."*

Providing opportunities and encouraging the client to contribute

If the first stage of achieving a shared understanding is to provide explanations that relate to the client's perspective, the second stage is discovering and addressing the client's thoughts and feelings about the information that you are in the process of giving. An essential element of this is providing opportunities for the client to ask questions, seek clarification or express doubts. Veterinarians have to be very explicit here – some clients are reluctant to express what they are thinking and are hesitant to ask questions. Unless positively invited to do so, clients may well leave the consultation with their questions unanswered and a reduced understanding and commitment to plans:

> Veterinarian: *"Is there something else you would like to discuss or something you would like to discuss further?"*

Then of course the veterinarian must respond appropriately – without validation and interest from the veterinarian, clients may think that their own views are unimportant and tend to revert to a more passive role:

> Veterinarian: *"Yes that is an important question – I'm glad you asked that – I'll try to answer it for you …"*

Picking up and responding to verbal and nonverbal cues

Another means of discovering the client's thoughts and feelings is to try to pick up the client's cues, both verbal and nonverbal. Remember that most people in medical contexts use indirect or oblique hints to express their doubts or questions rather than overt statements or questions. The veterinarian must therefore search for more subtle cues indicating that the client may wish to contribute information or ask questions, that they may be feeling overwhelmed with information or are becoming frustrated:

> Veterinarian: *"You look unsure – what are you thinking about in terms of the surgery option that I just mentioned for Kiwi?"*

Eliciting client's beliefs, reactions and concerns

In addition to picking up cues, it is important to actively seek out the client's reactions to the discussion that you are having by asking explicitly for their beliefs, reactions and concerns and then acknowledging and addressing them as necessary:

> Veterinarian: *"I'm not sure how that news has left you feeling ..."*
>
> or
>
> *"Does that leave you with concerns or doubts?"*
>
> or
>
> *"You have a lot to process and unfortunately, given your horse's condition, you have to do that quickly. If there are lingering doubts or concerns you have, it might be useful to bring them up in case they may be useful when we are deciding how to proceed."*

Planning: shared decision making

Following on from explanation comes planning. Not only have there been advances in how clinicians give information, there have also been considerable moves in human and recently veterinary medicine to involve human patients/clients more explicitly in planning and decision making. Researchers, educators, professional groups, insurance companies, industry, ethicists, and clinicians, clients and human patients themselves have increasingly advocated shared decision-making models incorporating partnership, negotiation and mutual collaboration. What is the evidence behind these initiatives?

Underlying concepts

Shared decision making is important to veterinary medicine. Nonetheless, this aspect of communication in veterinary medicine has not yet received the research attention it deserves. Therefore, in this section of the book we rely on concepts and research evidence drawn from the literature in human medicine. We invite veterinary students, educators and practitioners to weigh and consider the applicability of these concepts and findings to veterinary practice. Moreover, we invite researchers to consider, as well, the research questions and methods summarized here that might be usefully applied to research on shared decision making in veterinary medicine.

Many writers over the past 40 years have supported the concept of a collaborative approach to planning. For example, Brody (1980) suggests four steps necessary to encourage people to participate in decision making. These suggestions bring together many of the ideas that are advocated throughout this book. Although Brody framed these in terms of human medicine, we have taken the liberty of applying them to veterinary medicine, since they are equally applicable there:

1. Establishing an atmosphere conducive to participation where contributions are welcomed and where the clients' ideas and questions are actively sought.
2. Ascertaining the clients' reasons for seeing the veterinarian and their goals and expectations.
3. Giving appropriate information about the nature of the problem, including the veterinarian's rationale, possible alternatives, their advantages and disadvantages, and suggested recommendations (rather than directives).
4. Eliciting the client's suggestions and preferences and negotiating any disagreements.

Stewart et al. (1997) support mutuality, collaboration and partnership in their model of patient-centered medicine. So, too, does the Pew-Fetzer Task Force document (Tresolini and the Pew-Fetzer Task Force 1994) on relationship-centered care.

It's helpful to look at a few additional models on which shared decision making has been based. Roter and Hall (1992) in their book *Doctors Talking With Patients/ Patients Talking with Doctors* describe four possible models of the doctor–patient relationship that also relate to veterinary–client relationships (here and with the Charles et al. model that follows, we have taken the liberty to adapt the language to fit veterinary medicine):

- The *paternalistic model* is characterized by high veterinarian/low client control. The veterinarian makes decisions which they consider to be in the best interest of the client; the client cooperates with the advice and does as they are told. At certain times, this style of relationship is welcomed by the client, such as when there is a dire emergency.
- *Consumerism* is the other extreme. Here, there is low veterinarian/high client control. The veterinarian simply does whatever the client wants. There are problems here too, for example if the client's requests are outside normal practice or if they are not in the patient's best interests. In a system in which a) clients as consumers can exert their choice to go to another veterinarian until they find one who will accommodate their requests and b) the veterinarian's income is dependent on attracting more clients and performing more tasks, good medical practice can be sacrificed on the altar of consumerism and financial incentive.
- *Default or laissez faire* describes a model in which no one takes responsibility, where both veterinarian and client have low control and the relationship becomes aimless and unproductive for both parties.
- In the *mutuality model* there is both high veterinarian and high client control.

Clients' preferences are actively sought and compared explicitly to veterinarians' thoughts; veterinarians explain their reasoning in relation to clients' ideas. Open negotiation leads to a meeting of minds between two more equal parties and to the production of a mutually agreed upon collaborative plan. A client can openly explain which option they might prefer or why they might not be able to follow a particular course of action. Similarly, the veterinarian can openly discuss their own dilemmas, explain why a client's suggestion is not to the patient's advantage and why the veterinarian may not feel able to fulfill it. Often, both veterinarian and client perspectives can be accommodated with minor adjustment. In a more veterinarian-centered approach to planning, such doubts may not surface during the interview but appear later on, after the veterinarian has left.

Charles et al. (Charles et al. 1997, Charles et al. 1999a, Charles et al. 1999b) advocated a shared decision-making model. They contrasted three possible positions:

- The *paternalistic approach* as just described.
- *Informed choice* in which a partnership exists but is based on a strict division of labor – here the veterinarian's role is information giving only. The veterinarian goes first and provides sufficient information on all relevant treatment options, their benefits, and risks. Now it is the client's turn. At this point the client has both the information and the personal preferences required for decision making. The client deliberates alone and makes a choice.
- In contrast, the *shared decision making model* is more interactional in nature in that the veterinarian and the client share all stages in the decision-making process. In the shared decision model, there is instead a two-way exchange of information (including the technical information that *both* veterinarian and client bring to the interview and the client's ideas, concerns and expectations). Both parties talk about their treatment preferences and after discussion both agree on a decision to be implemented. Veterinarian and client alike have a legitimate investment in decisions made. As in the informed choice approach, the full sharing of information is essential but now leads on to a further stage of shared decision making – these are separate components of the explanation and planning phase of the interview requiring separate skills.

In the shared decision-making model, it is perfectly acceptable for the veterinarian to have a preference as long as they clearly signpost that the client's position is equally as important as the veterinarian's. However, as Elwyn et al. (2000) pointed out it is equally possible that the physician is in a position of "equipoise," and genuinely does not have a preference for which option the patient might choose. Whether in a position of equipoise or of preference, clinicians should not disapprove of the decision the patient/client eventually chooses – it is the discussion that is all important.

Although the research shows that shared decision making results in better adherence and follow-through, each of the approaches described above has its place depending on the context, preferences of the client and the needs of the animals. For example, there are times when shared decision making is not what is called for, such as when the animal's welfare is at stake and you as the clinician feel you must disapprove of certain options, where you want to take a more directive stance. Or initially during a life-threatening emergency when you must deal immediately with the animal. Your approach then may no longer be full-blown shared decision making, although even here you need to obtain consent before proceeding.

Referred to by a variety of different terms, the shared decision-making approach is beginning to take hold in veterinary medicine (Institute for Healthcare Communication, Veterinary Communication Project 2004; Cornell and Kopcha 2007; Coe et al. 2008; Jansen et al. 2010; Yeates and Main 2010) and is widely advocated in human medicine (Hope 1996; Braddock et al. 1997; Coulter et al. 1999; Elwyn et al. 1999a,b; Towle and Godolphin 1999; Holmes-Rovner et al. 2000; Edwards and Elwyn 2001a, b; Godolphin et al. 2001; Ford et al. 2003; Schofield et al. 2003; Trevena and Barratt 2003; Epstein et al. 2004; Makoul and Clayman 2006; Price et al. 2012).

Further approaches to encouraging patient/client participation and involvement have concentrated on the patient's and client's rather than the clinician's role and have used methods of enabling human patients and clients to prepare for or participate in the consultation (Tuckett et al. 1985; Kaplan et al. 1989; Middleton 1995; Health Canada 1996; Korsch and Harding 1997; Institute for Health Care Communication (1999); Fleissig et al. 2000; Cegala 2003; Dimoska et al. 2008) by, for instance:

- asking them to prepare lists of issues to discuss before the interview
- providing prompt cards or reminders of useful questions
- providing information about how to get the best out of the visit to the doctor
- asking them to fill in a diet history form
- asking them to keep a herd health plan.

Concordance – yet another approach to explanation, planning and decision making – is also worth considering here. Concordance emphasizes the reality that at the end of the day it is the patient (or client) who decides how or if they will follow through with medication or other treatment plans (Dowell et al. 2002; Britten 2003). Concordance is an attempt to admit that we might be colluding about what really is going to happen. In reality clients and patients make their own decisions about whether to follow recommendations or plans based on their beliefs, experiences and the information available to them at the time. They have their own rational discourse within themselves, based on their perceptions and experience and with others outside the medical arena that can be different and more wide-ranging than the particular focus of medicine. Concordance may resonate particularly well in veterinary contexts where, for example, euthanasia is an option that owners can request at any time or in the food animal industry where animals are often viewed as commodities or deemed property and owners make decisions to cull or keep them alive based on economic factors.

Industries in veterinary medicine, such as pharmaceutical companies and pet food companies, are highly engaged and possibly influential in terms of practice owner choices regarding what products to market and suggest to clients. For that matter many pressures are put upon clinicians that influence their decision making and recommendations regarding appropriate practice and treatment. These additional pressures may come from economic or business considerations, licensing bodies, insurers, and societal interests. Such external pressures may or may not be in line with what the client is thinking or prefers or what seems to be the best path from a medical perspective (Donovan 1995; Bonnett, pers. comm. 2015).

But do clinicians routinely engage in shared decision making or concordance? The evidence in human medicine suggests that current practice has not embraced these concepts. (Makoul et al. 1995; Stevenson et al. 2000; Elwyn et al. 2003b; Campion et al. 2002; Richard and Lussier 2003; Cohen and Britten 2003; Ford et al. 2006; Edwards et al. 2005; Young et al. 2008; Hanson 2008; Karnieli-Miller and Eisikovits 2009; Coulter 2009; Godolphin 2009; Sonntag et al. 2012). Indeed, based on a literature review and their own clinical and educational experience, Weiner and Roth (2006) point out that during discussions with patients and their families regarding goals of care near the end of life, some unintended but common physician communication behaviors may inadvertently impair shared decision making. Similarly in a study of veterinary–client communication about end-of-life decisions, Nogueira Borden et al. (2010) found that veterinarians often missed or inadvertently disregarded cues that clients gave about what the clients wanted to discuss, thereby potentially impairing decision making.

What research evidence do we have that demonstrates the efficacy of collaborative approaches to decision making?

In veterinary medicine, we know collaboration improves veterinarian and client satisfaction and agreement to proceed with dental or surgical procedures and that both of these elements are likely to enhance patient well-being and the economics of the practice (Coe 2008; Kanji et al. 2012; Shaw et al. 2012a). As discussed earlier in the chapter, a collaborative approach that includes the client's perspective influences client adherence and follow-through which in turn has an indirect effect on patient outcomes. Beyond these important findings, there is little outcome research on shared decision making in veterinary medicine. To highlight key messages, we present several relevant studies from human medicine here.

Further to their work on the relationship between eliciting patient expectations and subsequent patient satisfaction, Eisenthal et al. (1979) demonstrated that higher levels of negotiation and patient participation in the decision-making process are associated with both increased adherence and satisfaction. By a negotiated approach, the authors meant eliciting patients' expectations and requests for care, actively negotiating treatment plans and checking negotiated plans to see if the patient agrees with them. Veterinarians can use these same techniques with their clients.

Schulman (1979) found that hypertensive patients who were more actively involved in treatment programs had higher rates of adherence and more favorable treatment outcomes. Active involvement was defined as viewing themselves as collaborative partners, being involved in two-way communication and joint decision making, being informed of treatment rationales and being encouraged to voice opinions and report side effects.

In a series of studies, Kaplan et al. (1989, 1996) found that active patients (i.e. those who participated more actively in the consultation regarding their perspectives and ideas, asked questions, were involved in decision making, discussed their feelings, etc.) were consistently more likely to understand and follow through with recommendations, which then resulted in higher satisfaction and better health outcomes.

These findings confirm an earlier study by Roter (1977) which found that a simple 10-minute intervention prior to patients' consultations in primary care in which patients were helped to ask questions of their physicians led to a doubling of questions asked, a feeling of increased patient control and responsibility for their own health, and less drop-out from follow-up. Consider how little time it would take to coach clients to be more active during veterinary consultations.

Shepherd et al. (2011) tested the effect of a set of three simple questions asked by unannounced simulated patients to general practitioners. These questions were:

- What are my options?
- What are the possible benefits and harms of those options?
- How likely to occur are the benefits and harms of each option?

They demonstrated that asking these three questions improved information given by family physicians and increased physician facilitation of patient involvement without any increase in time.

In a review of evidence on patient–doctor communication, Stewart et al. (1999) found that the following aspects of communication about the management plan significantly influenced health outcomes:

- patient being encouraged to ask questions
- provision of clear information
- willingness of physician to share decision making
- agreement between patient and physician about the problem and the plan.

In a more recent selective review of the literature regarding patient engagement, including shared decision making, Coulter (2012) described 24 interventions that have been shown to support shared decision making and identified the evidence base behind those interventions. Based on her review of the literature she concluded that there is a compelling case for adapting medical practice styles to make it possible for patients to engage more actively in planning and shaping their healthcare.

Do all individuals want to be involved in shared decision making?

As with information giving, a proportion of people will not wish to have active involvement and will prefer to leave decisions to their clinicians. It is a mistake to assume that everyone wishes to be involved in a collaborative approach to planning (Cassileth et al. 1980; Strull et al. 1984; Blanchard et al. 1988; Ende et al. 1989; Sutherland et al. 1989; Beisecker and Beisecker 1990; Hack et al. 1994; Guadagnoli and Ward 1998; Levinson et al. 2005).

In Gattellari et al.'s (2001) study of cancer patients, mismatch between patients' preferred roles in decision making and what they perceived actually happened led to increased patient anxiety. However, whatever the preference of the patient prior to the interview, satisfaction with the consultation and the amount of information and emotional support received were all significantly greater for patients who reported a shared role. This gives support to the concept that as well as respecting individual differences in patient preference, part of the physician's role might include gentle encouragement of patients over time to take part in shared decision making. Patients may not understand the benefits they stand to gain from articulating their preferences to their clinician.

In their systematic review of 115 studies on patient preferences for shared decisions, Chewning et al. (2012) demonstrated that the number of patients who prefer participation in decision making has increased over the past three decades – patients preferred a role in decision making in 50% of studies before 2000, compared to 71% from 2000 and later. All of the studies in the review also identified a subset of patients who want to delegate decisions. However, the majority of patients still want to discuss options and receive information from their physician even though they may not wish to make the final decision.

Based on focus group discussions and survey interviews with 1068 patients in the USA, Novelli et al. (2012) found that 9 out of 10 patients agreed overall that they want to know all their options; nearly half strongly agreed that they wanted to discuss the option of doing nothing. However, far fewer people said that they were offered options in comparison to the number that wanted to discuss them. Patients reported a better experience when they were actively engaged. Similarly, the AAHA study (2003) of over 1000 pet owners that we described earlier in this chapter showed that 90% of pet owners wanted to know all their options.

The approach that we advocate here is not to make assumptions but to openly ask about clients' preferences for involvement in the process of shared decision making. Even if the client does not wish to be involved in decision making at the moment, such a discussion will alert the client that this is an option that they can return to in the future without criticism from the veterinarian. The question that we need to address is *how* to discover each client's individual wishes rather than making assumptions.

Although older patients, less educated patients and those with more serious illnesses have in past studies been more likely to prefer a non-participatory role (Degner and Sloan 1992; Belcher et al. 2006), many of them will choose to be informed and involved. In a qualitative study in 11 European countries, Bastiaens et al. (2007) demonstrated that older patients do want to be involved in their care but their definition of involvement is more focused on the "caring relationship," "person-centered approach" and "receiving information" than on "active participation in decision making." Older patients considered involvement as "taking time to elicit their preferences and needs and enabling them to take an active role in caring for their health accordingly." However, the authors also comment that older patients wish for involvement in decision making is highly heterogeneous so an individual approach for each patient in the ageing population is needed. In their focus group study looking at older adults' views on informed decision making (IDM), Price et al. (2012) found that participants overwhelmingly endorsed existing criteria for shared decision making and added the importance of also involving other people (family members, friends and others).

Since a patient's preferences for participation and information may vary depending on the nature or stage of the illness (Beaver et al. 1996; Chewning et al. 2012), preferences need to be discussed periodically over time and from situation to situation. Discovering someone's preference for participation in decision making is an ongoing task rather than a one-off assessment made at a single meeting.

What skills can we recommend to help veterinarians achieve shared decision making in planning?

A collaborative approach to planning requires the use of many skills throughout the consultation (Towle and Godolphin 1999; Elwyn et al. 2003b; Fallowfield 2008). A key challenge for veterinarians is to create an environment in which the client feels comfortable to engage in this collaborative process in the first place. The skills of relationship building and development of a partnership as discussed in Chapter 5 are therefore all important here. The discussion above has suggested a number of useful techniques to set the stage for shared decision making. But what additional specific skills can we use in this part of the consultation to enable the theory and research on shared decision making to be translated into clinical practice?

Sharing your own thinking as appropriate: ideas, thought processes and dilemmas

One specific skill that contributes to a more collaborative approach to planning is for veterinarians to share their thought processes, ideas and dilemmas as appropriate. Sharing your thinking offers advantages to veterinarian and client alike:

- Uncertainty is reduced and mutually understood common ground established. The client begins to understand the rationale behind the veterinarian's suggestions and what the dilemmas in a particular situation are. The client is not left guessing why you are proceeding along a certain path. Although close to half of the 100 veterinarians surveyed in a British study (Mellanby et al. 2007) thought that discussion about uncertainty would reduce client confidence, almost all of the 274 clients (95%) wanted to know about uncertainties that the veterinarian might have regarding diagnosis or treatment. Less than 20% of the clients indicated that they would have had less confidence in a veterinarian who expressed uncertainty.
- It encourages the client to contribute their views. Sharing your ideas is a signal that you might be interested in hearing your client's, thus encouraging more open communication, particularly if you make space for clients to participate.
- It forces you to organize your information giving. Veterinarians often skip over informing clients about diagnosis, etiology and prognosis and go straight to treatment – the sharing approach helps prevent the omission of logical steps or information that clients need if they are to participate effectively in decision making and follow through with plans made.

Veterinarian: *"Given the number of cows off feed and DAs [displaced abomasums] you've had this summer, I'm thinking it's time to take a closer look at your transition program and TMR [total mixed ration]. What do you think?"*

or

> "*There are dozens of causes of colic. Part of what our diagnostics do is help us clarify which of these causes might be the issue here. Right now, based on what we have found in terms of the reflux and pain level, the best treatment is a little murky. Some of the cases that act like this can be managed medically and do well while others will require surgery to improve. What I am thinking right now, based on what you have told me about your concerns and priorities, is that we have a few options*"

Involving the client

OFFERING SUGGESTIONS AND CHOICES RATHER THAN DIRECTIVES

In order to involve the client in the decision-making process, the veterinarian needs to outline the possible management options that they think are available, rather than proposing one particular course of action:

> Veterinarian: "*Given what you have said, I think there are two choices available for Lady that we ought to consider together – one is to try her on an allergy diet and eliminate all other forms of food to explore whether it is a food allergy causing her issues or, a second option is for me to refer you to a specialist for allergy testing which would explore a much broader range of possible allergies. What do you think?*"
>
> or
>
> "*We have a couple of different options for how to approach your goal of decreasing the number of respiratory cases we are seeing each month at the new feedlot. Obviously, what we decide on needs to fit within the management changes you are planning for the operation as a whole.*"

ENCOURAGING THE CLIENT TO CONTRIBUTE THEIR IDEAS AND SUGGESTIONS

The veterinarian can actively encourage the client to contribute their ideas and suggestions too. The client may well have options in mind that the veterinarian has not considered. Remember that many clients are reluctant to express their views directly to the veterinarian and need to be asked overtly. If the veterinarian signposts a clear interest in the client's comments, in future the client may be more confident in coming forth spontaneously with suggestions:

> Veterinarian: "*You have probably thought about this a lot, too – are those the choices as you see it? What are your own thoughts?*"
> Client: "*Well, to be honest I'm concerned about how much this will all cost, especially referral to a specialist. Do you think I could just change the food I get her from the grocery store?*"

> or
>
> Veterinarian: *"You're been in the industry a long time. What is your sense about the value of changing this vaccination protocol around?"*
> Client: *"We tried a similar protocol about ten years ago and did not think it was worth the expense, so you might have to work harder to convince me."*

Exploring management options with the client

Next, it is important for the veterinarian to explore the options available to the client in more depth and provide information about the risks and benefits of each, including the option of no treatment or action.

> Veterinarian: *"So to recap, we have identified three approaches we could take here. The first would be to refer you and Lady to a specialist for allergy testing; the second would be to try her on a special allergy diet and eliminate all other forms of food; and the third more conservative approach would be trying her on a different grocery store diet that uses a different form of protein and eliminating all other forms of food. Would it help if I ran through the pros and cons of each of these courses of action now?"*
>
> or
>
> *"Based on what we are seeing with the timing of the shipping fever, the approaches we can take are geared to decreasing the stress of the weaning process, increasing the amount of time between weaning to transport, and adjusting the vaccination protocol. I realize that some of these might be more practical than others based on your circumstances. Would it be useful to map out the resources needed to accomplish these changes and the benefits that might result to help you decide which of these are most feasible?"*

While discussion of goals and expectations starts during agenda setting at the beginning of the consultation, it is often necessary to re-open this conversation during discussion of management options. Your goals and/or the client's goals and expectations may change once an issue has been explored or a diagnosis has been reached. At this point the client has a better understanding of what they are dealing with, what their options are, what the costs might be, etc. All of these considerations may be influencing client goals and expectations that may therefore require further discussion.

Two other important areas in exploring options with clients have been the subject of considerable research in the last decade. The first is the issue of explaining risks in an objective fashion that clients can understand and use in their decision making. The second is the use of written information and decision aids to help clients understand the options available to them and choose between them. It is beyond the scope of this book to explore these complex areas in depth. We merely highlight the issues here.

RISK COMMUNICATION

A veterinary epidemiologist with years of experience, Brenda Bonnett (pers. comm. 2015) comments that in general veterinarians do not have access to good risk and outcome estimates for most conditions and situations. In the absence of these estimates, veterinarians are most likely to use non-quantitative words such as "common" or "rare," "likely" or "unlikely." There is poor consistency in the way veterinarians use these terms and it is difficult for clients to interpret what they mean.

Where numbers are available, several findings from human medicine may be useful (Gigerenzer 2002; Edwards et al. 2000; Mazur 2000; Edwards et al. 2002; Gigerenzer and Edwards 2003; Halvorsen et al. 2007; Apter et al. 2008; Gaissmaier and Gigerenzer 2008; Longman et al. 2012). These findings show that in the communication of risk estimates great care needs to be taken in the use of the following:

- the statistical presentation of risk: use of absolute and relative risk, numbers needed to treat (NNT) and natural frequencies
- framing effects: framing is defined as presenting logically equivalent information in different ways such as "a 98% chance of surviving an operation" as opposed to "a 2% chance of dying."

The most accessible way of presenting risk information to clients is by using natural frequencies rather than percentages. An example would be: *"If we were treating ten dogs with the same kind of cancer, we can expect that four will be alive in six months if we do nothing, and six would be alive in the same time frame if we treat with this new drug."*

Other aspects of the way that risk is represented also need to be taken into account:

- words versus numerical representation
- visual and graphic display formats.

Two potential problems here are that individuals vary greatly in the way they prefer to receive complex information (Edwards 2004) and in their level of literacy. It is therefore difficult to design formats that will suit everyone. Here again we underscore the value of developing a repertoire of skills and approaches so that you can be flexible when interacting with each individual.

In veterinary medicine, recognizing that each client has a different perception of risk is crucial to the explanation and planning phase of consultations where risk is a factor. For many conditions there is data available to guide the veterinarian in discussions of risk, even if that data is not definitive. Expected survival rates or complication rates of different procedures in specific contexts are available. Consider an equine surgeon discussing colic surgery with a client. An 80% chance of being alive in 1 year may be odds that the veterinarian considers to be quite good while the client may see this as too risky for the amount of investment. It becomes incumbent upon the veterinarian to understand the many factors that clients may consider in making their decision and to take these factors into consideration so as to arrive at the best plan for all involved. Specific understanding of the client's risk tolerance and how that relates to their decision making is important.

Another issue in veterinary medicine is that what little we know about risks and outcomes is often based on studies that are small and do not necessarily represent the profession as a whole. For instance, the outcome studies for equine dystocias have largely been done in Kentucky where the referral time is very short. If we use those statistics in places where our referral times are quite long in comparison, the numbers may not pertain. Moreover, we have to find a way to communicate such relative differences to clients or colleagues effectively.

There is great potential to provide biased information of risk by the selective use of statistics and/or the way that information is presented (the framing effect). Hudak et al. (2011) explore an example of this in their work regarding orthopedic surgeons' consultations in Canada. Although surgeons skillfully adapted their recommendations to the views and expectations of their patients, these efforts were counterbalanced by an overarching institutional bias favoring surgery over other treatment options.

Such bias can be unintentional or deliberate. This issue is particularly important when looking at risk communication in the context of shared decision making (Edwards and Elwyn 2001b). Statistics could easily be quoted that, while true, magnify the benefits and minimize the risks to any one individual of adopting a particular course. In such circumstances, relative risk has often been used to magnify, and absolute risk to minimize, effects. While this might be justified from the population viewpoint of public health with an eye to the well-being of the nation, from an individual's perspective the only acceptable outcome measure for risk communication is the provision of unbiased information leading to an increase in ability of the client/ human patient to come to an informed decision (Thornton et al. 2003).

In veterinary medicine, we may be unintentionally or even intentionally biasing recommendations based on the economic needs of the practice rather than on a more balanced combination of both good business and good medicine. Alternatively, we may be biasing recommendations based on a fear of complaints or disciplinary action or on a preference for the familiar or for an approach that we have favored in the past. This falls under the heading of how we use our perceptual skills – how aware are we of the basis upon which we make a given recommendation and what do we do with that awareness to ensure that we are giving our clients and patients the best care?

Longman et al. (2012) raise an additional concern regarding how risk estimates are presented. In a study of university students, they demonstrated that communicating uncertainty in risk estimates has the potential to negatively affect understanding, increase perceptions of risk and decrease perceived credibility.

DECISION AIDS

The field of decision aids is concerned with how to improve the quality of patients' and clients' decision making by supplementing face-to-face communication between professionals and clients with materials to help them make decisions (O'Connor and Edwards 2001; Robinson and Thomson 2001; Sepucha and Mulley 2003; O'Brien et al. 2009; Bunge et al. 2010; Elwyn 2011; Myers et al. 2011). Available in a variety of print and electronic formats, some decision aids are designed to be used by people on their own as a platform for discussions in further consultations and others are for use during consultations. Some decision aids provide information about possible choices and probabilities of different outcomes and provide guidance as to how to come to a decision, although there is debate about how effective these aids are (Nelson et al. 2007; Kaner et al. 2007). Decision aids in human medicine have been shown to:

- improve patients' knowledge of problems, options and outcomes
- reduce the number of patients who are uncertain what to do
- create more realistic expectations of outcomes
- reduce decisional conflict (uncertainty)
- stimulate patients to be more active in decision making without increasing their anxiety.

We have not seen research in veterinary medicine regarding the impact of decision aids but some research in human medicine shows that decision aids seem to have little effect on patient satisfaction and a variable effect on what decisions are eventually made (O'Connor et al. 1999; O'Connor et al. 2001; O'Connor et al. 2003). The words of caution that we included above regarding written information and patients who are functionally illiterate or whose eyesight is compromised apply here again. We also want to underscore here that decision aids cannot take the place of personalized face-to-face interaction.

Ascertaining the level of involvement the client wishes in making the decision at hand

One of the key aims of this part of the consultation should be to involve clients in decision making to the level that they wish. We have already seen that a large majority of patients and clients wish to be involved in making choices but a significant minority would prefer to leave decisions to their clinician. Therefore it is important for the veterinarians to ascertain each individual client's preferences for participation in making choices and to tailor their approach accordingly rather than make assumptions without checking. We have also seen that this preference can change over time for each individual client, so it is necessary to repeat this process periodically.

There are two ways that this can be achieved. Where genuine choice exists (and it often does), the veterinarian can gently encourage the client to become involved:

> *"So, there are several things we might try here. As we've discussed, each option has its own advantages and disadvantages. ... Do you have any clear preference?"*

The client may respond with either:

> *"Well, overall I don't like giving medications if they are not needed and given what you have said, I think I would prefer to hold off on medications for her diarrhea until we are sure we know what it is and know what we are treating."*

---

or

"I don't think I can get the drops into his eye three times a day, so I might need to consider leaving him here for a few days while we get this under control."

A more direct way of discovering the client's preference in making choices about their animal's care is to ask explicitly:

Veterinarian: *"Referrals like this can go in a number of different directions: we can work with both you and your regular veterinarian or we can work through what is the best approach and come back with a finished report complete with recommendations. What works best for you?"*

Client: *"I think this problem is too complex for you to work on without regular input from us. Would you mind if we met regularly with you during the process so that you, our regular veterinarian, and I are all on the same page with the plan moving forward?"*

or

Veterinarian: *"There are several options in managing or treating hyperthyroidism in cats: a diet option, medication or referral to a specialist for more advanced treatment. Some clients like to be involved in these decisions and I welcome that. Some prefer for the veterinarian to take the lead – how would you like to play this yourself at the moment?"*

Client: *"Well, I'd really like to know more about each option and then discuss the best choice with you."*

Negotiating a mutually acceptable plan

Next, the veterinarian and the client need to come to a decision that both can agree upon.

SIGNPOSTING POSITION OF EQUIPOISE OR OWN PREFERENCES

As we have said, in the shared decision-making model, it is perfectly acceptable for the veterinarian, having explored the possibilities, to state a preference as long as they clearly signpost this and also indicate that the client's position is just as important as the veterinarian's. It is equally possible that the veterinarian is in a position of "equipoise" and genuinely does not have a preference for which of several treatments the client might choose:

Veterinarian: *"In this particular instance and from a purely medical standpoint, I personally would come down on one side here – I think given your busy lifestyle and your concerns about long-term management, Optimist would be best off if we pursued*

> *referral for treatment by radioactive iodine or surgery. But we need to take your views into account here – it is still a balancing of the pros and cons."*

or

> *"Overall, in your circumstance I think starting with any of the options is fine and I don't have a strong feeling either way whether we pursue diet, medication or referral at this point. I've had situations where each option has worked well – I think it comes down to the relative importance you place on the various things we have discussed."*

or

> *"Based on my training in sports medicine, I tend to think about joint injections as the first line of treatment here with massage as an adjunctive therapy. Based on your interest in trying alternative therapies first, I think it is reasonable to start with the acupuncture treatments and reassess where we are in several weeks. If the lameness is not improving by that point, we can always try the injections then."*

DETERMINING THE CLIENT'S PREFERENCES

Note that there is a hierarchy of ways of making plans with clients, from paternalistic directives and orders ("you must do the following …") to consumerist handing over of all decision making to the client ("I'll do whatever you want"). In the shared decision-making process that this chapter espouses, both veterinarian and client have ample opportunity to express their views. Usually veterinarians need to be careful to offer their ideas as suggestions for consideration by the client and also to listen carefully to the client's ideas and responses:

> Veterinarian: *"What do you think – what would be your preference?"*

Epstein and Peters (2009) have written eloquently about the difficulties of establishing people's preferences and have explored not only the cognitive but also the emotional and relationship factors that affect how patients' preferences are constructed. Results of Weiner and Roth's (2006) thematic literature review on goals of care discussions with patients and families near the end of life also underscore the importance of including not only cognitive but also integral emotional and social elements of these difficult discussions.

The veterinarian can make it clear to the client that they wish to share the decision making, resolve differences and negotiate a mutually acceptable plan:

> Veterinarian: *"What I've suggested makes sense to me … but if it isn't right for you, we'll need to think again. Tell me how you feel about it."*
>
> or

> *"I do have some reservations about taking the approach you suggest – can I explain them to you and then perhaps we can try to find a solution that works for both of us?"*

Checking with the client

As a final check at the end of planning, it is good practice to confirm whether the client is happy with the decisions that have been made, whether they accept the plans and whether their concerns have been addressed:

> Veterinarian: *"Now, can I just check that you are happy with the plan?"*

Options in explanation and planning

The four sections of the Calgary–Cambridge Guides discussed above are common to all consultations featuring explanation and planning. We now discuss three optional sections that may or may not pertain to any given consultation:

- if offering opinion and discussing significance of problems
- if negotiating mutual plan of action
- if discussing investigations and procedures.

These options in explanation and planning include both process skills and content items.

If discussing opinions and significance of problems

As discussed in other parts of this chapter, clinicians and clients/patients tend to disagree about what they think is important to discuss and clients/patients are not always satisfied that they have been given enough information. We have also shown that client/patient understanding and commitment to management plans is often poor because clinicians seldom explain their rationales in any detail or provide explanations related to the perspectives of the client/patient.

So what specific skills help veterinarians to explain their opinion(s)? The following four key skills are useful:

- offering your opinion of what is going on and naming it if possible
- revealing your rationale for this opinion
- explaining causation, seriousness, expected outcome, short and long-term consequences
- eliciting client's beliefs, reactions and concerns, e.g. whether the opinion you have offered matches the client's thoughts, acceptability and feelings.

Common examples demonstrate these skills in action:

Veterinarian: *"Based on the sporadic occurrence of the problem and the cows this seems to affect, I think it is possibly Johne's disease. The reason why I think so is ... you are familiar with a few other operations that have encountered problems similar to what you have been experiencing. Does this fit with what you know? My suspicion about why we are seeing it more right now is ... and to get it under control we probably need to do ... What are your thoughts?"*

or

"Based on my assessment, the signs seem consistent with thiamine deficiency ... and the reason why I think this is because. ... Does that fit for you? All right, I think the reason why it might have come on is because ... it is important we start her on treatment right away and look into preventing it from showing up in the rest of the herd. What are your thoughts?"

If negotiating a mutual plan of action

The specific skills that we can use here are:

- discussing options, e.g. no action, investigation, medication or surgery, non-drug treatments (diet, exercise, behavioral counseling, massage, rehabilitation), preventive measures
- providing information on action or treatment offered:
  — name of the treatment or action
  — steps involved, how it works
  — benefits and advantages
  — possible side effects or disadvantages
- obtaining client's view of need for action, perceived benefits, barriers, motivation
- accepting client's views, advocating alternative viewpoint as necessary
- eliciting client's reactions and concerns about plans and treatments including acceptability
- taking client's lifestyle, beliefs, cultural background and abilities into consideration
- encouraging client to be involved in implementing plans, to take responsibility
- asking about client support systems, discussing other support available.

Discussing and offering options in management and treatment

Offering options is the first step in enabling client choice. How can a client whose horse has a painful back choose whether to try physiotherapy, osteopathy, medication relief, rest, or no treatment without having the possible options clearly explained first?

Providing information on action or treatment offered

Providing information about a proposed management or treatment is a highly skilled task. Take for example the scenario of a client seeking advice about what vaccinations to give to his indoor cat. Not only does the veterinarian have to give a clear explanation of the efficacy of various vaccinations and tailor their explanation to the client's understanding and the animal's needs, they must also describe the risks and benefits of the vaccinations accurately, taking into account the client's concerns about, for example, the relationship between vaccination and risks of fibrosarcoma.

Obtaining the client's view of need for action, perceived benefits, barriers and motivation

Balanced against the information that the veterinarian brings to the consultation are the knowledge, attitudes, values, priorities and beliefs of the client. These are equally important and valid in reaching a decision about the most appropriate way forward. The client's views about perceived benefits, barriers and motivations need to be elicited if a shared or negotiated decision regarding treatment is to be reached.

This is true for any decision in veterinary medicine. Kleen (2011) reminds us that the goals of production animal and small animal care are often different, so motivation for engagement with production animal medicine may be different from motivation for engagement in companion animal medicine. Certainly the actual substance of the goals is different, yet even though the content differs substantially, goals are important and need to be determined and discussed in all veterinary contexts.

Recently veterinarians have become particularly aware of barriers and motivation with respect to prevention and health promotion (Jansen et al. 2009; Lam et al. 2011; Garforth et al. 2013). These are increasingly important parts of veterinary practice.

Greene and Hibbard (2012) provide evidence linking human patient activation (i.e. knowledge, skills, beliefs and confidence for managing health and healthcare) with health outcomes. In a cross-sectional study of 25 047 patients in a Minnesota health service, they found that more activated patients were more likely to have received preventive care, less likely to smoke or have a high BMI and had better clinical indicators. The study found no evidence that socio-economic status affected the relationship between patient activation and outcomes. Might paying more attention to client activation in veterinary medicine prove as useful?

Priest and Speller (1991) cite three sets of perceptual skills physicians need in order to help patients change to healthier lifestyles:

- knowledge about risk factors
- awareness and understanding about the patient's attitude to the problem affecting their health
- knowledge and application of the skills involved in helping people to change.

The Jansen et al. (2010) research regarding Dutch dairy farmers and udder health management revealed that two communication strategies were successful in disseminating information to farmers and changing farmers' behavior:

- a media campaign on using milking gloves
- udder health study groups (continuing education programs) held on farm.

INFLUENCING CLIENTS' MOTIVATION TO CHANGE

How to influence what motivates people to change their health practices and use of health services has long been of interest in both human and veterinary medicine. Several models of change and motivation are helpful.

Decades ago Hochbaum (1958) developed the *Health Belief Model*, which helps us understand factors that influence a client's motivation to act. Figure 6.2 is a representation of the Health Belief Model as adapted by Janz (1984).

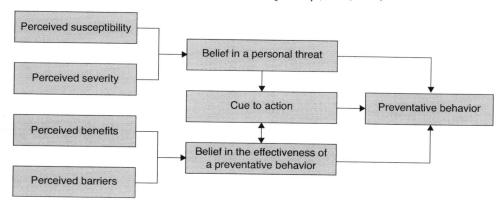

FIGURE 6.2 Health belief model. Janz (1984). Used with permission

As the diagram illustrates, what a client believes about a threat to the animals' health or their own well-being (including emotional or economic threat, etc.) is influenced by the client's perception of severity (how serious is this situation?) and susceptibility (how likely is my animal to be affected by this problem or by the sequelae of this problem, how vulnerable am I?). The client's belief in the effectiveness of a preventive behavior (e.g. vaccinations) or management plan is also influenced by the client's perception of benefits to reducing the perceived threat and/or barriers that the client must overcome in order to implement recommendations. The health belief model also takes into account the influence of clients' self-efficacy, i.e. their confidence in a preventive behavioral or management plan or in their ability to implement the plan. These factors on their own or as cues to action then motivate the client to engage in the preventive behavior or implement the management plan (Rosenstock et al. 1988; Jansen and Lam 2012).

Veterinary literature refers to additional theories that offer useful insights: the *theory of planned behavior* and the *theory of reasoned action* (Fishbein and Ajzen 1975; Ajzen and Fishbein 1980). In their study on owner attitudes and obesity in dogs Rohlf et al. (2010) used the theory of planned behavior and found that along with biological (age and breed) and environmental factors (other family members feeding the dog), owner attitudes, beliefs, intentions, mindfulness and motivation were factors contributing to obesity in their animals. The researchers concluded that all of these factors may be part of a complex causal model of obesity. Treating obesity effectively may require that all of these factors be taken into account. In large animal studies (Rehman et al. 2007; Alarcon et al. 2013), the theories of planned behavior and reasoned action focus attention on the connection between beliefs and behavior and highlight the variables involved in client decision making and motivation to act. Variables include the individual's positive or negative attitudes; perception of social norms, including the judgment of others, that pressure individuals to act in one way or another; perceived behavioral control and individual's need for control; beliefs about the consequences of a behavior; perception of ease or difficulty of performing a behavior; etc.

Another approach veterinary educators, researchers and practitioners use is called Motivational Interviewing and is based on the *"Stages of Change" model* shown in Figure 6.3. Prochaska and DiClemente (1986) originally designed the model for human medical contexts. The Stages of Change model describes a natural series of stages that people work through when considering change. It recognizes that at each of these stages people have different frames of mind and that professional intervention is more likely to be successful if tailored closely to whichever stage the individual is in at any given time. The clinician's role is to discover where the client is in the process of self-motivation and to encourage and support the client's efforts. Clients' levels of confidence (in their ability to make the change) and conviction (regarding

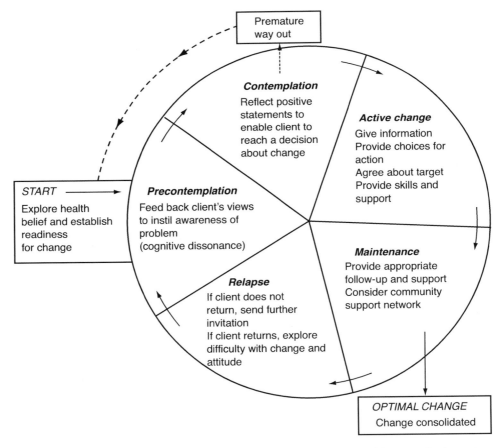

FIGURE 6.3 Interview process using the Stages of Change model. Adapted from Prochaska and DiClemente (1986)

how convinced they are that the change is important) will influence their success (Rollnick et al. 1997; Keller and Kemp-White 2001). Motivational interviewing attempts to empower clients to take responsibility for their own decisions by increasing their self-esteem and self-efficacy, by respecting their views and concerns and by negotiating suitable targets.

Note that motivational interviewing uses many of the core skills already discussed in this book: listening, exploring clients' beliefs, the use of open questions, reflection, summarizing, providing choices, negotiation, acceptance and support. Building on this model, Atkinson (2010b) proposes that in large animal veterinary practice the cycle of change also happens in stages, with farm team and veterinarian moving from contemplation to planning, experimenting and doing.

In contrast to most other models for behavior change which are complex and based on a longer consultation, Keller and Kemp-White (2001) created a model for influencing behavior that enables clinicians to have an impact on people's behavior in a brief office visit or other short interaction.

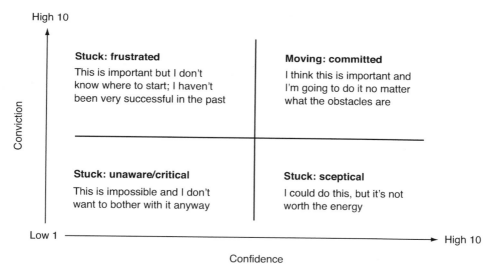

FIGURE 6.4 Confidence and Conviction Grid (Keller and Kemp-White 2001)

In the *Confidence and Conviction Grid* (Figure 6.3), the clinician assesses the client's readiness for change within two dimensions: conviction (does the client believe that making this change will enhance the health and well-being of their animals?) and confidence (does the client believe that they can make this change?). An intervention to increase the client's confidence, conviction, or both can then be applied to help the client move into a position of high conviction and high confidence. Keller and Kemp-White suggest specific strategies for working with clients who are low in both dimensions or high in one and low in the other. Used in both human and veterinary contexts, the model is applicable to a wide variety of client choices and actions from following medication regimes to changes in diet or housing.

We have found that one more model summarizes this discussion of motivation models and approaches usefully. Informally we have called this the *outcomes of change model*. It is easy to assume that we are successful only if clients (or in teaching contexts, learners) actually take action or accomplish a change in their behavior. In place of this somewhat limiting notion, it is helpful to consider the different outcomes or kinds of change that veterinarians (or teachers) can aim for. Rather than thinking only in terms of action, consider these four alternative outcomes:

Consideration (I am aware of and willing to consider the change)
Attitudes (I have a positive attitude toward the change)
Beliefs and Values (I believe the change is the best approach)
Action/Behavior (I change the way I act or behave in real life)

If we assess where in this progression clients (or learners) are, we can understand more precisely where to direct our efforts and what "next steps" to take to move forward. Of course, our ultimate aim is for clients (or learners) to take appropriate action regarding recommendations or treatment regimes for their animal, to achieve a change in behavior. But a more indirect approach often results in less defensiveness and proves more fruitful than trying to influence action immediately. If I am not yet even willing to consider a change, I am less likely to make a lasting change in behavior than if I already have a positive attitude toward the change. Thinking in terms of four outcomes instead of one (i.e. action) alters the way we assess our efforts and clients' (or learners') progress. It allows us to record advancement not only when we can see action or changes in behavior but also when we can see changes in what people are willing to consider, in their attitude or in what they believe and value.

Accepting clients' views and advocating an alternative viewpoint as necessary

In Chapter 5 we discussed the key concept of initially accepting and acknowledging the legitimacy of clients' ideas without necessarily agreeing with them. Non-judgmental acceptance allows you to offer your perspective of the problem later on in light of the client's beliefs, to discuss misperceptions, advocate a different approach if necessary and negotiate an agreed plan. But what if we feel that clients' attitudes or behaviors are seriously affecting the health of their animal(s) yet they brush aside our suggestions? How can we challenge a firmly held belief without denigrating the client?

CHALLENGING AND CONFRONTING SITUATIONS

Being honest in the consultation can present difficulties for the veterinarian, particularly when faced with clients who appear not to be dealing with an important issue. Conflict with clients is usually unproductive and can leave the client feeling both angry and unsupported.

Compare these comments from the veterinarian:

> *"I can't believe you still aren't vaccinating for this. How many people do you know have lost horses to this disease and you still aren't trying to prevent it?"*
>
> Compared to:
>
> *"There have been a number of cases of Potomac horse fever this year and several people have lost a number of horses from their herd. I know you can't afford that kind of loss. I am curious, what is keeping you from using the vaccine for your herd?"*
>
> or
>
> *"You must euthanize Riley today. He is suffering and there is nothing more you or I can do for him. This is animal cruelty."*
>
> Compared to:
>
> *"I know the thought of losing Riley is difficult … This has been an emotional journey for you and you are now faced with a very difficult decision … Unfortunately his condition has deteriorated quickly and there is no more you or I can do to make him comfortable at this point. I'm concerned he will continue to suffer if we don't make the difficult decision to let him die peacefully now with our assistance. It is something we can offer him at this point. What can I do to support you at this time?"*

Honesty and the ability to challenge beliefs in a constructive manner is an important part of enabling clients to change their points of view and to take different actions.

Eliciting clients' reactions and concerns about plans and treatments, including acceptability

> *"I've shared a lot of options with you, so I'm interested in knowing what thoughts or concerns you have at this point including which option seems most acceptable to you."*
>
> or
>
> *"I have suggested some pretty strong changes to how you manage your flock to help prevent an outbreak. At this point, what do you see as the benefits and barriers to implementing these changes?"*

Taking the client's lifestyle, beliefs, culture and abilities into consideration

> *"I appreciate you sharing with me your religious belief that euthanasia is not an acceptable option. I would like to respect your beliefs. Please do let me know if I say anything that further challenges them."*

or

"With your work schedule and concern about being able to get the medication into his eyes without getting hurt, I think it might be better to keep him here at the hospital while we get his uveitis under control. You can stop and visit on your way home from work and his treatments will be done by one of the technicians who is well trained in giving eye medication. That way Buster does not associate you with his treatments and you don't have to stress about leaving work early to get his medications given on time."

Encouraging the client to be involved in implementing plans and to take responsibility

"I am glad to hear that you want to work on getting Pooch down to a healthy weight. It will be important that you have a plan to get him out to exercise every day. Once the weather turns bad, it can be tempting to skip a few days. What you are probably going to find is that once Pooch starts to lose some of the weight, he will look forward to his walks and may be quite insistent upon getting out."

or

"Rocket's treatment will be twice a day and it'll be on going for the next two weeks. I know you mentioned you work long hours and live offsite. From your end of things, what thoughts do you have on how we can implement a plan to ensure he gets treated twice a day?"

Asking about the client's support network, discussing other support available

"It is incredibly important that after surgery Butch be watched closely for 24 hours. I know you said you had an important meeting on the day he is scheduled for surgery. Is there a neighbor who might be able to watch him for you during that time?"

or

"Ms Wright, I know you have had to make some very difficult and emotional decisions this afternoon; is there someone you would like me to call for you? Someone who can meet you here and take you home?"

If discussing investigations and procedures

During the consultation we often need to give information about investigations or procedures. Remember that what may seem to be trivial to the veterinarian may be quite alarming to the client. Watching a veterinarian draw blood may upset the client.

Waiting a week for the results of a biopsy can seem like forever. Listening, empathy and achieving a shared understanding are all important. Here are three key skills in this area of the consultation:

Providing clear information on procedures including what the animal might experience and how the client will be informed of results

What you would say regarding this skill is content driven and needs no further explanation or example.

Relating procedures to the treatment plan: value and purpose

> *"What the blood work will help us do is to make sure there is not something more going on with her other organ systems and to help me determine the most likely type of infection. When we look at the ... it tells us ... That helps us figure out how serious this is and what is likely to be our best course of action."*
>
> or
>
> *"When you are ready, I would like to draw some blood from one of Rory's front legs. The blood will give us information on his kidney function. If we find the values to be high we can discuss management options including a change to his diet to reduce the stress on his kidneys. If his kidneys are the issue, a diet change should allow him to live a longer and more comfortable life."*

Encouraging questions about and discussion of potential anxieties or negative outcomes

> *"This surgery requires a reasonable financial investment and it is not without risks. It is completely reasonable to have concerns and anxieties. I know I would.* (long pause to allow client to think). *What are your thoughts at this point?"*
>
> or
>
> *"I know all we have talked about today can be overwhelming. What questions or concerns do you have about Osa's situation at this time?"*

Summary: explanation and planning is an interactive process

In much of this chapter, we have advocated an interactive approach to explanation and planning: just giving information and dictating plans is clearly not enough. In Chapter 3, we discussed the limitations of direct, one-way transmission of information. If communication is viewed as a direct transmission process, the senders of messages assume that their responsibilities as communicators are fulfilled once they have formulated and sent a message. However, if communication is viewed as an interactive process, the interaction is complete only if the sender receives feedback about how the message is interpreted, whether it is understood and what impact it has on the receiver (Dance and Larson 1972).

We demonstrated that summarizing and checking are key skills which enable this interactive approach to be put into practice in the information-gathering phase of the interview by providing feedback to the client about what we think we have heard and understood. Now we have seen how further skills are required in the explanation and planning phase to ensure a similar degree of interaction. And we have seen again the significant role that relationship building plays – shared decision making and other interactive processes in the explanation and planning stages of the consultation are enhanced when a relationship conducive to collaboration and partnership between client and veterinarian has already been developed earlier in the interview.

In the explanation and planning phase, a one-sided speech can be counterproductive. To give information accurately, we need to check repeatedly whether we have made ourselves clear and whether the client understands our thoughts before proceeding to the next chunk of information. We have seen how:

- a two-way interaction enables us to discover what information we have not yet provided
- asking the client to restate the information they have just been told dramatically increases retention and understanding
- we need to give the client encouragement to ask questions, express doubts and seek clarification if we are to achieve a shared understanding and prevent non-adherence
- we need to understand our clients' ideas if we want to align our explanations to our clients' needs
- we need to involve the client in planning by allowing them to be part of the decision-making process and to voice their preferences.

We hope that this chapter has convinced you to continue the trend away from merely "giving" information to clients and toward "sharing" understanding and decision making. This shift promises not only more satisfying consultations for both clients and veterinarians but also better health outcomes for the animals.

CHAPTER 7

Closing the session

Communication problems at the end of the consultation often relate to time issues. Just as you think that you have satisfactorily completed the interview and are drawing the session to an end, the client introduces another major item. The dreaded "by the way, Doc" moment. The veterinarian wants to close things down and push on to the next appointment; the client seems eager to open things up again. Just as you begin to organize follow-up arrangements, the client asks a question that makes it clear that they have not understood your explanations so far or are unlikely to adhere to the plan. These unmatched agendas easily lead to conflict and frustration.

What skills can we recommend to help with these problems? First, difficulties in closure often emanate from communication issues occurring much earlier in the consultation, such as getting a complete list of problems and issues rather than a chief complaint, setting an agenda, asking about the client's perspectives. They can be avoided by attention to our use of communication skills during the beginning, information gathering, and explanation and planning phases of the interview. Once these have been addressed, problems in this part of the consultation tend to evaporate.

However, there are specific communication skills in the closing phase, too. Summarizing and clarifying plans made, and the next steps for both parties, establishing what the client should do if things do not go according to plan, checking that the client is comfortable with the follow-up arrangements, continuing to build the veterinarian–client–patient relationship – these are all essential elements of closing the consultation and contribute to improved adherence, satisfaction and health outcomes.

In this chapter we explore two separate but related questions:

1. What are the skills used throughout the rest of the consultation that can help closure to be more efficient?
2. What are the skills during closure itself that will help bring the consultation to a satisfactory end?

Objectives

Our objectives for this part of the interview may be summarized as follows:

- confirming the established plan of care
- clarifying the next steps veterinarian and client will take
- establishing contingency plans
- maximizing client adherence and animal health outcomes

- making efficient use of time in the consultation
- continuing to encourage the client to feel part of a collaborative process and to build the veterinarian–client–patient relationship for the future.

Again, these objectives encompass some of the tasks and checkpoints mentioned in other well known guides to the consultation: *see* Appendix C.

The process skills for closing the session

The following skills work together to help us achieve the objectives for this part of the consultation.

Box 7.1 Skills for closing the session

Forward planning
- **Contracting:** contracts with client regarding next steps for client and veterinarian
- **Safety netting:** safety nets appropriately – explains possible unexpected outcomes, what to do if plan is not working or complications occur, when and how to seek help and how urgently.

Ensuring appropriate point of closure
- **End summary:** summarizes session briefly and clarifies plan of care
- **Final checking:** checks that client agrees and is comfortable with plan and asks if there are any corrections, questions or other issues.

What to teach and learn about endings: the evidence for the skills

Before looking at the specific skills that contribute to effective endings, it is worth considering some of the issues that commonly arise at this point in the consultation and at some of the behaviors and skills from *earlier* in the interview that help prevent problems and aid effectiveness.

What actually happens in the closing section of the interview?

White et al. (1994) have looked specifically at closure and have attempted to separate this element of the consultation from the explanation and planning phase. Listening to audiotapes of primary care physicians in Oregon, they identified closure by looking for sentences which demonstrated a transition from the educational to the ending phase; for example, *"OK let's see you back in five months"* or *"We'll just see how it goes in the future."* Their results were as follows:

- Length of visits: av. 16.8 minutes
- Length of closure: av. 1.6 minutes (1–9 minutes range)
- Closure initiated by physician: in 86% of consultations

- New problems discussed not mentioned earlier in the visit: in 21% of closures
- Physician behaviors in closure:
  - clarifying the plan (75%)
  - orienting the patient to next steps (56%)
  - providing information about the condition or therapy (53%)
  - checking for understanding (34%)
  - asking whether more questions (25%).

Artemiou (pers. comm. 2016) conducted a pre- and post-training assessment of second-year veterinary students' communication skills. Her preliminary analysis showed that students improved in their ability to achieve agreement on next steps. However, safety netting was consistently missed in both pre and post interactions.

Jansen (2010) showed that the majority of the dairy veterinarians in her study did not summarize the visit or discuss plans for follow-up.

Bronshtein et al. (2006) showed in a study of Israeli specialists and family physicians, with consultation lengths averaging 9 minutes, that termination was never initiated by the patient in any of the 320 encounters observed, i.e. it is the physician's responsibility to close.

Rhodes et al. (2004) in a study in an academic medical centre emergency department in the USA showed that discharge instructions averaged 76 seconds. Only 16% of patients were asked whether they had questions, and there were no instances in which the provider confirmed patient understanding of the information.

What behaviors earlier in the visit prevent new problems arising during closure?

Problems with the end of the consultation can start with problems at the beginning. Recall the Dysart et al. (2011) study from Chapter 2 showing that the odds of a concern arising in the final moments were four times as great when the veterinarian did not solicit the client's concerns at the beginning of the consultation. Late-arising problems caused the veterinarian to choose between extending the appointment length, ignoring the concern or deferring these current concerns to another visit. In Chapter 2 we also described Beckman and Frankel's (1984) key research on how the physician's use of words and questions can easily and inadvertently direct the patient away from telling the physician their real reasons for coming to the office. Premature physician interruption and failure to screen for problems early on in the interview led to an increase in late-arising complaints.

White et al. (1994) found the following behaviors earlier in the visit tended to prevent new problems arising during closure in human medicine:

- using signposting to orientate people to the flow of the visit ("Now I'm going to [do a physical exam] and then we will have some time to discuss what's going on")
- giving more information about the therapeutic regimen
- patients talking more about the treatment plan
- asking for information about beliefs and being more responsive.

What communication skills can we recommend in the earlier sections of the consultation that will aid efficient and satisfactory closure of the session?

Initiating the consultation
- Attentive listening
- Screening to get problem list
- Agenda setting.

Information gathering
- Signposting
- Exploring client's ideas and concerns
- Addressing client's feelings, thoughts and emotions
- Discussing lifestyle and social issues.

Explanation and planning
- Information giving
- Involving clients in explanation and planning
- Checking for clients' understanding
- Asking for clients' questions.

What behaviors during closure are associated with inefficient endings?

Atkinson (2010a) notes that many veterinarians fall short of what he calls "reviewing and checking" back with the farmer once information and recommendations have been made, thus losing the opportunity to make sure the advice given is appropriate and to fine tune the plan if adjustments have to be made once the farmer has had a chance to comment.

White et al. (1994) discovered that the following behaviors during closure were associated with longer endings:

- Physicians asking open questions
- Physicians laughing or showing emotions, concern or responsiveness to patients
- Patients being friendly, dominant, responsive or in distress.

But are we trying to achieve a shorter closure? There is clearly a tension here between efficiency and completeness. If the veterinarian wishes to end the consultation more quickly, one option would be to behave in a more closed fashion. However, if the client has further questions or issues to discuss, closing them down will not maximize the full potential of the consultation (Dysart et al. 2011). It may instead add time both to the immediate interview and in the long term (Robinson 2001).

We need not abandon communicating in an open, collaborative and client-centered way during closure. Our previous behavior in the consultation will hopefully allow the client at this stage to say, *"No, I think you have answered all my questions"* or *"No, I don't have any other concerns."* Yet however well the consultation has proceeded, there will still be clients who leave their most worrying concern until the very end.

In a further qualitative study in human medicine, White et al. (1997) clarified this area further. They showed that 36% of closures were interrupted midstream, with new problems surfacing in 23% of visits; interruptions occurred even with open-ended beginnings and early physician requests for all of the patient's concerns. They surmised that interrupted closures which produce new agenda items may be less effective than others, increasing frustration for physicians and reducing patients' satisfaction with care. While recognizing that the medical visit is complicated and that physicians and patients can inadvertently forget things until the end or that physicians may empathize with patients late in the visit, the researchers observed three things about interrupted closures that may improve physician efficiency. Because these points seem equally relevant to veterinary practice, we have taken the liberty to contextualize them for veterinary medicine:

- Only when both client and veterinarian are ready to close the visit will they be able to do so successfully – listening and exploring clients' beliefs and concerns earlier in the visit will prepare the way for smooth closure later.
- Veterinarians should beware of asking *"Is there anything else?"* or *"Do you have some other concerns you want to discuss?"* so late in the interview that they are not expecting a positive reply. Veterinarians should ask for any final concerns *before* they start the process of closure rather than at the very end so that late-arising concerns can be meaningfully addressed. This screening for uncompleted business should therefore precede the move to closure.
- Clear signposting of the stages of the interview helps the client understand the process of the interview and what is happening at each stage – the optimal time for providing unstated concerns may then be more apparent to all. In our view, this would occur throughout the interview and include signaling that you are moving to closure, for example, by saying: *"I think we're just about finished ... is there something else you'd hoped to discuss?"*

It is important to consider a few additional circumstances in veterinary medicine that may require particular attention during closing. For example special attention is required when the person the veterinarian is talking to is not the person who will be responsible for following through with treatment plans. In this case, which may be similar to some human pediatric visits, it becomes important to explicitly discuss how that primary caregiver will be getting complete and accurate information regarding next steps and safety netting, including any follow-up calls from the practice. In large animal settings, the veterinarian may need to include a plan for (or even seek out) other people (such as the legal owner, hired hand, groom, milkers, calf treaters, etc.) who need to understand the information covered in the closing summary of treatment, follow-up plans, safety netting and to have an opportunity to ask questions.

Descriptions of the skills for closing the session
Forward planning
Contracting

Contracting about the next steps each party will take allows each person to identify their mutual roles and responsibilities (Stewart et al. 1997). The veterinarian may need to state explicitly how they will inform the client of test results and what the client should do in the meantime. The client may need to confirm their willingness to adhere to the agreed treatment plan.

> *"So, I'll drop off some medication later this afternoon that will help Sunshine's breathing – in the meantime if you would look into feeding her off the ground and reducing the amount of dust in the barn, that will also help her. I will then give you a call in a few days to see how things are going with her. Does that sound like a plan?"*

If you want the client to book for a recheck appointment or call the practice within a given period of time to let you know how things are going or if you are planning to telephone the client to check in with them later, then it is useful to make these plans a part of the closing contract.

Safety netting

Establishing contingency plans is a key step in closure. Explaining what the client should do if things do not go according to plan, how they should contact you and what certain developments might mean provides important back-up. As Neighbour (1987) described, explaining possible unexpected outcomes and when and how to seek help are important. In veterinary medicine this translates to being important for the safety of the animal, the peace of mind of the client, and the veterinarian–client relationship. For example, if a veterinarian prescribes antibiotics and anti-inflammatories for a dog with bacterial pneumonia without setting out a plan for follow-up, and if the dog does not improve, the client may be uncertain what to do or may feel the veterinarian has no further advice and therefore pursues a new line of treatment on their own without the veterinarian's knowledge. However, if the veterinarian requests that the client contact the practice if the dog continues to worsen or does not improve within a given period of time, then the client will know that there are other options and will feel empowered to contact the veterinarian if necessary. Alternatively, if the practice routinely makes follow-up calls, tell the client that someone from the practice will call to make sure everything is all right and clarify questions that have come up. Stoewen et al. (2014b) showed that clients of a teaching hospital oncology unit appreciated and expected the safety net of access to informational support 24 hours a day.

Ensuring appropriate point of closure
End summary

We have looked at the value of internal summary for information gathering and structuring the interview in Chapters 3, 4 and 6. Summary is an essential tool in this part of the consultation too. Summarizing the session briefly and clarifying the plan of care not only gives the veterinarian and client the chance to confirm their deliberations but can also act as a highly valuable facilitative tool allowing the client to question or amend the veterinarian's perceptions. Summarizing is an important aid to accuracy and hence to adherence. Remember to always leave space for the client to make corrections or additions.

> Veterinarian: *"So, just to recap, over the past year Otis has gained about 5 kg from where he was last year. You mentioned that you have not been able to get him out as often or for as long since your husband had his car accident nine months ago. Also, your husband has been home more the past nine months; therefore, Otis has likely gotten more 'extras'. Today we have agreed to put Otis on a weight management plan offered here by the clinic. This includes cutting out all table scraps as well as monitoring the number of other treats he receives outside of his regular diet. I will ask one of our technicians to discuss options for changing him over to a therapeutic weight loss diet with you and you plan to discuss with your family increasing each of his walks by five minutes. You or another member of your family will bring him in every other week to be weighed until we have him back down to where he was. Is that a reasonable summary of what we've agreed?"*
>
> Client: *"Yes, although it will have to be my daughter that brings him in every other week. It is too hard for me to leave work early on such a regular basis. She should be fine with bringing him in – she wants to be a veterinarian!"*

Final checking

As described above, it is important to check finally that the client agrees and is comfortable with the plans that have been made and to ask if they have any corrections or questions (Robinson 2001). Hopefully, the answer will be:

> *"No, that's just fine. Thanks so much for all of your help, you've answered all my questions."*

Summary

In this chapter, we have looked at the skills involved in closing the consultation. We have seen how the effectiveness of closure is related both to the appropriate use of communication skills in earlier sections of the consultation and also to the use of specific skills identified in this section of the Calgary–Cambridge Guides. Summarizing, contracting, safety netting and final checking all help to round off the interview safely, to establish mutually understood common ground, to reduce uncertainty for veterinarian and client about both what has happened and what is expected in the future, and to complete the process of sharing, collaboration and partnership which we have promoted throughout this book.

The skills of closure enable clients to feel comfortable with a mutually agreed plan, to be clear about what will happen next and to move on with more confidence. The same skills enable veterinarians to complete the consultation more effectively and to start the next interview with less unfinished business or anxieties to undermine their concentration. We have already mentioned that the beginning of the consultation is often the root cause of many of the problems of closure. Here we see that without care and attention, closure can be the root cause of difficulties at the beginning of the next consultation. Putting aside the last client and patient is an important prerequisite for focusing attention on the next.

Calgary–Cambridge Guides: Communication Process Skills feedback format for veterinary medicine[14]

Learner name _____ Observer _____ Date _____

INITIATING THE SESSION	COMMENTS
Preparation	
1. **Puts aside last task**, attends to self-comfort	
2. **Focuses attention** and prepares for this consultation	
Establishing initial rapport	
3. **Greets** client and patient and obtains names	
4. **Introduces** self, role and nature of visit; obtains consent if necessary	
5. **Demonstrates respect** and interest, attends to client's and patient's physical comfort	
Identifying the reason(s) for the consultation	
6. **Identifies problem list** or issues client wishes to address with appropriate **opening question** (e.g. "What would you like to discuss?" or "What questions did you hope to get answered today?")	
7. **Listens** attentively to the client's opening statement without interrupting or directing client's response	
8. **Confirms list and screens** for further problems (e.g. "So that's updating vaccinations and Max seems more tired than usual; anything else?" or "Do you have some other concerns you'd like to discuss today?")	
9. **Negotiates agenda** taking both client's and own perspectives into account	

GATHERING INFORMATION	COMMENTS

Exploration of problem(s)
 	
10. **Encourages client to tell story** of problem(s) from when first started to the present in own words (clarifying reason for presenting now)
 	
11. **Uses open and closed questioning** technique, appropriately moving from open to closed
 	
12. **Listens attentively,** allowing client to complete statements without interruption and leaving space for client to think before answering or go on after pausing
 	
13. **Facilitates client's responses verbally and nonverbally,** e.g. by using encouragement, silence, repetition, paraphrasing
 	
14. **Picks up verbal and nonverbal cues** (e.g. body language, facial expression); **checks out and acknowledges** as appropriate
 	
15. **Clarifies client's statements** that are unclear or need amplification (e.g. "Could you explain what you mean by sore?")
 	
16. **Periodically summarizes** to verify understanding of client's comments, invites client to correct interpretation or provide further information
 	
17. **Uses** concise, **easily understood questions and comments;** avoids or adequately explains jargon
 	
18. **Establishes dates and sequence of events**
 	
Additional skills for understanding the client's perspective
 	
19. **Actively determines and appropriately explores:**
  • Client's **ideas** (beliefs regarding cause)
  • Client's **concerns** (worries) regarding each problem
  • Client's **expectations** (goals, help client expects, cost issues, urgency)
  • **Effects on client's and animal's life**
  • **Relationship** between client, animal and others
 	
20. **Encourages client to express feelings**	

Additional comments:

PROVIDING STRUCTURE TO THE CONSULTATION	COMMENTS
Making organization overt	
21. **Summarizes at end of a specific line of inquiry** (e.g. current history) to confirm understanding and ensure no important data was missed; invites client to correct	
22. **Progresses** from one section to another **using signposting, transitional statements**; includes rationale for next section	
Attending to flow	
23. **Structures** consultation in **logical sequence**	
24. **Attends to timing** and keeping consultation on task	

BUILDING RELATIONSHIP – *facilitating client's involvement*	COMMENTS
Using appropriate nonverbal behavior	
25. **Demonstrates appropriate nonverbal behaviour** • eye contact, facial expressions • posture, position, gestures and other movement • vocal cues (e.g. rate, volume, intonation, pitch)	
26. **If reads, writes notes** or uses computer, does so **in a manner that does not interfere with dialogue or rapport**	
27. **Demonstrates** appropriate **confidence**	
Developing rapport	
28. **Accepts legitimacy** of client's views and feelings; **is not judgmental**	
29. **Uses empathy** to communicate understanding and appreciation of client's feelings or situation; overtly **acknowledges client's views and feelings**	
30. **Provides support**: expresses concern, understanding, willingness to help; acknowledges efforts and appropriate care; offers partnership	
31. **Deals sensitively with embarrassing or disturbing topics and animal's pain**, including when associated with physical examination	
Involving the client	
32. **Shares thinking** with client to encourage client's involvement (e.g. "What I am thinking now is …")	
33. **Explains rational** for questions or parts of physical examination that could appear to be non-sequiturs	
34. When **doing physical examination, explains process, findings**	

Additional comments:

EXPLANATION AND PLANNING	COMMENTS
Providing the correct amount and type of information	
35. **Chunks and checks**: gives information in manageable chunks; checks for understanding; uses client's response as a guide to how to proceed	
36. **Assesses client's starting point**: asks for client's prior knowledge early on when giving information; discovers extent of client's wish for information	
37. **Asks** client **what other information would be helpful** (e.g. etiology, prognosis)	
38. **Gives explanation at appropriate times**: avoids giving advice, information or reassurance prematurely	
Aiding accurate recall and understanding	
39. **Organizes explanation**: divides into discrete sections; develops logical sequence	
40. **Uses explicit categorization or signposting** (e.g. "There are three important things that I would like to discuss. 1st ... Now we shall move on to ...")	
41. **Uses reptition and summarizing** to reinforce information	
42. **Uses** concise, **easily understood language**, avoids or explains jargon	
43. **Uses visual methods of conveying information**: diagrams, models, written information and instructions	
44. **Checks client's understanding of information given** or plans made (e.g. by asking client to restate in own words; clarifies as necessary)	
Achieving shared understanding – incorporating the client's perspective	
45. **Relates explanations to client's perspective**: to previously elicited beliefs, concerns and expectations	
46. **Provides opportunities/encourages client to contribute**: to ask questions, seek clarification or express doubts, responds appropriately	
47. **Picks up, responds to verbal and nonverbval cues** (e.g. client's need to contribute information or ask questions, information overload, distress)	
48. **Elicits client's beliefs, reactions and feelings**: re: information given, decisions, terms used; acknowledges and addresses where necessary	

EXPLANATION AND PLANNING	COMMENTS
Planning: shared decision making	
49. **Shares own thoughts**: ideas, thought processes and dilemmas	

50. **Involves client**
  • offers suggestions and choices rather than directives
  • encourages client to contribute their own ideas, suggestions	

51. **Explores management options**	
52. **Ascertains** level of **involvement client wishes** regarding decision making	

53. **Negotiates mutually acceptable plan**
  • signposts own position of equipoise or preference re: available options
  • determines client's preferences	

54. **Checks with client**
  • if accepts plans
  • if concerns have been addressed	

Additional comments:

CLOSING THE SESSION	COMMENTS
Forward planning	
55. **Contracts with client** regarding steps for client and veterinarian	
56. **Safety nets**, explaining possible unexpected outcomes, what to do if plan is not working, when and how to seek help	
Ensuring appropriate point of closure	
57. **Summarizes session** briefly and clarifies plan of care	
58. **Final check** that client agrees and is comfortable with plan and asks if any correction, questions or other items to discuss	

OPTIONS IN EXPLANATION AND PLANNING	COMMENTS
If discussing opinion and significance of problem	
59. **Offers opinion** of what is going on and names if possible	
60. **Reveals rationale** for opinion	
61. **Explains** causation, seriousness, expected outcome, short and long term consequences	
62. **Elicits client's beliefs, reactions and concerns** (e.g. if opinion matches client's thoughts, acceptability, feelings)	
If negotiating mutual plan of action	
63. **Discusses options** (e.g. no action, investigation, medication, non-drug treatments, fluids, surgery, behavioral consult, preventative measures, euthanasia/cull)	
64. **Provides information** on action or treatment offered a) name b) steps involved, how it works c) benefits and advantages d) possible side effects, risks	
65. **Obtains client's view** of **need** for action, **benefits, barriers, motivation**; accepts and advocates alternative viewpoint as needed	
66. **Accepts** client's views; advocates alternative viewpoint as necessary	
67. **Elicits client's understanding, reactions and concerns** about plans and treatments, including acceptability	
68. **Takes client's lifestyle, beliefs**, cultural **background** and **abilities into consideration**	
69. **Encourages client to be involved** in implementing plans and **to follow through**	
70. **Asks about client support networks**, discusses other options	
If discussing investigations and procedures	
71. **Provides clear information on procedures** including what client might experience and how client will be informed of results	
72. **Relates procedure to treatment plan**: value and purpose	
73. **Encourages questions and expression of thoughts** regarding potential anxieties or negative outcome	

Additional comments:

APPENDIX B

Historical investigation pyramids: Beef, Dairy, Equine

Wilson J, Donszelmann D, Read E, Levy M, Krebs G, Pittman T, Atkins G, Leguillette R, Whitehead A and Adams CL (2012).

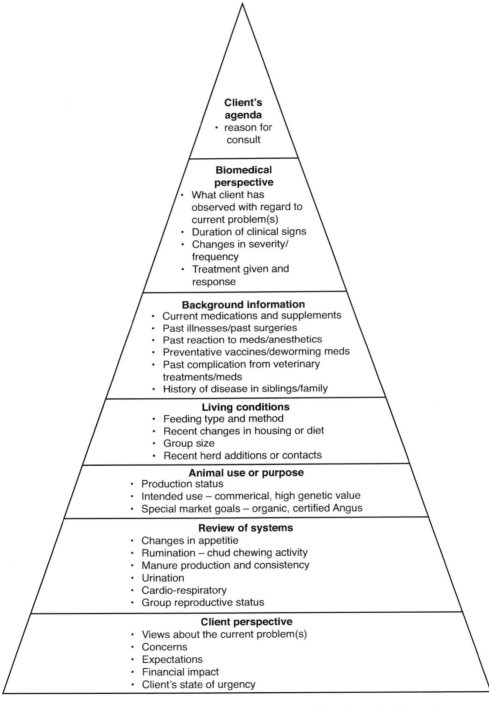

FIGURE B.1 Historical investigation pyramids: Beef. Wilson et al. (2012). Used with permission

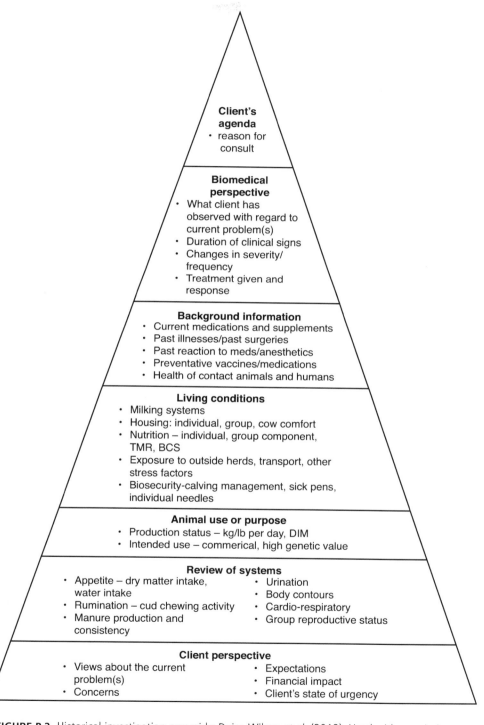

FIGURE B.2 Historical investigation pyramids: Dairy. Wilson et al. (2012). Used with permission

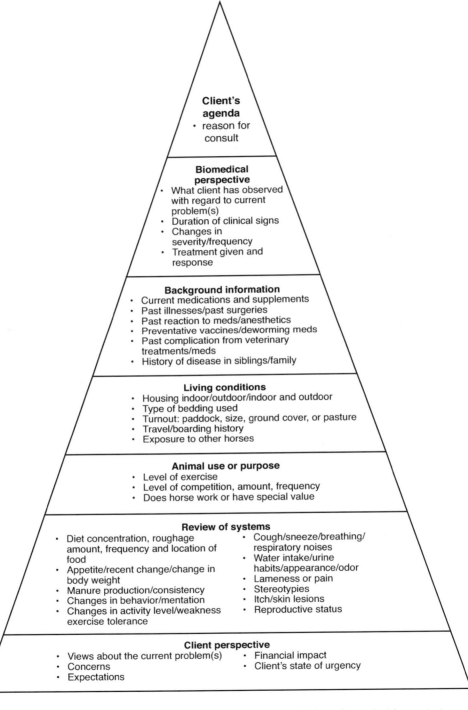

FIGURE B.3 Historical investigation pyramids: Equine. Wilson et al. (2012). Used with permission

Tasks and checkpoints mentioned in other guides

CHAPTER 3

- Pendleton et al. (1984, 2003)
  - To understand the reasons for the patient's attendance
    1. the nature and history of the problems
    2. their etiology
    3. the effects of the problems
    4. the patient's ideas, concerns and expectations
  - To establish or maintain a relationship with the patient that helps to achieve the other tasks.
- Neighbour (1987)
  - Connecting – establishing rapport with the patient
  - Summarizing – "Have I sufficiently understood why patient has come to see me?"
- AAPP 3-Function Model (Cohen-Cole 1991)
  - Gathering data to understand a patient's problems
  - Developing rapport and responding to patient's emotions.
- Bayer Institute for Health Care Communication E4 model (Keller and Carroll 1994)
  - Engaging the patient
  - Empathizing with the patient.
- The Four Habits Model (Frankel and Stein 1999; Krupat et al. 2006)
  - Elicit the patient's perspective.
- The SEGUE Framework for teaching and assessing communication skills (Makoul 2001)
  - Elicit information.
- The Maastricht Maas Global (van Thiel and van Dalen 1995)
  - Exploration
  - Clarification
  - Summarizations
  - Emotions.
- Essential Elements of Communication in Medical Encounters: Kalamazoo Consensus Statement (Participants in the Bayer-Fetzer Conference on Physician-Patient Communication in Medical Education 2001)
  - Gather information
  - Understand the patient's perspective.

- Patient-centered medicine (Stewart et al. 2003)
  - Exploring both the disease and the illness experience of the patient.
- The Model of the Macy Initiative in Health Communication (Kalet et al. 2004)
  - Gather
  - Elicit and understand patient's perspective.
- The Six Function Model (de Haes and Bensing 2009)
  - Gathering information.
- Institute for Healthcare Communication, Veterinary Communication Project (2004)
  - Engage the client.

CHAPTER 4

- Pendleton et al. (1984, 2003)
  - To use time and resources appropriately.
- Neighbour (1987)
  - Summarizing – "Have I sufficiently understood why this patient has come to see me?"
- AAPP 3-Function Model (Cohen-Cole 1991)
  - Gathering data:
    - ❯ survey of problems
    - ❯ negotiate priorities
    - ❯ summarizing.
- The Four Habits Model (Frankel and Stein 1999, Krupat et al. 2006)
  - Invest in the beginning
    - ❯ plan the visit with the patient.
- The Maastricht Maas Global (van Thiel and van Dalen 1995)
  - Summarizations
  - Ordering.
- Essential Elements of Communication in Medical Encounters: Kalamazoo Consensus Statement (Participants in the Bayer-Fetzer Conference on Physician-Patient Communication in Medical Education 2001)
  - Structure, clarify and summarize information.
- Patient-centered medicine (Stewart et al. 2003)
  - Enhancing the doctor–patient relationship: sharing power
  - Being realistic: time.
- The Model of the Macy Initiative in Health Communication (Kalet et al. 2004)
  - Manage flow.
- Institute for Healthcare Communication, Veterinary Communication Project (2004)
  - Engage the client
  - Negotiate agenda before exploring problems.

CHAPTER 5

- Pendleton et al. (1984, 2003)
  - To establish or maintain a relationship with the patient (client) that helps to achieve the other tasks.
- Neighbour (1987)
  - Connecting – establishing rapport with the patient.
- AAPP 3-Function Model (Cohen-Cole 1991)
  - Developing rapport and responding to patient's emotions.
- Bayer Institute for Health Care Communication E4 model (Keller and Carroll 1994)
  - Engaging the patient
  - Empathizing with the patient.
- The Four Habits Model (Frankel and Stein 1999; Krupat et al. 2006)
  - Demonstrate empathy.
- The SEGUE Framework for teaching and assessing communication skills (Makoul 2001)
  - Understand the patient's perspective.
- The Maastricht Maas Global (van Thiel and van Dalen 1995)
  - Emotions
  - Flexibility.
- Essential Elements of Communication in Medical Encounters: Kalamazoo Consensus Statement (Participants in the Bayer-Fetzer Conference on Physician-Patient Communication in Medical Education 2001)
  - Build a relationship.
- Patient-centered medicine (Stewart et al. 2003)
  - Enhancing the doctor–patient relationship.
- The Model of the Macy Initiative in Health Communication (Kalet et al. 2004)
  - Build a relationship.
- The Six Function Model (de Haes and Bensing 2009)
  - Fostering the relationship
  - Responding to emotions.
- Institute for Healthcare Communication, Veterinary Communication Project (2004)
  - Emphasize with the client.

CHAPTER 6

- Pendleton et al. (1984, 2003)
  - To enable the patient to choose an appropriate action for each problem
  - To achieve a shared understanding of the problems with the patient
  - To involve the patient in the management and encourage them to accept appropriate responsibility.
- Neighbour (1987)
  - Handing over – doctors' and patients' agendas; negotiating, influencing and gift-wrapping.

- AAPP 3-Function Model (Cohen-Cole 1991)
  - — Education, negotiation and motivation
  - — Developing rapport and responding to patient's emotions.
- Bayer Institute for Health Care Communication E4 model (Keller and Carroll 1994)
  - — Educating the patient
  - — Enlisting the patient in their own healthcare.
- The SEGUE Framework for teaching and assessing communication skills (Makoul 2001)
  - — Give information.
- The Maastricht Maas Global (van Thiel and van Dalen 1995)
  - — Information sharing
  - — Diagnosis
  - — Management.
- Essential Elements of Communication in Medical Encounters: Kalamazoo Consensus Statement (Participants in the Bayer-Fetzer Conference on Physician-Patient Communication in Medical Education 2001)
  - — Share information
  - — Reach agreement on problems and plans.
- The Four Habits Model (Frankel and Stein 1999; Krupat et al. 2006)
  - — Invest in the end
    - > deliver diagnostic information
    - > provide education
    - > involve patient in making decisions.
- Patient-centered medicine (Stewart et al. 2003)
  - — Finding common ground
  - — Incorporating prevention and health promotion.
- The Model of the Macy Initiative in Health Communication (Kalet et al. 2004)
  - — Patient education
  - — Negotiate and agree on plan.
- The Six Function Model (de Haes and Bensing 2009)
  - — Providing information
  - — Decision making.
- Institute for Healthcare Communication, Veterinary Communication Project (2004)
  - — Educate the client
  - — Enlist the client as a partner.

CHAPTER 7

- Pendleton et al. (1984, 2003)
  - — To use time and resources appropriately.
- Neighbour (1987)
  - — Safety netting: "What if?" – consider what the doctor might do in each case.

- AAPP 3-Function Model (Cohen-Cole 1991)
  - Education, negotiation and motivation
  - Developing rapport and responding to patient's emotions.
- Bayer Institute for Health Care Communication E4 model (Keller and Carroll 1994)
  - Educating the patient
  - Enlisting the patient in their own healthcare.
- The Four Habits Model (Frankel and Stein 1999; Krupat et al. 2006)
  - Invest in the end.
- The SEGUE Framework for teaching and assessing communication skills (Makoul 2001)
  - End the encounter.
- The Maastricht Maas Global (van Thiel and van Dalen 1995)
  - Management: determining who will do what and when.
- Essential Elements of Communication in Medical Encounters: Kalamazoo Consensus Statement (Participants in the Bayer-Fetzer Conference on Physician-Patient Communication in Medical Education 2001)
  - Provide closure.
- Patient-centered medicine (Stewart et al. 2003)
  - Time and timing.
- The Model of the Macy Initiative in Health Communication (Kalet et al. 2004)
  - Close.
- Institute for Healthcare Communication, Veterinary Communication Project (2004)
  - Close the visit.

References

Abdel-Tawab N and Roter D (2002) The relevance of client-centered communication to family planning settings in developing countries: lessons from the Egyptian experience. *Soc Sci Med.* **54**(9): 1357–68.

Abood SK (2008) Effectively communicating with your clients. *Topics in Comp Ani Med.* **23**(3): 143–7.

Accreditation Policies and Procedures of the AVMA Council on Education. Standard 11, Outcomes Assessment. AVMA Schaumburg, IL. 2012. Available at: www.avma.org/Professional.Development/Education/Accreditation/Colleges/Pages/coe-process.aspx.

Adams CL and Frankel RM (2007) It may be a dog's life but the relationship with her owners is also key to her health and well being: communication in veterinary medicine. *Vet Clinics of NA: SA Prac.* **37**(1): 1–17.

Adams CL and Kurtz SM (2006) Building on existing models from human medical education to develop a communication curriculum in veterinary medicine. *JVME* **33**(1): 28–37.

Adams CL and Kurtz SM (2012) Coaching and feedback: enhancing communication teaching and learning in veterinary practice settings. *JVME* **39**(3): 217–38.

Adams CL and Kurtz SM (2016) Communication in veterinary medical education In. J Hodgson and J Pelzer (eds) Veterinary Medical Education: A Practical Guide. Wiley Blackwell, Oxford. (in press)

Adams CL and Ladner LD (2004) Implementing a simulated client program: bridging the gap between theory and practice. *JVME.* **31**(2): 138–45.

Adams CL, Bonnett BN and Meek AH (2000) Predictors of owner response to companion animal death in 177 clients from 14 practices in Ontario. *Journal of the Amer Vet Med Assoc.* **217**(9): 1303–9.

Adams CL, Bonnett BN, Meek AH (1999) Owner response to companion animal death: development of a theory and practical implications. *The Can Vet J.* **40**(1): 33.

Adams CL, Conlon P and Long K (2004) Professional and veterinary competencies: addressing human relations and the human-animal bond in veterinary medicine. *JVME* **31**(1): 67–72.

Adams V, Campbell JR, Waldner CL, et al. (2005) Evaluation of client compliance with short-term administration of antimicrobials to dogs. *JAVMA.* **226**(4): 567–74.

Agledahl KM, Gulbrandsen P, Forde R and Wifstad A (2011) Courteous but not curious: how doctors' politeness masks their existential neglect; a qualitative study of video-recorded patient consultations. *J Med Ethics.* **37**(11): 650–4.

Aita V, McIlvain H, Backer E, McVea K and Crabtree B (2005) Patient-centered care and communication in primary care practice: what is involved? *Patient Educ Couns.* **58**(3): 296–304.

Ajzen I, Fishben M (1980) *Understanding attitudes and predicting social behaviour.* Prentice Hall, Englewood Cliffs, NJ.

Alamo MM, Moral RR and Perula de Torres LA (2002) Evaluation of a patient-centered approach in generalized musculoskeletal chronic pain/fibromyalgia patients in primary care. *Patient Educ Couns.* **48**(1): 23–31.

Alarcon P, Wieland B, Mateus ALP and Dewberry C (2013) Pig farmers' perceptions, attitudes, influences and management of information in the decision-making process for disease control. *Sci. Dir.* **116**: 223–42.

Als AB (1997) The desk-top computer as a magic box: patterns of behaviour connected with the desk-top computer; GPs' and patients' perceptions. *Fam Pract.* **14**(1): 17–23.

Ambady N, Koo J, Rosenthal R and Winograd CH (2002) Physical therapists' nonverbal communication predicts geriatric patients' health outcomes. *Psychol Aging.* **17**(3): 443–52.

American Animal Hospital Association (AAHA) (2003) *The path to high quality care, practical tips for improving compliance.* Lakewood, CO: AAHA.

American College of Veterinary Nutrition (2012) Nutrition related competencies of veterinarians. Available at: http://www.acvn.org/

Apter AJ, Paasche-Orlow MK, Remillard JT, Bennett IM, Ben-Joseph EP, Batista RM, Hyde J and Rudd RE (2008) Numeracy and communication with patients: they are counting on us. *J Gen Intern Med.* **23**(12): 2117–24.

Argyle M (1975) *Bodily Communication.* International Universities Press, New York, NY.

Arluke A (1997) Veterinary education: a plea and plan for sociological study. *Anthrozoos.* **10**: 3–7.

Artemiou E (2016) Personal communication with Cindy Adaams and Suzanne Kurtz.

Artemiou E, Adams CL, Hecker KG, Vallevand A, Violato C and Coe JB (2014) Standardized clients as assessors in a veterinary communication OSCE: a reliability and validity study. *Vet Rec.* **175**(20): 509. http://dx.doi.org/10.1136/vr.102633

Artemiou E, Adams CL, Toews L, Violato C and Coe JBE (2014) Informing web-based communication curricula in veterinary education: a systematic review of web-based methods used for teaching and assessing clinical communication in medical education. *JVME.* **41**(1): 45–54.

Artemiou E, Adams CL, Vallevand A, Violato C and Hecker KG (2013) Measuring the effectiveness of small-group and web-based training methods in teaching clinical communication: a case comparison study. *JVME.* **40**(3): 242–51.

Artemiou E, Hecker KG, Adams CL and Coe JB (2015) Does a rater's professional background influence communication skills assessment? *JVME.* **42**(4): 315–23.

Atkinson O (2010a) Communication in farm animal practice 1. Farmer–vet relationships. *In Practice.* **2**(3): 114–17.

Atkinson O (2010b) Communication in farm animal practice 1. Effecting change. *In Practice.* **32**(4): 163–5.

Audrey S, Abel J, Blazeby JM, Falk S and Campbell R (2008) What oncologists tell patients about survival benefits of palliative chemotherapy and implications for informed consent: qualitative study. *BMJ.* **337**: a752.

Azahar M, Fakri M, Pa M (2014) Associations between gender, year of study and empathy level with attitudes towards animal welfare among undergraduate doctor of veterinary medicine students in Universiti Putra Malaysia. *Education in Medicine.* **6**(4): 66–73.

Bachmann C, Abramovitch H, Barbu CG, Cavaco AM, Elorza RD, Haak R, Loureiro E, Ratajska A, Silverman J, Winterburn S and Rosenbaum M (2012) A European consensus on learning objectives for a core communication curriculum in health care professions. *Patient Educ Couns.* Epub Nov 28.

Bae SH and Fried MB (2010) Impact of nursing unit turnover on patient outcomes in hospitals. *J of Nurs Sch.* **42**(1): 40–9.

Baile WF and Beale EA (2001) Giving bad news to cancer patients: matching process and content. *J of Clin Onc.* **19**(9):2575–7.

Baillie S, Pierce S and May SA (2010) Fostering integrated learning and clinical professionalism using contextualized simulation in a small-group role-play. *JVME.* **37**(3): 248–53.

Baker LH, O'Connell D and Platt FW (2005) 'What else?' Setting the agenda for the clinical interview. *Ann Intern Med.* **143**(10): 766–70.

Baker SJ (1955) The theory of silences. *J Gen Psychol.* **53**(1): 145–67.

Barbour A (2000) Making Contact or Making Sense: functional and dysfunctional ways of relating. Humanities Institute Lecture 1999–2000 Series, University of Denver, Denver, CO.

Barnett PB (2001) Rapport and the hospitalist. *Am J Med.* **111**(9B): S31–5.

Barrows HS and Tamblyn RM (1980) *Problem-Based Learning: an approach to medical education.* Springer, New York, NY.

Barry CA, Bradley CP, Britten N, Stevenson FA and Barber N (2000) Patients' unvoiced agendas in general practice consultations: qualitative study. *BMJ.* **320**(7244): 1246–50.

Barry CA, Stevenson FA, Britten N, Barber N and Bradley CP (2001) Giving voice to the lifeworld. More humane, more effective medical care? A qualitative study of doctor–patient communication in general practice. *Soc Sci Med.* **53**(4): 487–505.

Barsky AJ 3rd (1981) Hidden reasons some patients visit doctors. *Ann Intern Med.* **94**(4 Pt. 1): 492–8.

Barter LS, Maddison JE, Watson ADJ (1996b) Comparison of methods to assess dog owners' therapeutic compliance *Australian Vet J.* **74**: 443–6.

Barter LS, Watson ADJ, Maddison JE (1996a) Owner compliance with short term antimicrobial medication in dogs. *Australian Vet J.* **74**: 277–80.

Bass LW and Cohen RL (1982) Ostensible versus actual reasons for seeking pediatric attention: Another look at the parental ticket of admission. *Pediatrics.* **70**(6): 870–4.

Bastiaens H, Van Royen P, Pavlic DR, Raposo V and Baker R (2007) Older people's preferences for involvement in their own care: a qualitative study in primary health care in 11 European countries. *Patient Educ Couns.* **68**(1): 33–42.

Bayer Institute for Health Care Communication (1999) *P.R.E.P.A.R.E. to be Partners (Program for Patients).* Bayer Institute for Health Care Communication, New Haven, CT.

Beach MC and Inui T (2006) Relationship-centered care: a constructive reframing. *J Gen Intern Med.* **21**(Suppl. 1): S3–8.

Beach MC, Roter DL, Wang NY, Duggan PS and Cooper LA (2006) Are physicians' attitudes of respect accurately perceived by patients and associated with more positive communication behaviors? *Patient Educ Couns.* **62**(3): 347–54.

Beaver K, Luker KA, Owens RG, Leinster SJ, Degner LF and Sloan JA (1996) Treatment decision making in women newly diagnosed with breast cancer. *Cancer Nurs.* **19**(1):8–19.

Beckman HB and Frankel RM (1984) The effect of physician behaviour on the collection of data. *Ann Intern Med.* **101**(5): 692–6.

Beckman HB and Frankel RM (1994) The use of videotape in internal medicine training. *J Gen Intern Med.* **9**(9): 517–21.

Beisecker A and Beisecker T (1990) Patient information-seeking behaviours when communicating with doctors. *Med Care.* **28**(1): 19–28.

Belcher VN, Fried TR, Agostini JV and Tinetti ME (2006) Views of older adults on patient participation in medication-related decision making. *J Gen Intern Med.* **21**(4): 298–303.

Bellet PS and Maloney MJ (1991) The importance of empathy as an interviewing skill in medicine. *JAMA.* **266**(13): 1831–2.

Bensing JM, Tromp F, van Dulmen S, van den Brink-Muinen A, Verheul W and Schellevis FG (2006) Shifts in doctor–patient communication between 1986 and 2002: a study of videotaped general practice consultations with hypertension patients. *BMC Fam Pract.* 7: 62.

Bergman L, Hart BL, Bain M and Cliff K (2002) Evaluation of urine marking by cats as a model for understanding veterinary diagnostic and treatment approaches and client attitudes. *JAVMA.* **221** (9): 1282–6.

Bertakis KD (1977) The communication of information from physician to patient: a method for increasing patient retention and satisfaction. *J Fam Pract.* **5**(2): 217–22.

Best C (2015) Exploring the role of interpersonal relationships in equine veterinary practice. PhD thesis, University of Guelph.

Blacklock (1977) The symptom of chest pain in family medicine. *J Fam Pract.* **4**(3): 429–33.

Blanchard CG, Labrecque MS, Ruckdeschel JC and Blanchard EB (1988) Information and decision making preferences of hospitalized adult cancer patients. *Soc Sci Med.* **27**: 1139.

Bland IM, Hill J (2011) Tackling dog obesity by tacking owner attitudes. *Perspectives in agriculture, veterinary science, nutrition and natural resources.* **6**: 1–7.

Blau PM and Duncan OD (1967) *The American Occupational Structure.* John Wiley & Sons, New York.

Bomzon L (1978) Short-term antimicrobial therapy: a pilot compliance study using ampicillin in dogs. BSAVA. *J Small Anim Pract.* **19**: 697–700.

Bonnett B (2015) Personal communication with Cindy Adams.

Bonvicini KA, Perlin MJ, Bylund CL, Carroll G, Rouse RA and Goldstein MG (2009) Impact of communication training on physician expression of empathy in patient encounters. *Patient Educ Couns.* **75**(1): 3–10.

Bonvicini KA. (2006) Tools for enhancing communication: an overview of risk management in equine practice. *AAEP.* **52**: 181–7.

Booth N, Kohannejad J and Robinson R (2002) *Information in the Consulting Room (iiCR) Final Project Report.* Sowerby Centre for Health, Newcastle upon Tyne.

Boreham P and Gibson D (1978) The informative process in private medical consultations: a preliminary investigation. *Soc Sci Med.* **12**(5A): 409–16.

Bourhis RY, Roth S and MacQueen G (1989) Communication in the hospital setting: a survey of medical and everyday language use amongst patients, nurses and doctors. *Soc Sci Med.* **28**(4): 339–46.

Bowen M (1985) *Family Therapy in Clinical Practice.* J. Aronson, New York.

Bowes P, Stevenson F, Ahluwalia S and Murray E (2012) I need her to be a doctor: patients' experiences of presenting health information from the internet in GP consultations. *Br J Gen Pract.* **62**(604): e732–8.

Braddock CH, Fihn SD, Levinson W, Jonsen AR and Pearlman RA (1997) How doctors and patients discuss routine clinical decisions: informed decision making in the outpatient setting. *J Gen Intern Med.* **12**(6): 339–45.

Bradshaw PW, Ley P, Kincey JA and Bradshaw J (1975) Recall of medical advice: comprehensibility and specificity. *Br J Soc Clin Psychol.* **14**: 55–62.

Branch WT and Malik TK (1993) Using 'windows of opportunities' in brief interviews to understand patients' concerns. *JAMA.* **269**(13): 1667–8.

Brandt JC and Bateman SW (2006) Senior Veterinary Students' perceptions of using role play to learn communication skills. *J of Vet Med Educ.* **31**(1): 76–80.

Bravo BN, Postigo JML, Segura LR, Selva JPS, Trives JJR, Córcoles MJ, López MN and Hidalgo JLT (2010) Effect of the evaluation of recall on the rate of information recalled by patients in primary care. *Patient Educ Couns.* **81**(2): 272–4.

Brennan ML and Christley RM (2013) Cattle producers' perceptions of biosecurity. *BMC Vet Res.* **9**: 71.

Briggs GW and Banahan BF (1979) A training workshop in psychological medicine for teachers of family medicine. Handouts 1–3: therapeutic communications. Society of Teachers of Family Medicine, Denver, CO.

Britten N (2003) Concordance and compliance. In: R Jones, N Britten, L Culpepper, D Gass, R Grol, D Mant and C Silagy (eds) *Oxford Textbook of Primary Medical Care.* Oxford University Press, Oxford.

Britten N, Stevenson FA, Barry CA, Barber N and Bradley CP (2000) Misunderstandings in prescribing decisions in general practice: qualitative study. *BMJ.* **320**(7233): 484–8.

Brody DS (1980) The patient's role in clinical decision-making. *Ann Intern Med.* **93**: 718–22.

Brody DS and Miller SM (1986) Illness concerns and recovery from a URI. *Med Care.* **24**(8): 742–8.

Bronshtein O, Katz V, Freud T and Peleg R (2006) Techniques for terminating patient-physician encounters in primary care settings. *Isr Med Assoc J.* **8**(4): 266–9.

Brown CE, Roberts NJ and Partridge MR (2007) Does the use of a glossary aid patient understanding of the letters sent to their general practitioner? *Clin Med.* **7**(5): 457–60.

Bryan J and Cary J (2010) Unpublished course materials for the clinical communication program, College of Veterinary Medicine, Washington State University. Used with permission.

Bryant C (1979) The zoological connection: animal-related human behavior. *Social Forces.* **58**(2): 399–421.

Buckman R (2002) Communications and emotions. *BMJ.* **325**(7366): 672.

Buller MK and Buller DB (1987) Physicians' communication style and patient satisfaction. *J Health Soc Behav.* **28**(4): 375–88.

Bunge M, Muhlhauser I and Steckelberg A (2010) What constitutes evidence-based patient information? Overview of discussed criteria. *Patient Educ Couns.* **78**(3): 316–28.

Buntain B, Allen-Scott L, North M, Rock M, Hatfield J (2015) Enabling academic one health environments in one health. In: Zinsstag J, Walter-Toews D, Whittaker M, Tanner M (eds). *One Health: the theory and practice of integrated approaches.* CABI Nosworthy Way, Oxfordshire, UK & CABI Chauncy Street, Boston MA, USA.

Burack RC and Carpenter RR (1983) The predictive value of the presenting complaint. *J Fam Pract.* **16**(4): 749–54.

Burton D, Blundell N, Jones M, Fraser A and Elwyn G (2010) Shared decision-making in cardiology: do patients want it and do doctors provide it? *Patient Educ Couns.* **80**(2): 173–9.

Butler C, Rollnick S and Stott N (1996) The practitioner, the patient and resistance to change: recent ideas on compliance. *CMAJ.* **154**(9): 1357–62.

Bylund CL and Makoul G (2002) Empathic communication and gender in the physician-patient encounter. *Patient Educ Couns.* **48**(3): 207–16.

Bylund CL and Makoul G (2005) Examining empathy in medical encounters: an observational study using the empathic communication coding system. *Health Commun.* **18**(2): 123–40.

Bylund CL, Gueguen JA, Sabee CM, Imes RS, Li Y and Sanford AA (2007) Provider-patient dialogue about Internet health information: an exploration of strategies to improve the provider-patient relationship. *Patient Educ Couns.* **66**(3): 346–52.

Byrne PS and Long BEL (1976) *Doctors Talking to Patients.* Her Majesty's Stationery Office, London.

Cake MA, Bell MA, Williams JC, Brown FJL, Dozier M, Rhind S and Baillie S (2016) Which professional (non-technical) competencies are most important to the success of graduate veterinarians? A best evidence medical education (BEME) systematic review: BEME Guide No. 38. Medical Teacher May 4: 1–14. (epub ahead of print)

Campion P, Foulkes J, Neighbour R and Tate P (2002) Patient centeredness in the MRCGP video examination: analysis of large cohort. Membership of the Royal College of General Practitioners. *BMJ.* **325**(7366): 691–2.

Campion PD, Butler NM and Cox AD (1992) Principle agendas of doctors and patients in general practice consultations. *Fam Pract.* **9**(2): 181–90.

Carmeli A and Gittell JH. (2010) High quality relationships, psychological safety and learning from failures in work organizations. *J Org Beh.* **30**(6): 709–29.

Carson CA (2007) Nonverbal communication in veterinary practice. (Effective Communication in Veterinary Practice.) *Vet Clin of NA, SA Pract.* **37**(1): 49–63.

Cary J and Kurtz S (2013) Integrating clinical communication with clinical reasoning and the broader medical curriculum. *Patient Ed. & Counseling.* **92**(3): 361–5.

Case DB (1988) Survey of expectations among clients of three small animal clinics. *JAVMA.* **192**(4): 498.

Cassata DM (1978) Health Communication theory and research: an overview of the communication specialist interface. In: BD Ruben (ed.) *Communication Yearbook.* Transaction Books, New Brunswick, NJ.

Cassileth B, Zupkis R and Sutton-Smith K (1980) Information and participation preferences among cancer patients. *Ann Intern Med.* **92**(6): 832–6.

Cegala DJ (1997) A study of doctors' and patients' communication during a primary care consultation: implications for communication training. *J Health Commun.* **2**(3): 169–94.

Cegala DJ (2003) Patient communication skills training: a review with implications for cancer patients. *Patient Educ Couns.* **50**(1): 91–4.

Cegala DJ and Post DM (2009) The impact of patients' participation on physicians' patient-centered communication. *Patient Educ Couns.* **77**(2): 202–8.

Charles C, Gafni A and Whelan T (1997) Shared decision-making in the medical encounter: what does it mean? (or it takes at least two to tango) *Soc Sci Med.* **44**(5): 681–92.

Charles C, Gafni A and Whelan T (1999a) Decision-making in the physician–patient encounter: revisiting the shared treatment decision-making model. *Soc Sci Med.* **49**(5): 651–61.

Charles C, Whelan T and Gafni A (1999b) What do we mean by partnership in making decisions about treatment? *BMJ.* **319**(7212): 780–2.

Chewning B, Bylund CL, Shah B, Arora NK, Gueguen JA and Makoul G (2012) Patient preferences for shared decisions: a systematic review. *Patient Educ Couns.* **86**(1): 9–18.

Chugh U, Agger-Gupta N, Dillmann E, Fisher D, Gronnerud P, Kulig JC, Kurtz S and Stenhouse A (1994) *The Case for Culturally Sensitive Health Care: a comparative study of health beliefs related to culture in six north-east Calgary communities.* Citizenship and Heritage Secretariat, Alberta Community Development & Calgary Catholic Immigration Society, Calgary, AB.

Chun R, Schaefer S, Lotta CC, Banning JA and Skochelak SE (2009) Didactic and experiential training to teach communication skills: the University of Wisconsin-Madison School of Veterinary Medicine collaborative experience. *JVME.* **36**(2): 196–201.

Coambs RB, Jensen P, Hoa Her M, Ferguson BS, Jarry JL, Wong JS and Abrahamsohn RV (1995) *Review of the Scientific Literature on the Prevalence, Consequences, and Health Costs of Noncompliance and Inappropriate Use of Prescription Medication in Canada.* Pharmaceutical Manufacturers Association of Canada (University of Toronto Press), Ottawa, ON.

Coe J (2008) Communication during veterinarian-client-patient interactions in companion animal practice. PhD thesis, University of Guelph.

Coe Jason B, Adams CL and Bonnett BN. (2008) A focus group study of veterinarians' and pet owners' perceptions of veterinarian-client communication in companion animal practice. *JAVMA.* **233**(7): 1072–80.

Coe JB, Adams CL and Bonnett BN (2007) A focus group study of veterinarians' and pet owners' perceptions of the monetary aspects of veterinary care. *JAVMA.* **231**(10): 1510–18.

Coe JB, Adams CL and Bonnett BN (2009) Prevalence and nature of cost discussions during clinical appointments in companion animal practice. *JAVMA.* **234**(11): 1418–24.

Cohen H and Britten N (2003) Who decides about prostate cancer treatment? A qualitative study. *Fam Pract.* **20**(6): 724–9.

Cohen-Cole SA (1991) *The Medical Interview: a three function approach*. Mosby-Year Book, St. Louis, MO.

Coleman C (2011) Teaching health care professionals about health literacy: a review of the literature. *Nurs Outlook*. **59**(2): 70–8.

Collins and Taylor (2002) Attributes of Australasian veterinary graduates: report of a workshop held at the veterinary conference centre, Faculty of Veterinary Science, University of Sydney, January 28–29, *JVME*. **29**: 71–2.

Cornell KK and Kopcha M (2007) Client-veterinarian communication: skills for client centered dialogue and shared decision making. *Vet Clin N Am Sm An*. **37**(1): 37–47.

Coulehan JL, Platt FW, Egener B, Frankel R, Lin CT, Lown B and Salazar WH (2001) 'Let me see if I have this right ...': words that help build empathy. *Ann Intern Med*. **135**(3): 221–7.

Coulter A (1999) Paternalism or partnership? Patients have grown up: and there's no going back. *BMJ*. **319**(7212): 719–20.

Coulter A (2002) After Bristol: putting patients at the centre. *BMJ*. **324**(7338): 648–51.

Coulter A (2009) *Implementing Shared Decision Making in the UK*. Health Foundation, London.

Coulter A (2012) Patient engagement: what works? *J Ambul Care Manage*. **35**(2): 80–9.

Coulter A, Entwistle V and Gilbert D (1999) Sharing decisions with patients: is the information good enough? *BMJ*. **318**(7179): 318–22.

Cox A (1989) Eliciting patients' feelings. In: Stewart M and Roter D (eds) *Communicating with Medical Patients*. Sage Publications, Newbury Park, CA.

Cox A, Hopkinson K and Rutter M (1981a) Psychiatric interviewing techniques II: naturalistic study. *Br J Psychiatry*. **138**: 283–91.

Cox A, Rutter M and Holbrook D (1981b) Psychiatric interviewing techniques V: experimental study. *Br J Psychiatry*. **139**: 29–37.

Cox ME, Yancy YS, Coffman CJ, Ostbye T, Tulsky JA, Alexander SC, Brouwer RJ, Dolor RJ and Pollak KI (2011) Effects of counseling techniques on patients' weight-related attitudes and behaviors in a primary care clinic. *Patient Educ Couns*. **85**(3): 363–8.

Croom A, Wiebe DJ, Berg CA, Lindsay R, Donaldson D, Foster C, Murry M and Swinyard MT (2011) Adolescent and parent perceptions of patient-centered communication while managing type 1 diabetes. *J Pediatr Psychol*. **36**(2): 206–15.

Cummings J, Vickers L and Marbaugh J. (1995) *Evaluation of Veterinary Dispensing Records to Measure "Clinical Compliance" with recommended heartworm prevention programs*. Proceedings of the heartworm symposium 1995 Batavia, IL. American Heartworm Society. pp. 183–86.

Dance FEX (1967) Toward a theory of human communication. In: FEX Dance (ed.) *Human Communication Theory: original essays*. Holt, Rhinehart & Winston, New York, NY.

Dance FEX and Larson CE (1972) *Speech Communication: concepts and behaviour*. Holt, Rinehart & Winston, New York, NY.

Davis MA, Hoffman JR and Hsu J (1999) Impact of patient acuity on preference for information and autonomy in decision making. *Acad Emerg Med*. **6**(8): 781–5.

De Haes H and Bensing J (2009) Endpoints in medical communication research, proposing a framework of functions and outcomes. *Patient Educ Couns*. **74**(3): 287–94.

De Morgan SE, Butow PN, Lobb EA, Price MA and Nehill C (2011) Development and pilot testing of a communication aid to assist clinicians to communicate with women diagnosed with ductal carcinoma in situ (DCIS). *Support Care Cancer*. **19**(5): 717–23.

Deber R (1994) The patient-physician partnership: changing roles and the desire for information. *CMAJ*. **151**(2): 171–6.

Degeling C. (2012) Narrative medicine: learning through stories. *Veterinary Record*. **170**(20): 522.

Degner LF and Sloan JA (1992) Decision making during serious illness: what role do patients really want to play? *J Clin Epidemiol*. **45**(9): 941–50.

Degner LF, Kristjanson LJ, Bowman D, Sloan JA, Carriere KC, O'Neil J, Bilodeau B, Watson P and Mueller B (1997) Information needs and decisional preferences in women with breast cancer. *JAMA*. **277**(18): 1485–92.

Del Piccolo L, Mazzi MA, Dunn G, Sandri M and Zimmermann C (2007) Sequence analysis in multilevel models: a study on different sources of patient cues in medical consultations. *Soc Sci Med*. **65**(11): 2357–70.

Derbyshire B (2015) Personal communication with Cindy Adams,.

Derks M, vanWoudenbergh B, Boender M, Kremer W, vanWerven T and Hodeveen H. (2013) Veterinarian awareness of farmer goals and attitudes to herd health management in The Netherlands. *Veterinary Journal.* **198**(1): 224–8.

DeVito JA (1988) *Human Communication: the basic course* (4th ed). Harper & Row, New York, NY.

DiMatteo MR (2004) The role of effective communication with children and their families in fostering adherence to pediatric regimens. *Patient Educ Couns.* **55**(3): 339–44.

DiMatteo MR, Hays RD and Prince LM (1986) Relationship of physicians' nonverbal communication skill to patient satisfaction, appointment noncompliance and physician workload. *Health Psychol.* **5**(6): 581–94.

DiMatteo MR, Taranta A, Friedman HS and Prince LM (1980) Predicting patient satisfaction from physicians' nonverbal communication skill. *Med Care.* **18**(4): 376–87.

Dimoska A, Tattersall MHN, Butow PN, Shepherd H and Kinnersley P (2008) Can a 'prompt list' empower cancer patients to ask relevant questions? *Cancer.* **113**(2): 225–37.

Dinsmore J and McConnell D (1992) Communication to avoid malpractice claims. *JAVMA.* **201**(3): 383–7.

Donovan JL (1995) Patient decision making: the missing ingredient in compliance research. *Int J Technol Assess Health Care.* **11**(3): 443–55.

Donovan JL and Blake DR (2000) Qualitative study of interpretation of reassurance among patients attending rheumatology clinics: 'just a touch of arthritis, doctor?' *BMJ.* **320**(7234): 541–4.

Dornan T and Carroll C (2003) Medical communication and diabetes. *Diabet Med.* **20**(2): 85–7.

Dowell J, Jones A and Snadden D (2002) Exploring medication use to seek concordance with 'non-adherent' patients: a qualitative study. *Br J Gen Pract.* **52**(474): 24–32.

Duke P, Reis S and Frankel RMA (2013) A skills-based approach for integrating the electronic health record and patient-centered communication into the medical visit. *Teach Learn Med.* **25**(4): 358–65.

Dunn SM, Butow PN, Tattersall MH, Jones QJ, Sheldon JS, Taylor JJ and Sumich MD (1993) General information tapes inhibit recall of the cancer consultation. *J Clin Oncol.* **11**(11): 2279–85.

Dysart LMA, Coe JB and Adams CL (2011) Analysis of solicitation of client concerns in companion animal practice. *JAVMA.* **238**(12): 1609–15.

Edwards A (2004) Flexible rather than standardised approaches to communicating risks in health care. *Qual Saf Health Care.* **13**(3): 169–70.

Edwards A and Elwyn G (2001a) *Evidence-Based Patient Choice: inevitable or impossible?* Oxford University Press, Oxford.

Edwards A and Elwyn GJ (2001b) Risks: listen and don't mislead. *Br J Gen Pract.* **51**(465): 259–60.

Edwards A, Elwyn G and Mulley A (2002) Explaining risks: turning numerical data into meaningful pictures. *BMJ.* **324**(7341): 827–30.

Edwards A, Elwyn G, Wood F, Atwell C, Prior L and Houston H (2005) Shared decision making and risk communication in practice: a qualitative study of GPs' experiences. *Br J Gen Pract.* **55**(510): 6–13.

Edwards A, Hood K, Matthews E, Russell D, Russell I, Barker J, Bloor M, Burnard P, Covey J, Pill R, Wilkinson C and Stott N (2000) The effectiveness of one-to-one risk communication interventions in health care: a systematic review. *Med Decis Making.* **20**(3): 290–7.

Egan G (1990) *The Skilled Helper: a systematic approach to effective helping.* Brooks/Cole, Pacific Grove, CA.

Eggins S, Slade D and Geddes F (2016), *Effective Communication in Clinical Handover From Research to Practice.* Walter de Gruyter, Berlin.

Eide H, Graugaard P, Holgersen K and Finset A (2003) Physician communication in different phases of a consultation at an oncology outpatient clinic related to patient satisfaction. *Patient Educ Couns.* **51**(3): 259–66.

Eisenthal S and Lazare A (1976) Evaluation of the initial interview in a walk-in clinic: the patient's perspective on a 'customer approach'. *J Nerv Mental Dis.* **162**(3): 169–76.

Eisenthal S, Emery R, Lazare A and Udin H (1979) 'Adherence' and the negotiated approach to parenthood. *Arch Gen Psych.* **36**(4): 393.

Eisenthal S, Koopman C and Stoeckle JD (1990) The nature of patients' requests for physicians. *Help Acad Med.* **65**(6): 401–5.

Ekman P, Friesen WV and Ellsworth P (1972) *Emotion in the Human Face: guidelines for research.* Pergamon, New York, NY.

Ellis-Iversen (2009) Perceptions, circumstances and motivators that influence implementation of zoonotic control programs on cattle farms. *Prev Vet Med.* **93**: 276–85.

Elstein AS and Schwarz A. (2002) Clinical problem solving and diagnostic decision making: selective review of the cognitive literature. *BMJ.* **324**: 729–32.

Elwyn G, Edwards A and Kinnersley P (1999b) Shared decision-making in primary care: the neglected second half of the consultation. *Br J Gen Pract.* **49**(443): 477–82.

Elwyn G, Edwards A, Gwyn R and Grol R (1999a) Towards a feasible model for shared decision making: focus group study with general practice registrars. *BMJ.* **319**(7212): 753–6.

Elwyn G, Edwards A, Kinnersley P and Grol R (2000) Shared decision making and the concept of equipoise: the competences of involving patients in healthcare choices. *Br J Gen Pract.* **50**(460): 892–9.

Elwyn G, Edwards A, Mowle S, Wensing M, Wilkinson C, Kinnersley P and Grol R (2001a) Measuring the involvement of patients in shared decision-making: a systematic review of instruments. *Patient Educ Couns.* **43**(1): 5–22.

Elwyn G, Edwards A, Wensing M, Hood K, Atwell C and Grol R (2003) Shared decision making: developing the OPTION scale for measuring patient involvement. *Qual Saf Health Care.* **12**(2): 93–9.

Elwyn G, Joshi H, Dare D, Deighan M and Kameen F (2001b) Unprepared and anxious about 'breaking bad news': a report of two communication skills workshops for GP registrants. *Educ Gen Pract.* **12**: 34–40.

Elwyn G, Kreuwel I, Durand MA, Sivell S, Joseph-Williams N, Evans R and Edwards A (2011) How to develop web-based decision support interventions for patients: a process map. *Patient Educ Couns.* **82**(2): 260–5.

Ely JW, Levinson W, Elder NC, Mainous AG 3rd and Vinson DC (1995) Perceived causes of family physicians' errors. *J Fam Pract.* **40**(4): 337–44.

Ende J, Kazis L, Ash AB and Moskovitz MA (1989) Measuring patients' desire for autonomy. *J Gen Intern Med.* **4**: 23–30.

Englar RE, Williams M and Weingand K (2016) Applicability of the Calgary-Cambridge Guide to dog and cat owners for teaching veterinary clinical communication. *JVME.* April **13**: 1–27. (epub ahead of print)

Epstein RM (2000) The science of patient-centered care. *J Fam Pract.* **49**(9): 805–7.

Epstein RM and Peters E (2009) Beyond information: exploring patients' preferences. *JAMA.* **302**(2):195–7.

Epstein RM, Alper BS and Quill TE (2004) Communicating evidence for participatory decision making. *JAMA.* **291**(19): 2359–66.

Everitt S, Pilnick A, Waring J and Cobb M (2013) The structure of the small animal consultation. *J Sm An Pract.* **54**(9): 453–8.

Faden RR, Becker C, Lewis C et al. (1981) Disclosure of information to patients in medical care. *Med Care.* **19**: 718–33.

Fallowfield LJ (2008) Treatment decision-making in breast cancer: the patient-doctor relationship. *Breast Cancer Res Treat.* **112**(Suppl. 1): 5–13.

Fink AS, Prochazka AV, Henderson WG, Bartenfeld D, Nyirenda C, Webb A, Berger DH, Itani K, Whitehill T, Edwards J, Wilson M, Karsonovich C and Parmelee P (2010) Enhancement of surgical informed consent by addition of repeat back: a multicenter, randomized controlled clinical trial. *Ann Surg.* **252**(1): 27–36.

Fishbein M and Ajzen I (1975) *Belief, Attitude, Intention and Behavior: an introduction to theory and research.* Addison-Wesley, Reading, MA.

Fleissig A, Glasser B and Lloyd M (2000) Patients need more than written prompts for communication to be successful. *BMJ.* **320**(7230): 314–15.

Fogassi L (2011) The mirror neuron system: how cognitive functions emerge from motor organization. *J of Eco Behav Org.* **77**: 66–75.

Ford S, Schofield T and Hope T (2003) What are the ingredients for a successful evidence-based patient choice consultation? A qualitative study. *Soc Sci Med.* **56**(3): 589–602.

Ford S, Schofield T and Hope T (2006) Observing decision-making in the general practice consultation: who makes which decisions? *Health Expect.* **9**(2): 130–7.

Francis V, Korsch B and Morris M (1969) Gaps in doctor-patient communication. *N Engl J Med.* **280**(10): 535–40.

Frankel R and Stein T (1999) Getting the most out of the clinical encounter: the four habits model. *Permanente Journal.* **3**(3): 79–88.

Frankel R, Altschuler A, George S, Kinsman J, Jimison H, Robertson NR and Hsu J (2005) Effects of exam-room computing on clinician-patient communication: a longitudinal qualitative study. *J Gen Intern Med.* **20**(8): 677–82.

Frankel RM (2006) Pets, vets and frets: what relationship centered care research has to offer veterinary medicine. *JVME.* **33**(1): 20–7.

Frankel RM (2009) Empathy research: a complex challenge. *Patient Educ Couns.* **75**(1): 1–2.

Freidson E (1970) *Professional Dominance.* Atherton Press, Chicago Il.

Friedman EH (1985) *Generation to Generation: family process in church and synagogue.* Guilford Press, New York.

Friedman HS (1979) Nonverbal communication between patient and medical practitioners. *J Soc Issues.* **35**(1): 82–99.

Gabay F, Moskowitz HR, Rotondo KJ, Aspros DG (2013) Understanding the mind of the pet owner for veterinary services. *Services Marketing Quarterly.* **35**(1): 1–18.

Gafaranga J and Britten N (2003) 'Fire away': the opening sequence in general practice consultations. *Fam Pract.* **20**(3): 242–7.

Gaissmaier W and Gigerenzer G (2008) Statistical illiteracy undermines informed shared decision making. *Z Evid Fortbild Qual Gesundhwes.* **102**(7): 411–13.

Garden R (2009) Expanding clinical empathy: an activist perspective. *J Gen Intern Med.* **24**(1): 122–5.

Garforth CJ, Bailey AP and Tranter RB (2013) Farmers' attitudes to disease risk management in England: a comparative analysis of sheep and pig farmers. *Preventive Vet Med.* **110**(3–4): 456–66.

Gates MC and Nolan TJ (2010) Factors influencing heartworm, flea, and tick preventative use in patients presenting to a veterinary teaching hospital. *Preventive Vet Med.* **93**(2–3):193–200.

Gattellari M, Butow PN and Tattersall MH (2001) Sharing decisions in cancer care. *Soc Sci Med.* **52**: 1865–78.

Gauthier JL and Richardson DJ. (2002) Knowledge and attitudes about zoonotic helminths: A survey of Connecticut pediatricians and veterinarians. *Compend Contin Educ Pract Vet.* **24**: 4–9.

Gazda GM, Asbury FR, Balzer FJ, Childers WC, Phelps RE and Walters RP (1995) *Human Relations Development: a manual for educators* (5th ed). Allyn & Bacon, Boston, MA.

Gibb JR (1961) Defensive communication. *J Commun.* **11**(3): 141–8.

Gick ML (1986) Problem-solving strategies. *Educ Psychol.* **21**(1–2): 99–120.

Giger R, Carruthers TD, Ribble CS and Townsend HGG. (1994) A survey of veterinarian and producer perceptions of herd health services in the Saskatoon milkshed *Can Vet J.* **35**: 359–66.

Gigerenzer G (2002) *Reckoning with Risk.* Penguin Books, London.

Gigerenzer G and Edwards A (2003) Simple tools for understanding risks: from innumeracy to insight. *BMJ.* **327**(7417): 741–4.

Gittell J (2003) How relational coordination works in other industries: the case of health care. In: *The Southwest Airlines Way: using the power of relationships to achieve high performance.* McGraw-Hill, New York, NY.

Gittell J, Fairfield K, Beirbaum B, Head W, Jackson R, Kelly M, Laskin R, Lipson S, Siliski J, Thornhill T and Zuckerman J (2000) Impact of relationship coordination on quality of care, post-operative pain and functioning and the length of stay: a nine-hospital study of surgical patients. *Med Care.* **38**(8): 807–19.

Gittell JH (2009) *High Performance Healthcare: using the power of relationships to achieve quality, efficiency and resilience.* McGraw Hill, New York.

Gittell JH, Fairfield K, Bierbaum B et al. (2000) Impact of relational coordination on quality of care, post-operative pain and functioning, and length of stay: a nine hospital study of surgical patients. *Medical Care.* **38**(8): 807–19.

Gittell JH, Weinberg D, Bennett A et al. (2008b) Is the doctor in? A relational approach to job design and the coordination of work. *Hum Resour Manag J.* **47**(4): 729–55.

Gittell JH, Weinberg DB, Pfefferle S, et al. (2008a) Impact of relational coordination on job satisfaction and quality outcomes: study of nursing homes. *Hum Resour Manag J.* **18**(2): 154–70.

Godolphin W (2009) Shared decision-making. *Health Q.* 12 Spec No Patient; e186–90.

Godolphin W, Towle A and McKendry R (2001) Evaluation of the quality of patient information to support informed shared decision making. *Health Expect.* **4**: 235–42.

Goldberg D, Steele JJ, Smith C and Spivey L (1983) *Training Family Practice Residents to Recognize Psychiatric Disturbances*. National Institute of Mental Health, Rockville, MD.

Goleman D (2011) *The Brain and Emotional Intelligence: new insights*. More Than Sound, Northampton, MA.

Good MJD and Good BJ (1982) *Patient Requests in Primary Care Clinics*. D Reidel, Boston, MA.

Goodwin C (1981) *Conversation Organization: interaction between speakers and hearers*. Academic Press, New York, NY.

Grandin T (2005) Maintenance of good animal welfare standards in beef slaughter plants by use of auditing programs. *JAVMA*. **226**: 370–73.

Grandin T (2010) Auditing animal welfare at slaughter plants. *Meat Sci*. **86**(1): 56–65.

Grandin T (2013) Making slaughterhouses more humane for cattle, pigs and sheep. *Annu Rev Anim Biosci*. **Jan 1**: 491–512.

Grandin T and Shivley C (2005) How farm animals react and perceive stressful situations such as handling, restraint, and transport. *Animals*. **15**(4): 1233–51.

Grant S and Olsen DW (1999) Preventing zoonotic diseases in immune-compromised persons: the role of physicians and veterinarians. *Emerg Infec Dis*. **5**: 159–63.

Grave K and Tanem H. (1999) Compliance with short-term oral antibacterial drug treatment in dogs. *J of SA Prac*. **40**: 158–62.

Gray C and Moffett J (2010) *Handbook of Veterinary Communication Skills*. Wiley-Blackwell, New Jersey.

Gray CA, Blaxter AC, Johnston PA, Latham CE, May S, Philips CA, Turnbull N and Yamagishi B. (2006) Communication education in veterinary in the United Kingdom and Ireland: the NUVACS project coupled to progressive individual school endeavors. *JVME*. **33**(1): 85–92.

Greatbach D, Luff P, Heath C and Campion P (1993) Interpersonal communication and human-computer interaction: an examination of the use of computers in medical consultations. *Interact Comput*. **5**(2): 193–216.

Greene J and Hibbard JH (2012) Why does patient activation matter? An examination of the relationships between patient activation and health-related outcomes. *J Gen Intern Med*. **27**(5): 520–6.

Greenfield S, Kaplan SH and Ware JE (1985) Expanding patient involvement in care. *Ann Intern Med*. **102**(4): 520–8.

Greenhill N, Anderson C, Avery A and Pilnick A (2011) Analysis of pharmacist-patient communication using the Calgary-Cambridge guide. *Patient Educ Couns*. **83**(3): 423–31.

Griffin SJ, Kinmonth AL, Veltman MW, Gillard S, Grant J and Stewart M (2004) Effect on health-related outcomes of interventions to alter the interaction between patients and practitioners: a systematic review of trials. *Ann Fam Med*. **2**(6): 595–608.

Groopman J (2007) *How Doctors Think*. Houghton Mifflin, Boston, MA.

Guadagnoli E and Ward P (1998) Patient participation in decision-making. *Soc Sci Med*. **47**(3): 329–39.

Gunn GJ, Heffernan C, Hall M, McLeod A and Hovi M (2008) Measuring and comparing constraints to improved biosecurity amongst GB farmers, veterinarians and the auxiliary industries. *Pre Vet Med*. **84**: 310–23.

Hack TF, Degner LF and Dyck DG (1994) Relationship between preferences for decision control and illness information among women with breast cancer. *Soc Sci Med*. **39**: 279–89.

Hack TF, Pickles T, Bultz BD, Ruether JD and Degner LF (2007) Impact of providing audiotapes of primary treatment consultations to men with prostate cancer: a multi-site, randomized, controlled trial. *Psychooncology*. **16**(6): 543–52.

Hafen M Jr, Rush BR and Nelson SC (2009) Utilizing filmed authentic student-client interactions as a communication teaching tool. *JVME*. **36**(4): 429–35.

Hafen M, Drake AA, Rush BR and Nelson, SC (2013) Using authentic client interactions in communication skills training: predictors of proficiency. JVME. 40(4): 318–26.

Hall J and Wapenaar W (2012) Opinions and practices of veterinarians and dairy farmers towards herd health management in the UK. *Veterinary Record*. **170**(17): 441.

Hall JA, Harrigan JA and Rosenthal R (1995) Nonverbal behaviour in clinician-patient interaction. *Appl Prev Psychol*. **4**(1): 21–35.

Hall JA, Roter DL and Katz NR (1987) Task versus socioemotional behaviour in physicians. *Med Care*. **25**(5): 399–412.

Hall JA, Roter DL and Katz NR (1988) Meta-analysis of correlates of provider behaviour in medical encounters. *Med Care.* **26**(7): 657–75.

Hall JA, Roter DL and Rand CS (1981) Communication of affect between patient and physician. *J Health Soc Behav.* **22**(1): 18–30.

Halvorsen PA, Selmer R and Kristiansen IS (2007) Different ways to describe the benefits of risk-reducing treatments: a randomized trial. *Ann Intern Med.* **146**(12): 848–56.

Hamood WJ, Chur-Hansen A and McArthur ME (2014) A qualitative study to explore communication skills in veterinary medical education. *Inter J Med Ed.* **5**: 193–8.

Hampton JR, Harrison MJ, Mitchell JR, Prichard JS and Seymour C (1975) Relative contributions of history-taking, physical examination and laboratory investigation to diagnosis and management of medical outpatients. *Br Med J.* **2**(5969): 486–9.

Hannawa AF (2012) 'Explicitly implicit': examining the importance of physician nonverbal involvement during error disclosures. *Swiss Med Wkly.* **142**: w13576.

Hanson JL (2008) Shared decision making: have we missed the obvious? *Arch Intern Med.* **168**(13): 1368–70.

Harrigan JA, Oxman TE and Rosenthal R (1985) Rapport expressed through nonverbal behaviour. *J Nonverbal Behav.* **9**(2): 95–110.

Harvey JB, Roberts JM and Shantz PM (1991) Survey of veterinarians' recommendations for treatment and control of intestinal parasites in dogs: Public health implications. *JAVMA* **199**(6): 702–07.

Haskard K, Williams S, DiMatteo M, Heritage J and Rosenthal R (2008) The provider's voice: patient satisfaction and the content-filtered speech of nurses and physicians in primary medical care. *J Nonverbal Behav.* **32**(1)1–20.

Hay MC, Cadigan RJ, Khanna D, Strathmann C, Lieber E, Altman R, McMahon M, Kokhab M and Furst DE (2008) Prepared patients: internet information seeking by new rheumatology patients. *Arthritis Rheum.* **59**(4): 575–82.

Haynes RB, McKibbon KA and Kanani R (1996) Systematic review of randomized trials of interventions to assist patients to follow prescriptions for medications. *Lancet.* **348**(9024): 383–6.

Haynes RB, Scakett OC, Guyatt GH et al. (2005) *Clinical epidemiology: how to do clinical practice research (Clinical Epidemiology (Sackett)) third edition.* Lippincott, Williams and Wilkins, Philadelphia.

Haynes RB, Taylor DW and Sackett DL (1979) *Compliance in Health Care.* Johns Hopkins University Press, Baltimore, MD.

Headache Study Group of the University of Western Ontario, The (1986) Predictors of outcome in headache patients presenting a family physicians: a one year prospective study. *Headache.* **26**(6): 285–94.

Health Canada (1996) *It Helps to Talk.* Health Canada, Ottawa, ON.

Heath C (1984) Participation in the medical consultation: the co-ordination of verbal and nonverbal behaviour between the doctor and the patient. *Social Health Illn.* **6**(3): 311–38.

Heath T (1996) Teaching communication skills to veterinary students. *JVME.* **23**: 2–7.

Hecker KG, Adams CL and Coe JB (2012) Assessment of first-year veterinary students' communication skills using an objective structured clinical examination: the importance of context. *JVME.* **39**(3): 304–10.

Heffernan C, Nielsen L, Thomson K and Gunn G (2008) An exploration of the drivers to bio-security collective action among a sample of UK cattle and sheep farmers. *Preventive Veterinary Medicine.* **87**(3–4): 358–72.

Helman CG (1978) Free a cold, starve a fever: folk models of infection in an English suburban community and their relation to medical treatment. *Cult Med Psychiatry.* **2**(2): 107–37.

Heritage J (2011) The interaction order and clinical practice: some observations on dysfunctions and action steps. *Patient Educ Couns.* **84**(3): 338–43.

Heritage J and Robinson JD (2006) The structure of patients' presenting concerns: physicians' opening questions. *Health Commun.* **19**(2): 89–102.

Heritage J, Robinson JD, Elliott MN, Beckett M and Wilkes M (2007) Reducing patients' unmet concerns in primary care: the difference one word can make. *J Gen Intern Med.* **22**(10): 1429–33.

Hewson CJ (2007) Factors affecting Canadian veterinarians' use of analgesics when dehorning beef and dairy calves. *CJV.* **48**: 1129–36.

Hochbaum G (1958) Public participation in medical screening programs: A sociopsychological study. *Public Health Serv Publ.* **572**.

Hodgson JL, Pelzer J and Inzana K (2013). Beyond NAVMEC: competency-based veterinary education and assessment of the professional competencies. *NVME.* **40**(2): 102–18.

Hofmeister, EH, Thompson BF, Brainard BM, Kegge S, Kube S, Egger CM, Jehn C, Green B (2008) Survey of academic veterinarians' clinical practice in cardiopulmonary-cerebral resuscitation. *J Vet Emerg Crit Care.* **8**(2): 142–52.

Hojat M, Vergare MJ, Maxwell K, Brainard G, Herrine SK, Isenberg GA, Veloski J and Gonnella JS (2009) The devil is in the third year: a longitudinal study of erosion of empathy in medical school. *Acad Med.* **84**(9): 1182–91.

Holmes-Rovner M, Valade D, Orlowski C, Draus C, Nabozny-Valerio B and Keiser S (2000) Implementing shared decision-making in routine practice: barriers and opportunities. *Health Expect.* **3**(3): 182–91.

Hope T (1996) *Evidence-Based Patient Choice.* King's Fund Publishing, London.

Hsu I, Saha S, Korthuis PT, Sharp V, Cohn J, Moore RD and Beach MC (2012) Providing support to patients in emotional encounters: a new perspective on missed empathic opportunities. *Patient Educ Couns.* **88**(3): 436–42.

Hudak PL, Clark SJ and Raymond G (2011) How surgeons design treatment recommendations in orthopedic surgery. *Soc Sci Med.* **73**(7): 1028–36.

Institute for Healthcare Communication (2004) Veterinary Communication Project. New Haven, CT. Available from www.healthcarecomm.org.

Inui TS, Yourtee EL and Williamson JW (1976) Improved outcomes in hypertension after physician tutorials. *Ann Intern Med.* **84**: 646–51.

Jansen and Lam (2012) The role of communication in improving udder health. *Veterinary Clinics of North America – Food Animal Practice.* **28**(2): 363–79.

Jansen J (2010) Mastitis and farmer mindset towards effective communication strategies to improve udder health management on Dutch dairy farms. PhD Thesis, Wageningen University.

Jansen J, Butow PN, van Weert JC, van Dulmen S, Devine RJ, Heeren TJ, Bensing JM and Tattersall MH (2008) Does age really matter? Recall of information presented to newly referred patients with cancer. *J Clin Oncol.* **26**(33): 5450–7.

Jansen J, Rene RJ and Lam TJGM (2010) Evaluation of two communication strategies to improve udder health management. *J Dairy Sci.* **93**(2): 604–12.

Jansen J, Van Den Borne BHP, Renes RJ, et al. (2009) Explaining mastitis incidence in Dutch dairy farming: the influence of farmers' attitudes and behaviour. *Preventive Vet Med.* **92**(3): 210–23.

Janz NK and Becker MH (1984) The health belief model: a decade later, *Health Education Quarterly.* **11**(1): 1–47.

Jenkins V, Fallowfield L and Saul J (2001) Information needs of patients with cancer: results from a large study in UK cancer centres. *Br J Cancer.* **84**(1): 48–51.

Jenkins V, Solis-Trapala I, Langridge C, Catt S, Talbot DC and Fallowfield LJ (2011) What oncologists believe they said and what patients believe they heard: an analysis of phase I trial discussions. *J Clin Oncol.* **29**(1): 61–8.

Johnson R and Ellis L. (2006) Personal communication with Suzanne Kurtz.

Joos SK, Hickam DH and Borders LM (1993) Patients' desires and satisfaction in general medical clinics. *Public Health Rep.* **108**(6): 751–9.

Joos SK, Hickam DH, Gordon GH and Baker LH (1996) Effects of a physician communication intervention on patient care outcomes. *J Gen Int Med.* **11**(3): 147–55.

Kalet A, Pugnaire MP, Cole-Kelly K, Janicik R, Ferrara E, Schwartz MD, Lipkin M Jr and Lazare A (2004) Teaching communication in clinical clerkships: models from the Macy Initiative in Health Communication. *Acad Med.* **79**(6): 511–20.

Kaner E, Heaven B, Rapley T, Murtagh M, Graham R, Thomson R and May C (2007) Medical communication and technology: a video-based process study of the use of decision aids in primary care consultations. *BMC Med Inform Decis Mak.* **7**: 2.

Kanji N, Coe JB, Adams CL, and Shaw JR. (2012) Effect of veterinarian-client-patient interactions on client adherence to dentistry and surgery recommendations in companion-animal practice. *JAVMA.* **240**(4): 427–36.

Kaplan CB, Siegel B, Madill JM and Epstein RM (1997) Communication and the medical interview: strategies for learning and teaching. *J Gen Intern Med.* **12**(Suppl.2):S49–55.

Kaplan SH, Greenfield S and Ware JE (1989) Assessing the effects of physician-patient interactions on the outcomes of chronic disease. *Med Care.* **27**(3 Suppl): S110–27.

Kaplan SH, Greenfield S, Gandek B, Rogers WH and Ware JE (1996) Characteristics of physicians with participatory decision-making styles. *Ann Intern Med.* **124**: 497–504.

Karnieli-Miller O and Eisikovits Z (2009) Physician as partner or salesman? Shared decision-making in real-time encounters. *Soc Sci Med.* **69**(1): 1–8.

Kassirer JP (1983) Teaching clinical medicine by iterative hypothesis testing. *N Engl J Med.* **309**(15): 921–3.

Kassirer JP and Gorry GA (1978) Clinic Keithley J and Marsh G (1995) *Counselling in Primary Health Care.* Oxford Medical Publications, Oxford University Press, Oxford.

Kedrowicz A (2015) Clients and veterinarians as partners in problem solving during cancer management: implications for veterinary education. *JVME.* **42**(4): 373–82.

Keller VF and Carroll JG (1994) A new model for physician-patient communication. *Patient Educ Couns.* **23**(2): 131–40.

Keller VF and Kemp-White M (2001) Choices and changes: a new model for influencing patient health behavior. *J Clin Outcomes Manag.* **4**(6, Special publication): 33–6.

Kemp EC, Floyd MR, McCord-Duncan E and Lang F (2008) Patients prefer the method of 'tell back-collaborative inquiry' to assess understanding of medical information. *J Am Board Fam Med.* **21**(1): 24–30.

Kessel N (1979) Reassurance. *Lancet.* **1**(8126): 1128–33.

Kindelan K and Kent G (1987) Concordance between patients' information preferences and general practitioners" perceptions. *Psychol Health.* **1**(4): 399–409.

Kinmonth AL, Woodcock A, Griffin S, Spiegal N and Campbell MJ (1998) Randomized controlled trial of patient centered care of diabetes in general practice: impact on current wellbeing and future disease risk. Diabetes Care from Diagnosis Research Team. *BMJ.* **317**(7167): 1202–8.

Kinnison T, May SA and Guile D (2014) Inter-professional practice from veterinarian to the veterinary team. *JVME.* **41**(2): 172–8.

Kleen JL, Atkinson O and Noordhuizen JP. (2011) Communication in production animal medicine: modelling a complex interaction with the example of dairy herd health medicine. *IVJ.* **64**(1): 8.

Kleinman A, Eisenberg L and Good B. (1978) Culture, illness, and care: clinical lessons from anthropologic and cross-cultural research. *Ann Intern Med.* **88**(2): 251–8.

Klingborg J. (2011) *Exam Room Communication for Veterinarians: the science and art of conversing with clients.* AAHA Press, Lakewood, CO.

Koch R (1971) The teacher and nonverbal communication. *Theory Pract.* **10**(4): 231–42.

Kogan LR, Goldwaser G, Stewart SM and Schoenfeld-Tacher R (2008) Sources and frequency of use of pet health information and level of confidence in information accuracy, as reported by owners visiting small animal veterinary practices. *JAVMA.* **232**(10): 1536–42.

Kogan LR, Schoenfeld-Tacher R and Viera AR (2012) The Internet and health information: differences in pet owners based on age, gender, and education. *J Med Libr Assoc.* **100**(3): 197–204.

Kogan LR, Schoenfeld-Tacher R, Gould L, Viera AR and Hellyer PW (2014) Providing an information prescription in veterinary medical clinics: a pilot study. *J Medical Lib Assoc.* **102**(1): 41–6.

Korsch B and Harding C (1997) *The Intelligent Patient's Guide to the Doctor-Patient Relationship.* Oxford University Press, New York, NY.

Korsch BM, Gozzi EK and Francis V (1968) Gaps in doctor-patient communication. *Pediatrics.* **42**(5): 855–71.

Kravitz RL, Cope DW, Bhrany V and Leake B (1994) Internal medicine patients' expectations for care during office visits. *J Gen Intern Med.* **9**(2): 75–81.

Kripalani S and Weiss BD (2006) Teaching about health literacy and clear communication. *J Gen Intern Med.* **21**(8): 888–90.

Kristensen E and Enevoldsen C. (2008) A mixed methods inquiry: how dairy farmers perceive the value(s) of their involvement in an intensive dairy herd health management program. *Acta Vet Scand.* **50**: 50.

Krupat E, Frankel R, Stein T and Irish J (2006) The Four Habits Coding Scheme: validation of an instrument to assess clinicians' communication behavior. *Patient Educ Couns.* **62**(1): 38–45.

Kuiper D, Jansen J, Renes RJ, Leeuwis C and Zwagg van der Henk (2005). Social factors related to mastitis control practices: the role of dairy farmers' knowledge, attitude, values, behaviour and networks. Conference paper. Wageningen Academic Publishers, Wageningen, Gelderland, The Netherlands.

Kupst M, Dresser K, Schulman JL and Paul MH (1975) Evaluation of methods to improve communication in the physician-patient relationship. *Am J Orthopsychiatry*. **45**(3): 420.

Kurtz S (2016) Clinical communication education for surgeons. In SJ White and JA Cartmill (eds) *Communication in Surgical Practice*. Equinox Publishing, Sheffield UK and Bristol, CT.

Kurtz S, Silverman J and Draper J (1998) *Teaching & Learning Communication Skills in Medicine*. 1st ed. Radcliffe Medical Press, Oxford.

Kurtz S, Silverman J and Draper J (2005) *Teaching and Learning Communication Skills in Medicine*. 2nd ed. CRC Press, Boca Raton, FL.

Kurtz S, Silverman J, Benson J and Draper J (2003) Marrying content and process in clinical method teaching: enhancing the Calgary–Cambridge Guides. *Acad Med*. **78**(8): 802–9.

Kurtz SM (1989) Curriculum structuring to enhance communication skills development. In: M Stewart and D Roter (eds) *Communicating with Medical Patients*. Sage Publications, Newbury Park, CA.

Kurtz SM (2006) Teaching and learning communication in veterinary medicine. *JVME*. **33**(1): 11–19.

Kurtz SM and Adams CL (2009) Essential education in communication skills and cultural sensitivities for global public health in an evolving veterinary world. *Revue Scientifique et Technique*. **28**(2): 635–47.

Lam TJ, Jansen J, van den Borne BH, Renes RJ and Hogeveen H. (2011) What veterinarians need to know about communication to optimise their role as advisors on udder health in dairy herds. *NZ Vet J*. **59**(1): 8–15.

Lang F, Floyd MR and Beine KL (2000) Clues to patients' explanations and concerns about their illnesses: a call for active listening. *Arch Fam Med*. **9**(3): 222–7.

Lang F, Floyd MR, Beine KL and Buck P (2002) Sequenced questioning to elicit the patient's perspective on illness: effects on information disclosure, patient satisfaction and time expenditure. *Fam Med*. **34**(5): 325–30.

Langewitz W, Denz M, Keller A, Kiss A, Ruttimann S and Wossmer B (2002) Spontaneous talking time at start of consultation in outpatient clinic: cohort study. *BMJ*. **325**(7366): 682–3.

Larsen KM and Smith CK (1981) Assessment of nonverbal communication in the patient-physician interview. *J Fam Pract*. **12**(3): 481–8.

Latham CE and Morris A (2007) Effects of formal training in communication skills on the ability of veterinary students to communicate with clients. *Veterinary Record*. **160**: 181–6.

Lazare A, Eisenthal S and Wasserman L (1975) The customer approach to patienthood: attending to patient requests in a walk-in clinic. *Arch Gen Psychiatry*. **32**(5): 553–8.

Lazarus RS and Folkman S. (1984) *Stress, Appraisal, and Coping*. Springer, New York.

Levenstein JH, Belle Brown J, Weston WW, Stewart M, McCracken EC and McWhinney I (1989) Patient centred clinical interviewing. In. M Stewart and D Roter (eds). Communicating with medical patients. Sage Publications, Newbury Park CA.

Levinson W and Pizzo PA (2011) Patient-physician communication: it's about time. *JAMA*. **305**(17): 1802–3.

Levinson W, Gorawara-Bhat R and Lamb J (2000) A study of patient clues and physician responses in primary care and surgical settings. *JAMA*. **284**(8): 1021–7.

Levinson W, Kao A, Kuby A and Thisted RA (2005) Not all patients want to participate in decision making. A national study of public preferences. *J Gen Intern Med*. **20**(6): 531–5.

Levinson W, Roter DL, Mullooly JP, Dull VT and Frankel RM (1997) Physician-patient communication: the relationship with malpractice claims among primary care physicians and surgeons. *JAMA*. **277**(7): 553–9.

Levinson W, Stiles WB, Inui TS and Engle R (1993) Physician frustration in communicating with patients. *Med Care*. **31**(4): 285–95.

Ley P (1988) *Communication with Patients: improving satisfaction and compliance*. Croom Helm, London.

Lipkin M Jr (1987) The medical interview and related skills. In: WT Branch (ed.) *The Office Practice of Medicine*. WB Saunders, Philadelphia, PA.

Loftus L (2011) Review of current wound-care protocol and dressing choice in equine veterinary practice. *Vet Nurs J.* 26(9): 309–313.

Loftus L (2012) The non-compliant client. *Vet Nurs J.* 27(8): 294–7.

Logue DN (2004) Constraints on reproduction in dairy cattle: a veterinary viewpoint. *BCVA.* **12**: 51–6.

Longman T, Turner RM, King M and McCaffery KJ (2012) The effects of communicating uncertainty in quantitative health risk estimates. *Patient Educ Couns.* **89**(2): 252–9.

Lue TW, Patenburg DP and Crawford PM. (2008) Impact of the owner-pet and client-veterinarian bond on the care that pets receive. *JAVMA.* **232**(4): 531–40.

Lussier MT and Richard C (2008) Because one shoe doesn't fit all: a repertoire of doctor-patient relationships. *Can Fam Physician.* **54**(8): 1089–92, 1096–9.

Macdonald J and Gray C (2014) 'Informed consent' – how do we get it right? *Vet Nurs J.* **29**(3): 101–3.

MacDonald K (2009) Patient-clinician eye contact: social neuroscience and art of clinical engagement. *Postgrad Med.* **121**(4): 136–44.

MacMartin C, Coe JB and Adams CL (2014) Treating distressed animals as participants: I know responses in veterinarians' pet-directed talk. *Res Language and Social Interaction.* **47**(2): 151–74.

MacMartin C, Wheat HC, Coe JB and Adams CL (2015) Effect of question design on dietary information solicited during veterinarian–client interactions *JAVMA.* **246**(11): 1203–14.

MacMartin C (2015) Personal communication with Cindy Adams.

Maddison JE (2011) Medication compliance in small animal practice. *Vet Ireland J.* **64**(1): 39–43.

Maddison JE, Volk HA and Church DB (2015) *Clinical Reasoning in Small Animal Practice.* Wiley Blackwell, Oxford.

Maguire P and Rutter D (1976) History-taking for medical students: 1. Deficiencies in performance. *Lancet.* **2**(7985): 556–8.

Maguire P, Fairbairn S and Fletcher C (1986) Consultation skills of young doctors: II. Most young doctors are bad at giving information. *BMJ.* **292**(6535): 1576–8.

Maguire P, Faulkner A, Booth K, Elliott C and Hillier V (1996) Helping cancer patients disclose their concern. *Eur J Cancer.* **32**A(1): 78–81.

Makoul G (2001) The SEGUE Framework for teaching and assessing communication skills. *Patient Educ Couns.* **45**(1): 23–34.

Makoul G (2003) The interplay between education and research about patient-provider communication. *Patient Educ Couns.* **50**(1): 79–84.

Makoul G and Clayman ML (2006) An integrative model of shared decision making in medical encounters. *Patient Educ Couns.* **60**(3): 301–12.

Makoul G and Schofield T (1999) Communication teaching and assessment in medical education: an international consensus statement. Netherlands Institute of Primary Health Care. *Patient Educ Couns.* **37**(2): 191–5.

Makoul G, Arnston P and Scofield T (1995) Health promotion in primary care: physician-patient communication and decision about prescription medications. *Soc Sci Med.* **41**(9):1241–54.

Makoul G, Curry RH and Tang PC (2001) The use of electronic medical records: communication patterns in outpatient encounters. *J Am Med Inform Assoc.* **8**(6): 610–15.

Mandin H, Jones A, Woloshuk W and Harasym P (1997) Helping students learn to think like experts when solving clinical problems. *Acad Med.* **72**(3): 173–9.

Manning P and Ray GB (2002) Setting the agenda: an analysis of negotiation strategies in clinical talk. *Health Commun.* **14**(4): 451–73.

Martin F and Taunton A (2006) Perceived importance and integration of the human-animal bond in private veterinary practice. *JAVMA.* **228**(4): 522–7.

Marvel MK, Epstein RM, Flowers K and Beckman HB (1999) Soliciting the patient's agenda: have we improved? *JAMA.* **281**(3): 283–7.

Mauksch LB, Dugdale DC, Dodson S and Epstein R (2008) Relationship, communication and efficiency in the medical encounter: creating a clinical model from a literature review. *Arch Intern Med.* **168**(13): 1387–95.

Mazur DJ (2000) Information disclosure and beyond: how do patients understand and use the information they report they want? *Med Decis Making.* **20**(1): 132–4.

Mazzullo JM, Lasagna L and Griner PF (1974) Variations in interpretation of prescription instructions. *JAMA.* **227**(8): 929–31.

McArthur ML and Fitzgerald JR (2013) Companion animal veterinarians' use of clinical communication skills. *Australian Vet J.* **91**(9): 374–80.

McConnell D, Butow PN and Tattersall MH (1999) Audiotapes and letters to patients: the practice and views of oncologists, surgeons and general practitioners. *Br J Cancer.* **79**(11–12): 1782–8.

McCroskey JC, Larson CE and Knapp ML (1971) *An Introduction to Interpersonal Communication.* Prentice Hall, Englewood Cliffs, NJ.

McDermott MP, Tischler V, Cobb MA, Robbé IJ, Dean RS (2015) Veterinarian-client communication skills: current state, relevance, and opportunities for improvement. *JVME.* **42**(4): 305–14.

McGrath JM, Arar NH and Pugh JA (2007) The influence of electronic medical record usage on non-verbal communication in the medical interview. *Health Inform J.* **13**(2): 105–18.

McKinlay JB (1975) Who is really ignorant: physician or patient? *J Health Soc Behav.* **16**(1): 3–11.

McKinley RK and Middleton JF (1999) What do patients want from doctors? Content analysis of written patient agendas for the consultation. *Br J Gen Pract.* **49**(447): 796–800.

McMillan F (2002) Development of a mental wellness program for animals. *JAVMA.* **220**(7): 965–72.

McWhinney I (1989) The need for a transformed clinical method. In: M Stewart and D Roter (eds) *Communicating with Medical Patients.* Sage Publications, Newbury Park, CA.

Meagher DM (2005) A review of equine malpractice claims. *AAEP.* **51**: 508–14.

Mehrabian A (1972) *Nonverbal Communication.* Aldine Atherton, Chicago, IL.

Mehrabian A and Ksionsky S (1974) *A Theory of Affiliation.* Lexington Books, DC Health, Lexington, MA.

Meichenbaum D and Turk DC (1987) *Facilitating Treatment Adherence: a practitioner's guidebook.* Plenum Press, New York, NY.

Mellanby RJ, Crisp J, De Palma G, Spratt D P, Urwin D, Wright MJH and Zago S (2007) Perceptions of veterinarians and clients to expressions of clinical uncertainty. *J Sm Anim Prac.* **48**(1): 26–31.

Mellanby RJ, Rhind SM, Bell C, Shaw DJ, Gifford J, Fennell D, Manser C, Spratt DP, Wright MJH, Zago S and Hudson NPH (2011). Perceptions of clients and veterinarians on what attributes constitute 'a good vet'. *Veterinary Record.* **168**(23): 616.

Middleton JF (1995) Asking patients to write lists: feasibility study. *BMJ.* **311**(6996): 34.

Miller SM and Mangan CE (1983) Interacting effects of information and coping style in adapting to gynecologic stress: should the doctor tell all? *J Pers Soc Psychol.* **45**(1): 223–36.

Mills JN (1997) Use of drama in teaching the human side of veterinary practice. *Australian Vet J.* **75**(7): 497–9.

Mills JN, Irwin P, Baguley J, Meehan M, Austin H, Fitzpatrick L, Parry B and Heath T (2006) Development of veterinary communication skills at Murdoch University and in other Australian veterinary schools. *JVME.* **33**(1) 93–9.

Minhas R (2007) Does copying clinical or sharing correspondence to patients result in better care? *Int J Clin Pract.* **61**(8): 1390–5.

Mishel MH (1983) Parents' perceptions of uncertainty concerning their hospitalized child. *Nurs Res* **2**: 324–30.

Mishel MH (1981) The measurement of uncertainty in illness. *Nurs Res.* **30**: 258–63.

Mishel MH (1997) Uncertainty in acute illness. *Ann Rev Nursing Research.* New York, NY: Springer Publishing, **15**: 57–80.

Mishler EG (1984) *The Discourse of Medicine: dialectics of medical interviews.* Ablex, Norwood, NJ.

Mitchell E and Sullivan F (2001) A descriptive feast but an evaluative famine: systematic review of published articles in primary care computing during 1980–97. *BMJ.* **322**(7281): 279–82.

Mjaaland TA, Finset A, Jensen BF and Gulbrandsen P (2011a) Patients' negative emotional cues and concerns in hospital consultations: a video-based observational study. *Patient Educ Couns.* **85**(3): 356–62.

Mjaaland TA, Finset A, Jensen BF and Gulbrandsen P (2011b) Physicians' responses to patients' expressions of negative emotions in hospital consultations: a video-based observational study. *Patient Educ Couns.* **84**(3): 332–7.

Moore DA, Sischo WM, Kurtz S, Siler JD, Pereira RV, Warnick LD and Davis MA (2016) Improving dairy organizational communication from the veterinarian's perspective: results of a continuing veterinary medical education pilot program. *JVME.* **43**(1): 33–40.

Moore IC (2016) Personal communication with Cindy Adams.

Moore IC, Coe JB, Adams CA, Conlon PD and Sargeant JM (2014) The role of veterinary team effectiveness in job satisfaction and burnout in companion animal veterinary clinics. *JAVMA.* **245**(5): 513–24.

Moore IC, Coe JB, Adams CL, Conlon PD and Sargeant JM (2015) Exploring the impact of toxic attitudes and a toxic environment on the veterinary healthcare team. *Frontiers in Vet Sci.* **2**(78): 1–9.

Morris P (2012) Managing pet owners' guilt and grief in veterinary euthanasia encounters. *J Contemp Ethnogr.* **41**(3): 337–65.

Morse DS, Edwardsen EA and Gordon HS (2008) Missed opportunities for interval empathy in lung cancer communication. *Arch Intern Med.* **168**(17): 1853–8.

Myers RE, Daskalakis C, Kunkel EJ, Cocroft JR, Riggio JM, Capkin M and Braddock CH 3rd (2011) Mediated decision support in prostate cancer screening: a randomized controlled trial of decision counseling. *Patient Educ Couns.* **83**(2): 240–6.

NAVMEC Board of Directors. (2011) The North American Veterinary Medical Education Consortium (NAVMEC) looks to veterinary education for the future: roadmap for veterinary medical education in the 21st century: responsive, collaborative, flexible. *JVME.* **38**(4): 320–7.

Neighbour R (1987) *The Inner Consultation: how to develop an effective and intuitive consulting style.* MTP Press, Lancaster, England.

Nekolaichuk CL and Bruera E. (1998) On the nature of hope in palliative care. *J Pallliat Care.* **14**: 36–42.

Nelson WL, Han PK, Fagerlin A, Stefanek M and Ubel PA (2007) Rethinking the objectives of decision aids: a call for conceptual clarity. *Med Decis Making.* **27**(5): 609–18.

Neumann M, Bensing J, Mercer S, Ernstmann N, Ommen O and Pfaff H (2009) Analyzing the 'nature' and 'specific effectiveness' of clinical empathy: a theoretical overview and contribution towards a theory-based research agenda. *Patient Educ Couns.* **74**(3): 339–46.

Newton BW, Barber L, Clardy J, Cleveland E and O'Sullivan P (2008) Is there hardening of the heart during medical school? *Acad Med.* **83**(3): 244–9.

Nielsen-Bohlman L, Panzer AM and Kindig DA (eds) (2004) *Health Literacy: a prescription to end confusion.* Institute of Medicine of the National Academies of Practice, Committee on Health Literacy. Board of Neuroscience and Behavioral Health. National Academies Press, Washington DC. www.nap.edu.

Nogueira Borden LJ, Adams CL, Bonnett BN, Shaw JR and Ribble CS (2010) Use of the measure of patient-centered communication to analyze euthanasia discussions in companion animal practice. *JAVMA.* **237**(11): 1275–87.

Noordman J, Verhaak P, van Beljouw I and van Dulmen S (2010) Consulting room computers and their effect on general practitioner-patient communication. *Fam Pract.* **27**(6): 644–51.

Norfolk T, Birdi K and Walsh D (2007) The role of empathy in establishing rapport in the consultation: a new model. *Med Educ.* **41**(7): 690–7.

Norman G (2005) Research in clinical reasoning: past history and current trends. *Med Educ.* **39**: 418–27.

Norring M, Wilman I, Hokkanen AH, Kujala MV and Hanninen L (2014) Empathic veterinarians score cattle pain higher. *The Vet J.* **200**: 186–190.

Novelli WD, Halvorson GC and Santa J (2012) Recognizing an opinion: findings from the IOM Evidence Communication Innovation Collaborative. *JAMA.* **308**(15): 1531–2.

Nunalee M and Weedon G (2004) Modern trends in veterinary malpractice: how our evolving attitudes toward non-human animals will change veterinary medicine. *Animal Law.* **10**(125): 125–61.

Nunes PW, Williams S, Sa B, Stevenson K (2011) A study of empathy decline in students from five health disciplines during their first year of training. *IJME.* **2**: 12–17.

O'Brien MA, Whelan TJ, Villasis-Keever M, Gafni A, Charles C, Roberts R, Schiff S and Cai W (2009) Are cancer-related decision aids effective? A systematic review and meta-analysis. *J Clin Oncol.* **27**(6): 974–85.

O'Connor AM and Edwards A (2001) The role of decision aids in promoting evidence-based patient choice. In: A Edwards and G Elwyn (eds) *Evidence-Based Patient Choice.* Oxford University Press, Oxford.

O'Connor AM, Legare F and Stacey D (2003) Risk communication in practice: the contribution of decision aids. *BMJ.* **327**(7417): 736–40.

O'Connor AM, Rostom A, Fiset V, Tetroe J, Entwistle V, Llewellyn-Thomas H, Holmes-Rovner M,

Barry M and Jones J (1999) Decision aids for patients facing health treatment or screening decisions: systematic review. *BMJ.* **319**(7212): 731–4.

O'Connor AM, Stacey D, Rovner D, Holmes-Rovner M, Tetroe J, Llewellyn-Thomas H, Entwistle V, Rostom A, Fiset V, Barry M and Jones J (2001) Decision aids for people facing health treatment or screening decisions. *Cochrane Database Syst Rev.* **3**: CD001431.

Orth JE, Stiles WB, Scherwitz L, Hennrikus D and Vallbona C (1987) Patient exposition and provider explanation in routine interviews and hypertensive patients' blood pressure control. *Health Psychol.* **6**(1): 29–42.

Osborne CA (2005) 'Damn-It' acronym offers practical diagnostic aid. *dvm360.* 1 Mar. Available at: http://veterinarynews.dvm360.com/damn-it-acronym-offers-practical-diagnostic-aid

Osborne CA (2010) The 'Damn-It acronym': are you using this practical diagnostic aid? *dvm360.* 1 Dec. Available at: http://veterinarynews.dvm360.com/damn-it-acronym-are-you-using-practical-diagnostic-aid

Osborne CA (1983) The problem oriented medical system. *Vet Clinics of NA – SA.* **13**(4): 745–90.

Osborne CA, Ulrich LK and Nwaokorie EE (2013) Reactive versus empathic listening: what is the difference? *JAVMA.* **242**(4): 460–62.

Owens N (2015) Protecting the self: veterinarians' perspectives on dealing with people. *Society & Animals.*1–23.

Oxtoby C, Ferguson E, White K and Mossop L (2015) We need to talk about error: cause and types of error in veterinary practice. *Veterinary Record.* **177**(17): 438–44.

Panksepp J (2011) The basic emotional circuits of mammalian brains: do animals have affective lives? *Neurosci Biobehav Rev.* **35**(9): 1791–804.

Panksepp J and Panksepp JB (2013) Toward a cross-species understanding of empathy. *Trends Neurosci.* **36**(8): 48–96.

Participants in the Bayer-Fetzer Conference on Physician-Patient Communication in Medical Education (2001) Essential elements of communication in medical encounters: the Kalamazoo consensus statement. *Acad Med.* **76**(4): 390–3.

Paul ES (2015) Empathy with animals and with humans: are they linked? *Anthrozoos.* **13**(4): 194–202.

Paul ES and Podberscek AL (2000) Veterinary education and students' attitudes towards animal welfare. *Vet Record.* **146**: 269–72.

Paul M (2012) Lead the way: 7 steps to boost acceptance of your medical recommendations. *dvm360.* Available at: http://veterinarymedicine.dvm360.com/lead-way-7-steps-boost-acceptance-your-medical-recommendations

Pearce C, Trumble S, Arnold M, Dwan K and Phillips C (2008) Computers in the new consultation: within the first minute. *Fam Pract.* **25**(3): 202–8.

Peltenburg M, Fischer JE, Bahrs O, van Dulmen S and van den Brink-Muinen A (2004) The unexpected in primary care: a multicenter study on the emergence of unvoiced patient agenda. *Ann Fam Med.* **2**(6): 534–40.

Pendleton D, Schofield T, Tate P and Havelock P (1984) *The Consultation: an approach to learning and teaching.* Oxford University Press, Oxford.

Pendleton D, Schofield T, Tate P and Havelock P (2003) *The New Consultation.* Oxford University Press, Oxford.

Peppiatt R (1992) Eliciting patients' views of the cause of their problem: a practical strategy for GPs. *Fam Pract.* **9**(3): 295–8.

Peräkylä A (2002) Agency and authority: extended responses to diagnostic statements in primary care encounters. *Res Lang Soc Interact.* **35**(2): 219–47.

Peterson MC, Holbrook J, VonHales D, Smith NL and Staker LV (1992) Contributions of the history, physical examination and laboratory investigation in making medical diagnoses. *West J Med.* **156**(2): 163–5.

Pfizer Animal Health/Zoetis (2015) "Frank" communication training workshop, Colorado State University Fort Collins Colorado. Available from: http://csu-cvmbs.colostate.edu/academics/clinsci/veterinary-communication/Pages/frank-workshops.aspx.

Pilgram MD (2010) Communicating social support to grieving clients: the veterinarians' view. *Death Studies.* **34**(8): 699–714.

Pilnick A and Dingwall R (2011) On the remarkable persistence of asymmetry in doctor/patient interaction: a critical review. *Soc Sci Med.* **72**(8): 1374–82.

Pinder R (1990) *The Management of Chronic Disease: patient and doctor perspectives on Parkinson's disease*. MacMillan Press, London.

Platt FW and Keller VF (1994) Empathic communication: a teachable and learnable skill. *J Gen Intern Med*. **9**(4): 222–6.

Platt FW and McMath JC (1979) Clinical hypocompetence: the interview. *Ann Intern Med*. **91**(6): 898–902.

Platt FW and Platt CM (2003) Two collaborating artists produce a work of art. *Arch Intern Med*. **163**(10): 1131–2.

Platt FW, Gaspar DL, Coulehan JL, Fox L, Adler AJ, Weston WW, Smith RC and Stewart M (2001) 'Tell me about yourself': The patient-centered interview. *Ann Intern Med*. **134**(11): 1079–85.

Pollard-Williams S, Doyle RE and Freire R (2014) The influence of workplace learning on attitudes toward animal welfare in veterinary students. *J Vet Med Educ*. **41**(3): 253–7.

Poole AD and Sanson-Fisher RW (1979) Understanding the patient: a neglected aspect of medical education. *Soc Sci Med Med Psychol Med Sociol*. **13A**(1): 37–43.

Prescott J, Beadle R and Ferguson D (1994) Communication skills in veterinary education. *J Am Vet Med Assoc*. **204**: 189–90.

Price EL, Bereknyei S, Kuby A, Levinson W and Braddock CH 3rd (2012) New elements for informed decision making: a qualitative study of older adults' views. *Patient Educ Couns*. **86**(3): 335–41.

Priest V and Speller V (1991) *The Risk Factor Management Manual*. Radcliffe Medical Press, Oxford.

Prochaska JO and DiClemente CC (1986) Towards a comprehensive model of change. In: R Miller and N Heather (eds) *Treating Addictive Behaviours*. Plenum Press, New York, NY.

Putnam SM, Stiles WB, Jacob MC and James SA (1988) Teaching the medical interview: an intervention study. *J Gen Intern Med*. **3**(1): 38–47.

Quilligan S and Silverman J (2012) The skill of summary in clinician-patient communication: a case study. *Patient Educ Couns*. **86**(3): 354–9.

Radford A, Stockley P, Silverman J, Taylor I, Turner R and Gray C (2006) Development, teaching and evaluation of a consultation structure model for use in veterinary education. *J Vet Med Educ*. **33**(1): 38–44.

Radford AD, Stockley P, Taylor IR, Turner R, Gaskell CJ, Kaney S, Humphris G and Magrath C (2003) Use of simulated clients in training veterinary undergraduates in communication skills. *Veterinary Record*. **152**(14): 4212–27.

Rehman T, McKemey K, Yates CM et al (2007) Identifying and understanding factors influencing the uptake of new technologies on dairy farms in SW England using the theory of reasoned action. *Science Direct*. **94**(2): 281–93.

Reilly S and Muzarkara B (1978) *Mixed Message Resolution by Disturbed Adults and Children. Behavioral Sciences Clinical Research Center. Philadelphia State Hospital*. Paper presented at the International Communication Association Annual Conference, Chicago, Illinois, April 1978.

Rhodes KV, Vieth T, He T, Miller A, Howes DS, Bailey O, Walter J, Frankel R and Levinson W (2004) Resuscitating the physician-patient relationship: emergency department communication in an academic medical center. *Ann Emerg Med*. **44**(3): 262–7.

Riccardi VM and Kurtz SM (1983) *Communication and Counseling in Health Care*. Charles C Thomas Publisher, Springfield, IL.

Richard C and Lussier MT (2006) MEDICODE: an instrument to describe and evaluate exchanges on medications that occur during medical encounters. *Patient Educ Couns*. **64**(1–3): 197–206.

Richard C and Lussier MT (2007) Measuring patient and physician participation in exchanges on medications: dialogue ratio, preponderance of initiative and dialogical roles. *Patient Educ Couns*. **65**(3): 329–41.

Richard R and Lussier MT (2003) *Dialogic Index: a description of physician and patient participation in discussions of medications*. Paper presented at the National Association of Primary Care Research Group Annual Conference, Banff, Alberta, 21–25 October 2003.

Ritter C, Kwong GPS, Wolf R, Pickel C, Slopm M, Flaig J, Mason S, Adams CL, Kelton DF, Jansen J, DeBuck J and Barkema HW (2015) Factors associated with participation of Alberta dairy farmers in a voluntary, management-based Johne's disease control program. *American Dairy Science Assoc*. **98**(11): 7831–45.

Roberts F (2004) Speaking to and for animals in a veterinary clinic: a practice for managing interpersonal interaction. *Research on Language & Social Interaction*. **37**(4): 421–46.

Robins L, Witteborn S, Miner L, Mauksch L, Edwards K and Brock D (2011) Identifying transparency in physician communication. *Patient Educ Couns.* **83**(1): 73–9.

Robinson A and Thomson R (2001) Variability in patient preferences for participating in medical decision making: implication for the use of decision support tools. *Qual Health Care.* **10**(Suppl, 1): i34–38.

Robinson J (2001) Soliciting patients' presenting concerns. In: J Heritage and D Maynard (eds) *Practicing Medicine: structure and process in primary care encounters.* Cambridge University Press, Cambridge.

Robinson JD (1998) Getting down to business: talk, gaze and body organization during openings of doctor patient consultations. *Health Commun.* **25**(1): 97–123.

Robinson JD (2001) Closing medical encounters: two physician practices and their implications for the expression of patients' unstated concerns. *Soc Sci Med.* **53**(5): 639–56.

Robinson JD and Heritage J (2006) Physicians' opening questions and patients' satisfaction. *Patient Educ Couns.* **60**(3): 279–85.

Roche SM, Jones-Bitton A, Meehan M and VonMasso M Kelton DF (2016) A qualitative exploration of Ontario dairy producer and veterinarian perceptions of barriers and motivators to adopting on-farm management practices for control of John's disease. *Pre Vet Med.* (in review)

Rock M and Babinec P (2010) Prototypes connect human diabetes with feline and canine diabetes in the context of animal human bonds: an anthropological analysis *Anthrozoos: A Multidisciplinary Journal of the Interactions of People & Animals.* **23**(1): 5–20.

Rock M, Buntain BJ, Hatfield JM and Hallgrimsson B (2009) Animal-human connections. *Soc Sci & Med.* **68**(6): 991–95.

Rodriguez HP, Anastario MP, Frankel RM, Odigie EG, Rogers WH, von Glahn T and Safran DG (2008) Can teaching agenda-setting skills to physicians improve clinical interaction quality? A controlled intervention. *BMC Med Educ.* **8**: 3.

Rogers CR (1980) *A Way of Being.* Houghton-Mifflin, Boston, MA.

Rohlf VI, Toukhsati S, Colejman GJ, Bennett PC. (2010) Dog obesity: can dog caregivers', owners' feeding and exercise intentions and behaviors be predicted from attitudes? *J Appl Anim Welf Sci.* **13**: 213–36.

Rohrbach BW, Odoi A and Patton S. (2011) Survey of heartworm prevention practices among members of a national hunting dog club. *JAAHA.* **47**(3): 161–9.

Rollnick S, Butler CC and Stott N (1997) Helping smokers make decisions: the enhancement of brief intervention for general medical practice. *Patient Educ Couns.* **31**(3): 191–203.

Rosenstock IM, Strecher VJ, and Becker MH (1988) Social learning theory and the health belief model. *Health Ed Q.* **15**(2): 175–83.

Roshier AL and McBride EA (2013) Canine behaviour problems: discussions between veterinarians and dog owners during annual booster consultations. *Vet Rec.* **172**(9):235.

Roter D (2000) The enduring and evolving nature of the patient-physician relationship. *Patient Educ Couns.* **39**(1): 5–15.

Roter DL (1977) Patient participation in the patient-provider interaction: the effects of patient question asking on the quality of interaction, satisfaction and compliance. *Health Education Monographs.* **5**(4): 281–315.

Roter DL and Hall JA (1987) Physicians' interviewing styles and medical information obtained from patients. *J Gen Intern Med.* **2**(5): 325–9.

Roter DL and Hall JA (1992) *Doctors Talking with Patients/Patients Talking with Doctors.* Auburn House, Westport, CT.

Roter DL and Hall JA. (2006) *Doctors Talking with Patients/Patients Talking with Doctors: improving communication in medical visits.* Auburn House, Westport, CT.

Roter DL, Frankel RM, Hall JA and Sluyter D (2006) The expression of emotion through nonverbal behavior in medical visits: mechanisms and outcomes. *J Gen Intern Med.* **21**(Suppl. 1): S28–34.

Roter DL, Hall JA, Kern DE, Barker R, Cole KA and Roca RP (1995) Improving physicians' interviewing skills and reducing patients' emotional distress. *Arch Intern Med.* **155**(17): 1877–84.

Roter DL, Stewart M, Putnam SM, Lipkin M Jr, Stiles W and Inui TS (1997) Communication patterns of primary care physicians. *JAMA.* **277**(4): 350–6.

Rowe MB (1986) Wait time: slowing down may be a way of speeding up. *J Teach Educ.* **37**(1): 43–50.

Ruiz Moral R, Parras RJM and Perula De Torres LA (2006) Is the expression 'Oh, by the way …' a problem that arises in the early moments of a consultation? *Eur J Gen Pract.* **12**(1):40–1.

Rutter M and Cox A (1981) Psychiatric interviewing techniques I: methods and measures. *Br J Psychiatry.* **138**: 273–82.

Ruusuvuori J (2001) Looking means listening: coordinating displays of engagement in doctor-patient interaction. *Soc Sci Med.* **52**(7): 1093–108.

Sackett DL, Straus SE, Richardson ES, Rosenberg W and Haynes RB (2000) *Evidence-Based Medicine: how to practice and teach EBM.* Wiley & Sons, New York.

Salmon P, Dowrick CF, Ring A and Humphris GM (2004) Voiced but unheard agendas: qualitative analysis of the psychosocial cues that patients with unexplained symptoms present to general practitioners. *Br J Gen Pract.* **54**(500): 171–6.

Sanders CR (1994) Annoying owners: Routine interactions with problematic clients in a general veterinary practice. *Qual Sociol.* **17**(2): 159–70.

Sandler G (1980) The importance of the history in the medical clinic and the cost of unnecessary tests. *Am Heart J.* **100**(6Pt1): 928–31.

Schein E (2011) *Helping: how to offer, give, and receive help.* Berrett-Koehler Publishers, Inc. CA.

Schibbye A (1993) The role of 'recognition' in the resolution of a specific interpersonal dilemma. *J Phenomenol Psychol.* **24**(2): 175–89.

Schmidt HG, Norman GR and Boshuizen HP (1990) A cognitive perspective on medical expertise: theory and implication. *Acad Med.* **65**(10): 611–21.

Schoenfeld-Tacher R, Kogan Lori R, Meyer-Parsons, Royal Kenneth D and Shaw Jane R (2015) Educational Research Report: changes in students' levels of empathy during the didactic portion of a veterinary program. *JVME.* **15**; **42**(3): 194–205.

Schofield T, Elwyn G, Edwards A and Visser A (2003) Shared decision making. *Patient Educ Couns.* **50**(3): 229–30.

Schulman BA (1979) Active patient orientation and outcomes in hypertensive treatment. *Med Care.* **17**: 267–81.

Scott JT, Entwistle VA, Sowden AJ and Watt I (2001) Giving tape recordings or written summaries of consultations to people with cancer: a systematic review. *Health Expect.* **4**(3): 162–9.

Sepucha KR and Mulley AG (2003) Extending decision support: preparation and implementation. *Patient Educ Couns.* **50**(3): 269–71.

Shachak A and Reis S (2009) The impact of electronic medical records on patient–doctor communication during consultation: a narrative literature review. *J Eval Clin Pract.* **15**(4): 641–9.

Shachak A, Hadas-Dayagi M, Ziv A and Reis S (2009) Primary care physicians' use of an electronic medical record system: a cognitive task analysis. *J Gen Intern Med.* **24**(3): 341–8.

Shadle C (2011) *Communication Case Studies: building interpersonal skills in the veterinary practice.* AAHA Press, Lakewood CO.

Shaw DH and Ihle SL. (2006) Communication skills training at the Atlantic Veterinary College, University of Prince Edward Island. *JVME.* **33**(1): 100–4.

Shaw JR, Adams CL, Bonnett BN, Larson S and Roter DL (2012a) Veterinarian satisfaction with companion animal visits. *JAVMA.* **240**(7): 832–41.

Shaw JR, Bonnett BN, Roter DL, Adams CL and Larson S (2012b) Gender differences in veterinarian-client-patient communication in companion animal practice. *JAVMA.* **241**(1): 81–8.

Shaw JR, Bonnett BN, Adams CL, Roter DL (2006) Veterinarian-client-patient communication patterns used during clinical appointments in companion animal practice. *JAVMA.* **228**(5): 714–721.

Shaw JR, Adams CL and Bonnett BN (2004a) What can veterinarians learn from studies of physician-patient communication about veterinarian-client-patient communication? *JAVMA.* **224**(5): 676–84.

Shaw JR, Adams CL, Bonnet BN, Larson S and Roter DL (2008) Veterinarian-client-patient communication during wellness appointments versus appointments related to a health problem in companion animal practice. *JAVMA.* **233**(10): 1576–86.

Shaw JR, Adams CL, Bonnett BN, Larson S and Roter DL (2004b) Use of the roter interaction analysis system to analyze veterinarian-client-patient communication in companion animal practice. *JAVMA.* **225**(2): 222–9.

Shaw JR, Barley GE, Hill AE, Larson S and Roter DL (2010) Communication skills education onsite in a veterinary practice. *Patient Educ Couns.* **80**(3): 337–44.

Shepherd HL, Barratt A, Trevena LJ, McGeechan K, Carey K, Epstein RM, Butow PN, Del Mar CB,

Entwistle V and Tattersall MHN (2011) Three questions that patients can ask to improve the quality of information physicians give about treatment options: a cross-over trial. *Patient Educ Couns.* **84**(3): 379–85.

Silverman J (2009) Teaching clinical communication: a mainstream activity or just a minority sport? *Patient Educ Couns.* **76**(3): 361–7.

Silverman J and Kinnersley P (2010) Doctors' non-verbal behaviour in consultations: look at the patient before you look at the computer. *Br J Gen Pract.* **60**(571): 76–8.

Silverman J, Deveugele M, de Haes H and Rosenbaum M (2011) Unskilled creativity is counterproductive. *Med Educ.* **45**(9): 959–60; author reply 961–2.

Silverman J, Kurtz S and Draper J (1998) *Skills for Communicating with Patients.* 1st ed. Radcliffe Medical Press, Oxford.

Silverman J, Kurtz S and Draper J (2005) *Skills for Communicating with Patients.* 2nd ed. Radcliffe Publishing, Oxford.

Silverman J, Kurtz S and Draper J (2013) *Skills for Communication with Patients.* 3rd ed. CRC Press, Boca Raton, FL.

Simpson M, Buckman R, Stewart M, Maguire P, Lipkin M, Novack D and Till J (1991) Doctor-patient communication: the Toronto consensus statement. *BMJ.* **303**(6814): 1385–7.

Sischo WM, Periera R, Moore DA, Kurtz S, Kinder D, Heaton K, Siler J and Davis MA (2016) Who's talking when setting goals and protocols for dairy calf care. (research in progress)

Skelton JR (2005) Everything you were afraid to ask about communication skills. *Br J Gen Pract.* **55**(510): 40–6.

Slade D, Scheeres H, Manidis M, Iedema R, Dunston R, Stein-Parbury J, Matthiessen C, Herke M and McGregor J (2008) Emergency communication: the discursive challenges facing emergency clinicians and patients in hospital emergency departments. *Discourse Commun.* **2**(3): 271–98.

Slade D, Manidis M, McGregor J, Scheeres H, Chandler E, Stein-Parbury J, Dunston R, Herke M and Matthiesen C (2015) Communicating in Hospital Emergency Departments. Springer-Verlag, Berlin, Heidelberg.

Sluyter D (2004). Personal communication with Suzanne Kurtz.

Smith RC and Hoppe RB (1991) The patient's story: integrating the patient and physician-centred approaches to interviewing. *Ann Intern Med.* **115**(6): 471–7.

Sonntag U, Wiesner J, Fahrenkrog S, Renneberg B, Braun V and Heintze C (2012) Motivational interviewing and shared decision making in primary care. *Patient Educ Couns.* **87**(1): 62–6.

Sorge U, Kelton D, Lissemore K, Godkin A, Hendrick S and Wells S (2010) Attitudes of Canadian dairy farmers toward a voluntary Johne's disease control program. *J. Dairy Sci.* **93**: 1491–9.

Sowden AJ, Forbes C, Entwistle V and Watt I (2001) Informing, communicating and sharing decisions with people who have cancer. *Qual Health Care.* **10**(3): 193–6.

Spiro H (1992) What is empathy and can it be taught? *Ann Intern Med.* **116**(10): 843–6.

Starfield B, Wray C, Hess K, Gross R, Birk PS and D'Lugoff BC (1981) The influence of patient-practitioner agreement on outcome of care. *Am J Public Health.* **71**(2): 127–31.

Steele DJ and Hulsman RL (2008) Empathy, authenticity, assessment and simulation: a conundrum in search of a solution. *Patient Educ Couns.* **71**(2): 143–4.

Steihaug S, Gulbrandsen P and Werner A (2012) Recognition can leave room for disagreement in the doctor-patient consultation. *Patient Educ Couns.* **86**(3): 316–21.

Stepien KA and Baernstein A (2006) Educating for empathy: a review. *J Gen Intern Med.* **21**(5): 524–30.

Steptoe A, Sutcliffe I, Allen B and Coombes C (1991) Satisfaction with communication, medical knowledge and coping style in patients with metastatic cancer. *Soc Sci Med.* **32**(6): 627–32.

Stevenson FA, Barry CA, Britten N, Barber N and Bradley CP (2000) Doctor-patient communication about drugs: the evidence for shared decision making. *Soc Sci Med.* **50**(6): 829–40.

Stewart M (2001) Towards a global definition of patient centered care. *BMJ.* **322**(7284): 444–5.

Stewart M and Roter D (eds) (1989) *Communicating with Medical Patients.* Sage Publications, Newbury Park, CA.

Stewart M, Belle Brown J, Donner A, McWhinney IR, Oates J and Weston W (1997) *The Impact of Patient-centered Care on Patient Outcomes in Family Practice.* Thames Valley Family Practice Research Unit, London, ON.

Stewart M, Brown JB, Boon H, Galajda J, Meredith L and Sangster M (1999) Evidence on patient-doctor communication. *Cancer Prev Control.* **3**(1): 25–30.

Stewart M, Brown JB, Donner A, McWhinney IR, Oates J, Weston WW and Jordan J (2000) The impact of patient-centered care on outcomes. *J Fam Pract.* **49**(9): 796–804.

Stewart MA (1985) *Comparison of Two Methods of Analyzing Doctor Patient Communication.* Paper presented at the North American Primary Care Research Group Conference, Seattle, 14–17 April 1985.

Stewart MA, Belle Brown J, Wayne Weston W, McWhinney I, McWilliam C and Freeman T (1995) *Patient-Centred Medicine: transforming the clinical method.* Sage, Thousand Oaks, CA.

Stewart MA, Brown JB, Weston WW, McWhinney IR, McWilliam CL and Freeman TR (2003) *Patient-Centered Medicine: transforming the clinical method.* 2nd ed. Radcliffe Medical Press, Oxford.

Stewart MA, McWhinney IR, Buck CW (1979) The doctor/patient relationship and its effect upon outcome. *The J Royal Coll Gen Practitioners.* **29**(199): 77.

Stiles WB, Putnam SM, James SA and Wolf MH (1979) Dimensions of patient and physician roles in medical screening interviews. *Soc Sci Med.* **13A**(3): 335–41.

Stivers T (1998) Prediagnostic commentary in veterinarian-client interaction. *Research on Language and Social Interaction.* **31**(2): 241–77.

Stoewen D (2012) Clients' service expectations and practitioners' treatment recommendations in veterinary oncology. PhD thesis, University of Guelph.

Stoewen DL (2014a) Qualitative study of the information expectations of clients accessing oncology care at a tertiary referral center for dogs with life-limiting cancer. *JAVMA.* **245**(7): 773–83.

Stoewen DL (2014b) Qualitative study of the communication expectations of clients accessing oncology care at a tertiary referral center for dogs. *JAVMA.* **245**(7): 785–95.

Strand (2006) Enhanced communication by developing a non-anxious presence: a key attribute for the successful veterinarian. *AAVMC.* **33**(1): 65–70.

Street RL Jr, Makoul G, Arora NK and Epstein RM (2009) How does communication heal? Pathways linking clinician-patient communication to health outcomes. *Patient Educ Couns.* **74**(3): 295–301.

Strull WM, Lo B and Charles G (1984) Do patients want to be participate in medical decision making? *JAMA.* **252**: 2990–4.

Stull JW, Carr AP, Chomel BB et al. (2007) Small animal deworming protocols, client education and veterinarian perception of zoonotic parasites in western Canada. *CVJ.* **48**: 269–76.

Suchman A, Deci E, McDaniel S and Beckman H (2002) *Relationship Centered Administration.* In TE Quill, RM Frankel and SH McDaniel (eds) *The Biopsychosocial Approach: past, present and future.* University of Rochester Press, Rochester, NY.

Suchman A, Sluyter DM and Williamson PR (2011) *Leading Change in Healthcare: transforming organizations using complexity, positive psychology and relationship-centered care.* Radcliffe Publishing, Oxford.

Suchman AL (2001) The influence of health care organizations on well-being. *West J Med.* **174**(1): 43–7.

Suchman AL (2003) Research on patient-clinician relationships: celebrating success and identifying the next scope of work. *J Gen Intern Med.* **18**(8): 677–8.

Suchman AL, Markakis K, Beckman HB and Frankel R (1997) A model of empathic communication in the medical interview. *JAMA.* **277**(8): 678–82.

Suchman AL, Williamson PR (2003) Personal communication with Suzanne Kurtz.

Sudore RL and Schillinger D (2009) Interventions to improve care for patients with limited health literacy. *J Clin Outcomes Manag.* **16**(1): 20–9.

Sullivan HS (1953) *The Interpersonal Theory of Psychiatry.* North, New York.

Sutherland HJ, Llewellyn-Thomas HA, Lockwood GA, Tritchler DL and Till JE (1989) Cancer patients: their desire for information and participation in treatment decisions. *J R Soc Med.* **82**(5): 260–3.

Svarstad BL (1974) *The Doctor-Patient Encounter: an observational study of communication and outcome.* Doctoral dissertation, University of Wisconsin, Madison.

Swayden KJ, Anderson KK, Connelly LM, Moran JS, McMahon JK and Arnold PM (2012) Effect of sitting vs. standing on perception of provider time at bedside: a pilot study. *Patient Educ Couns.* **86**(2): 166–71.

Tait I (1979) The history and function of clinical records. Unpublished MD dissertation thesis, University of Cambridge.

Takemura Y, Atsumi R and Tsuda T (2007) Identifying medical interview behaviors that best elicit information from patients in clinical practice. *Tohoku J Exp Med.* **213**(2): 121–7.

Takeuchi Y, Houpt KA and Scarlett JM. (2000) Evaluation of treatments for separation anxiety in dogs. *JAVMA.* **217**(3): 342–45.

Tamblyn R, Abrahamowicz M, Dauphinee D, Wenghofer E, Jacques A, Klass D, Smee S, Blackmore D, Winslade N, Girard N, Du Berger R, Bartman I, Buckeridge DL and Hanley JA (2007) Physician scores on a national clinical skills examination as predictors of complaints to medical regulatory authorities. *JAMA.* **298**(9): 993–1001.

Tattersall MH, Butow PN and Ellis PM (1997) Meeting patients' information needs beyond the year 2000. *Support Care Cancer.* **5**(2): 85–9.

Teherani A, Hauer KE and O'Sullivan P (2008) Can simulations measure empathy? Considerations on how to assess behavioral empathy via simulations. *Patient Educ Couns.* **71**(2): 148–52.

Thorne SE, Hislop TG, Stajduhar K and Oglov V (2009) Time-related communication skills from the cancer patient perspective. *Psychooncology.* **18**(5): 500–7.

Thornton H, Edwards A and Baum M (2003) Women need better information about routine mammography. *BMJ.* **327**(7406): 101–3.

Toews L (2011) The information infrastructure that supports evidence-based veterinary medicine: a comparison with human medicine. *JVME.* **38**(2): 123–34.

Towell TL, Hampe S, Wayner C (2010) Referring veterinarians' opinions and veterinary teaching hospital veterinarians' perceptions of those opinions regarding communication and nutritional product recommendations. *JAVMA.* **237**(5): 513–518.

Towle A and Godolphin W (1999) Framework for teaching and learning informed shared decision making. *BMJ.* **319**(7212): 766–71.

Tresolini CP and the Pew-Fetzer Task Force (1994) *Health Professions Education and Relationship-centred Care.* Pew-Fetzer Task Force on Advancing Psychosocial Health Education, Pew Health Professions Commission and the Fetzer Institute, San Francisco, CA.

Trevena L and Barratt A (2003) Integrated decision making: definitions for a new discipline. *Patient Educ Couns.* **50**(3): 265–8.

Truax CB and Carkhuff RR (1967) *Towards Effective Counseling and Psychotherapy.* Aldine, Chicago.

Tuckett D, Boulton M, Olson C and Williams A (1985) *Meetings between Experts: an approach to sharing ideas in medical consultations.* Tavistock, London.

Van der Meulen N, Jansen J, van Dulmen S, Bensing J and van Weert J (2008) Interventions to improve recall of medical information in cancer patients: a systematic review of the literature. *Psychooncology.* **17**(9): 857–68.

Van Thiel J and van Dalen J (1995) *MAAS-Globaal criterialijst, versie voor de vaardigheidstoets Medisch Basiscurriculum.* Maastricht University, Netherlands.

Ventres W, Kooienga S and Marlin R (2006) EHRs in the exam room: tips on patient-centered care. *Fam Pract Manag.* **13**(3): 45–7.

Verderber RF and Verderber KS (1980) *Inter-Act: using interpersonal communication skills.* Wadsworth, Belmont, CA.

Verker MJ, van Stokrom M and Endenburg N (2008) How can veterinarians optimize owner compliance with medication regimes. *EJCAP.* **18**(1): 73–9.

Volk JO, Felsted KE, Thomas JG, Siren CW (2011a) Executive summary of the Bayer veterinary care usage study. *JAVMA.* **238**(10): 1275–82.

Volk JO, Felsted KE, Thomas JG, Siren CW (2011b) Executive summary of phase 2 of the Bayer veterinary care usage study. *JAVMA.* **239**(10): 1311–16.

Volk JO, Felsted KE, Thomas JG, Siren CW (2014) Executive summary of phase 3 of the Bayer veterinary care usage study. *JAVMA.* **244**(7): 799–802.

Von Fragstein M, Silverman J, Cushing A, Quilligan S, Salisbury H and Wiskin C (2008) UK consensus statement on the content of communication curricula in undergraduate medical education. *Med Educ.* **42**(11): 1100–7.

Waitzkin H (1984) Doctor-patient communication: clinical implications of social scientific research. *JAMA.* **252**(17): 2441–6.

Waitzkin H (1985) Information giving in medical care. *J Health Soc Behav.* **26**(2): 81–101.

Walsh DA, Klosterman ES and Kass PH (2009) Approaches to veterinary education-tracking versus a final year broad clinical experience. Part 2 installed values. *Rev Sci Tech Off.* **28**(2): 811–22.

Wasserman RC, Inui TS, Barriatua RD, Carter WB and Lippincott P (1984) Pediatric clinicians' support for parents makes a difference: an outcome based analysis of clinician-parent interaction. *Pediatrics.* **74**(6): 1047–53.

Watzlawick P, Beavin J and Jackson D (1967) *Pragmatics of Human Communication.* WW Norton, New York.

Wear D and Varley JD (2008) Rituals of verification: the role of simulation in developing and evaluating empathic communication. *Patient Educ Couns.* **71**(2): 153–6.

Weiner JS and Roth J (2006) Avoiding iatrogenic harm to patient and family while discussing goals of care near the end of life. *J Palliat Med.* **9**(2): 451–63.

Wessels R, Lam T and Jansen J (2014) *Communication in Practice: the vet's manual on clienthusiasm.* Communication in Practice, The Netherlands.

White J, Levinson W and Roter D (1994) 'Oh, by the Way': the closing moments of the medical interview. *J Gen Int Med.* **9**: 24–8.

White JC, Rosson C, Christensen J, Hart R and Levinson W (1997) Wrapping things up: a qualitative analysis of the closing moments of the medical visit. *Patient Educ Couns.* **30**(2): 155–65.

White SJ, Stubbe MH, Macdonald LM, Dowell AC, Dew KP and Gardner R (2013) Framing the consultation: the role of the referral in surgeon-patient consultations. *Health Commun.* Epub Feb 12.

Williams D and Jewell J (2012) Family-centred veterinary medicine: learning from human pediatric care. *Veterinary Record.* **170**(3): 79–80.

Williamson PR (2011) Appendix 1: a 4–step model of relationship-centered communication. In: A Suchman, DM Sluyter and PR Williamson (eds) *Leading Change in Healthcare: transforming organizations using complexity positive psychology and relationship-centered care.* Radcliffe Publishing, Oxford.

Wilson J, Donszelmann D, Read E, Levy M, Krebs G, Pittman T, Atkins G, Leguillette R, Whitehead A and Adams CL (2012) Historical investigation pyramids-beef, diary, equine, small animal, Unpublished course materials for the Clinical Communication Program – Professional Skills, University of Calgary Veterinary Medicine. Used with permission.

Windish DM, Price EG, Clever SL, Magaziner JL and Thomas PA (2005) Teaching medical students the important connection between communication and clinical reasoning. *J Gen Intern Med.* **20**(12): 1108–13.

Winnicott DW (1986) *Home is Where We Start From: essays by a psychoanalyst.* Morton, New York.

Wissow LS, Roter DL and Wilson MEH (1994) Pediatrician interview style and mothers' disclosure of psychosocial issues. *Pediatrics.* **93**(2): 289–95.

Yeates J and Main DCJ (2010) The ethics of influencing clients. *JAVMA.* **237**(3): 263–7.

Young HN, Bell RA, Epstein RM, Feldman MD and Kravitz RL (2008) Physicians' shared decision-making behaviors in depression care. *Arch Intern Med.* **168**(13): 1404–8.

Zak, PJ (2011) The physiology of moral sentiments. *J Econ Behavior & Organization.* **77**: 53–65.

Zandbelt LC, Smets EM, Oort FJ, Godfried MH and de Haes HC (2007) Patient participation in the medical specialist encounter: does physicians' patient-centred communication matter? *Patient Educ Couns.* **65**(3): 396–406.

Zimmermann C, Del Piccolo L and Finset A (2007) Cues and concerns by patients in medical consultations: a literature review. *Psychol Bull.* **133**(3): 438–63.

Zoetis F (2015) Communication Series (Internet). Zoetis, Florham Park, NJ (cited 2014 Dec 29). Available from: www.zoetis.com/solutions/pages/frank/frank_veterinarian.aspx.

Zolnierek KBH and DiMatteo MR (2009) Physician communication and patient adherence to treatment: a meta-analysis. *Med Care.* **47**(8): 826–34.

Index

Entries in **bold** denote boxes; entries in *italics* denote figures.

Author Index

Made in the USA
Columbia, SC
24 August 2017